Neural Dynamics of
Neurological Disease

Neural Dynamics of Neurological Disease

Christopher A. Shaw

Department of Ophthalmology and Visual Sciences,
University of British Columbia,
Canada

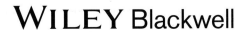

Library of Congress Cataloging-in-Publication Data

Names: Shaw, Christopher A. (Christopher Ariel), author.
Title: Neural dynamics of neurological disease / Christopher A. Shaw.
Description: Hoboken, New Jersey : John Wiley & Sons, Inc., [2017] | Includes
  bibliographical references and index.
Identifiers: LCCN 2016051232 (print) | LCCN 2016051536 (ebook) | ISBN
  9781118634578 (cloth) | ISBN 9781118634479 (pdf) | ISBN 9781118634738
  (epub)
Subjects: | MESH: Central Nervous System Diseases | Disease Progression |
  Aging–physiology
Classification: LCC RC346 (print) | LCC RC346 (ebook) | NLM WL 301 | DDC
  616.8–dc23
LC record available at https://lccn.loc.gov/2016051232

Cover credit: © Karen Santos 2015
Cover design: Wiley

Set in 10/12pt Warnock by SPi Global, Chennai, India
Printed and bound in Malaysia by Vivar Printing Sdn Bhd

10 9 8 7 6 5 4 3 2 1

For my parents, my children, and for all peregrinos.

Contents

Preface

"Babylon in all its desolation is a sight not so awful as that of the human mind in ruins."

Scrope Berdmore Davies[1]

"I can face death, but I cannot face watching myself disappear from within...I don't know who I am anymore."

Claude Jutra[2]

Each annual meeting of the Society for Neuroscience (SfN) is, for me, once more a reminder just how reductionist the field of neuroscience has been, continues to be, and apparently is destined to remain.

Anyone who has gone to this conference, or any similar type of large meeting, cannot help but be overwhelmed by the sheer quantity of the information on display. During the three and a half days of the main SfN meeting, some 30 000 participants will present over 15 000 posters along with almost 13 000 talks of various lengths. These numbers were the projected figures for the 2014 conference in Washington, DC, but other SfN conferences of the recent past will have been much the same in size. Future conferences will likely be even larger.

Most of the talks at the meeting occur in the so-called "mini"- and "nano"-symposia which feature 15-minute-long presentations, each usually containing a small body of data and its preliminary interpretation. However, the poster sessions really show the true dimensions of the conference: seven 4-hour-long sessions, each filling an area the size of several football fields.

Each poster, or mini-talk, contains a snippet of information – almost all of it, as noted, preliminary – a lot of which will turn out to be conceptually flawed in design or experimentally incorrect. Much of the time, as the lack of later publications bears out, the work is simply not reproducible. This outcome is in accord with studies by various scholars who have noted a lack of reproducibility in experimental data of all kinds, perhaps particularly often in the biomedical sciences.

Multiply these numbers by the additional numbers of people and presentations at conferences in neurology or more specialist neurological diseases, multiply again by the number of years these conferences have all been going on, and one likely gets billions of words and millions of tons of paper in a virtual tidal wave of information, which, combined with endless time spent by a great variety of otherwise quite talented scientists, actually produces what, at the end of the day, amounts to relatively little useful information about neurological diseases. Further, very little of this information is actually sorted, compiled, or cross-checked internally or externally with the previous decades of results from all of the similar meetings.

What then are the outcomes for neurological disease remediation? First, the field still does not understand the etiology of most neurological diseases, and, as a consequence, it has only a very limited means of translating what it thinks it knows into treatments that actually halt the progression of – never mind "cure" – these diseases.

The problem here is therefore obviously not one of quantity, or even in many cases of quality. Rather, the problem is that the field still cannot answer some really fundamental questions about the diseases in question and therefore cannot come up with treatments that make a lot of sense mechanistically or, at the very least, do what they are intended to do. Maybe what this really means is that the field of neurological disease research is not asking the right questions, or that it does not know how to interpret the answers.

For me, the question is not how to (over) simplify the nervous system and its diseases, but rather how to understand them in their entirety. Admittedly, the task of understanding the former has proven quite difficult. The second goal clearly depends on accomplishing the first.

As other authors have pointed out in different contexts, attempts to "atomize" a subject of study into ever smaller bits without any context to their inter-relationships can be enormously detrimental (see, for example, Gould and Lewontin, 1979). Further, should the field really expect that a system as complex as the nervous system will break down in a simple way, or should it expect that its pieces will, in some measure, reflect its overall innate complexity? Almost for sure, it is the latter. At least, this is the perspective I will take in the pages that follow. I should acknowledge here that my bias against overusing reductionist approaches when considering neurological disease origins in as complex a system as the human central nervous system (CNS) is very much the polar opposite to the tack taken by Dr. Christof Koch, one of the foremost theorists on human consciousness (see Koch, 2012). The latter subject is surely as complex as the breakdown of the CNS in neurological diseases, but there may be some common ground (see Chapter 14).

As will be discussed in this book, the origin, function, and diseases of the nervous system are, by their very nature, complex, and are highly interconnected amongst the various types of cells and regions affected. The concept of biosemiosis, or biological signaling, is in this context highly relevant, and it will be highlighted in much of the discussion that follows. Moreover, the diseases upon which this book will focus are "progressive," meaning that they continue to get worse in terms of nervous system pathology and functioning over time. They are also age-related and somewhat sex-dependent, are complicated by the added complexities of genetic variations, individual microbiomes, and a host of other likely contributing factors.

How all of these aspects combine to produce any neurological disease is actually something that neurological disease research has not really begun to understand. If the nervous system is constructed as a complex system both developmentally and functionally, which it decidedly is, then it is surely so when it malfunctions. In brief, those of us in what can broadly be described as the neurological disease "field," a term that will be used throughout the book, are in rather dire need of a conceptual frame shift.

Many scientists are hard at work to accomplish such a shift, but they are swimming against a powerful tide of overwhelming amounts of data, which, as noted earlier, are often incorrect. How, then, is one to sort the wheat from the chaff, the valid from the invalid?

This book is intended to help the process along. Inevitably, in so doing, it will annoy some of my neuroscience colleagues as it may seem to imply that all their myriad experiments – often with amazingly spectacular methodologies – are not going to get the field to any answers without reframing the questions. Techniques are, after all, merely the equivalent of tactics in a military setting, simply, in this case, the means to accomplish the larger strategic goal of understanding these diseases. The strategic goal is aimed at an end state of prevention (or of effective treatment, as the second-best option).

Understanding this end state is actually critical to our collective wellbeing, because these various diseases are threatening to overwhelm the medical systems of the developed nations. (As for the developing countries, their medical systems are in many cases in poor enough shape as is, and hardly need the added burden of increased neurological diseases.)

My hope is that *Neural Dynamics of Neurological Disease* will spark debate. Time will tell if this hope has been realized. While desirable, indeed essential, from my perspective, such an outcome is decidedly a long shot. Scientific journals and meetings such as the SfN have become major industries, and are often mired in dogma, with an apparently dominant philosophy that "more equates to better."

It is clear from the work of Prof. John Ioannidis and others that more is not necessarily better if the data are incorrect or interpreted incorrectly and/or are not verified by replication, or at least convergent forms of information. Thus, of the approximately 28 000 talks and poster presentations at SfN, some two-thirds (or more) will be incorrect, and virtually none will be replicated. This is a vastly larger problem than most of those in the field realize, and I will touch upon it further in Chapter 8.

It is reasonable to assume that much of what follows in this book will be controversial, not so much because the data are contested (although in many cases they are) but because the way I have chosen to put them together in particular categories leads to certain conclusions. Other authors, ordering the subjects in different ways, might reach very different outcomes. In this sense, the process of writing a book is a lot like museum curatorship in that what one chooses to put on display versus what one leaves in the basement will provide very different narratives. When writing about neurological diseases, how one collates and arranges the key subjects and lesser items shapes the presentation, and thus the conclusions. And, needless to say, all authors have their own assumptions, prejudices for or against certain hypotheses and data, and ways of viewing any particular field of study.

Given this, it seems only fair at the outset for me to state my own assumptions. These are listed in a sequence from what I hope will be the least controversial, "motherhood" sorts of assertions to those that perhaps deviate to a lesser or greater extent from mainstream concepts of the nervous system in disease. Each will be bolstered by the relevant literature in the appropriate places in the book's chapters.

One point to be addressed first, however, is the following: the terms "disease" and "disorder" tend to be used synonymously when speaking of those conditions that afflict the human nervous system. This consideration applies particularly to those diseases that are the main focus of this book, namely Parkinson's disease, amyotrophic lateral sclerosis (ALS) (colloquially called Lou Gerhig's disease, although it might just as well have been termed Charcot's disease, as it sometimes has been), and Alzheimer's disease. Is it correct to term these conditions "diseases"? The difference between the two words can be subtle. "Disease" is normally used in the sense of sickness or illness. These neurological conditions fit this definition, and hence their names are appropriate. In addition, there is some evidence – not particularly strong, but evidence nevertheless – that they actually arise as part of an infectious process. Hence, calling them "diseases" is even more correct. In regard to the word "disorder," various dictionaries define it to mean "an illness that disrupts normal physical or mental functions." These conditions definitely do both, so it is equally correct to refer to them as "disorders." Therefore, with apologies to the purists amongst the readers, the terms "neurological disease" and "neurological disorder" will be used interchangeably in the chapters that follow. When speaking of specific conditions (e.g., Alzheimer's disease), the word "disease" will always be used.

With that out of the way, I want to introduce the central theses to be addressed, not necessarily in the following order:

1) The human CNS is complex. It contains something on the order of 86 billion neurons, organized into multiple subsystems, surrounded by 85 billion supporting glial cells. Neurons are totally dependent on these support cells for their normal functions. Each neuron connects to multiple other neurons for an estimated 94 trillion synaptic connections. There should be nothing particularly controversial about anything in this paragraph for anyone in neuroscience/neurological disease research.

2) The complexity of the nervous system arises due to the interplay between genetic programs and environmental influences. This complexity includes the interactions that lead to neurodegeneration. Gene defects in the germ cell line and in the early developing CNS are likely to be fatal or result in profoundly disturbed neuronal functions. Environmental impacts on the CNS depend crucially on the stage of development: prenatal ones are likely to be of greater impact than those occurring in postnatal life, while early postnatal ones will be more impactful than those later in life. The concept of the "fetal basis of adult disease" used in other fields of study likely applies to neurological disease just as strongly (or even more so) to those disorders with which it is more conventionally associated. Environmental impacts also crucially depend on the number of CNS levels impacted (e.g., from genome to the whole CNS).

3) It is almost certain that gene defects/mutations alone will not explain most types of age-related neurological disease. Nor, for that matter, will obvious environmental stressors/toxins be found to be solely responsible in most cases. Hence, gene–toxin interactions are the likely source of most such diseases, acted upon by a number of other variables across the lifespan.

4) Neuronal compensation for genetic or environmental insults to the CNS will be limited by the type of insult and the stage(s) at which they occurs. Early gene defects, if not rapidly fatal, may be compensated for by redundancy of function of other genes. Environmental impacts, if they do not cross too many levels of organization, may allow for neuronal compensation by unaffected cells or regions. "Neuronal plasticity" is not a simple process, nor one strictly limited to the stage of neuronal development.

5) For all of these reasons, neurological diseases that are age-related (e.g., Parkinson's disease, ALS, Alzheimer's disease, and others) are going to be complex as well. The same applies to neuronal disorders at the other end of the age spectrum (e.g., autism spectrum disorder (ASD)).

6) At least for Parkinson's disease, ALS, Alzheimer's disease, there is only one, possibly two, real neurological clusters with a sufficient number of afflicted patients to allow effective epidemiology. The first cluster is ALS–parkinsonism dementia complex (ALS-PDC) of the Western Pacific. This includes the islands of Guam and Rota (where it was first described), Irian Jaya, and perhaps the Kii Peninsula of Japan (whether the CNS disorders in Kii are related to the others is an area of some controversy). The second possible cluster is the form of parkinsonism associated with consumption of the soursop fruit on the French Caribbean island of Guadeloupe.

7) The gene–toxin interactions leading to neurological diseases are not CNS-specific, but impact other organ systems as well. They may not be the cause of death or nervous system dysfunction, but ignoring these other organ impacts misses a number of crucial clues to disease etiology.

8) Still other organ systems are likely significantly involved in neurological diseases. A good example is the immune system in which autoimmune reactions may be a primary player in the onset and progression of some neurological diseases. The immune system also plays important roles in normal neuronal development.

9) Because of the complexity and interconnectedness of the CNS, damage at any level must necessarily cascade to other levels (e.g., cell to circuit, circuit to a particular region, etc.). So-called "cascading failures" will, at some point, trigger a total system collapse. Thus, after such a critical stage is reached, no effective therapy will be possible. For this reason, therapies designed to target late stages of disease, namely most at the "clinical" diagnosis stage, will inevitably fail and may simply exacerbate rather than relieve underlying pathological processes. The concepts from biosemiosis of the "true narrative representation" (TNR) apply here.

10) Any models of neurological diseases, no matter what kind of model or for which disease, are at best a limited means of understanding the complexity of the particular disease. They are even less effective in developing therapeutic approaches to early or late disease states.

11) Many of the data in the literature in any of the subfields of neurological disease research are likely to be wrong and thus highly misleading. Each subfield needs a thorough review to cull such incorrect material. This is not likely to happen.

12) Each of the sporadic/gene-susceptibility age-dependent neurological diseases represents not one entity but a spectrum of related disease states. Each case is therefore individual. Against such individual (and thus, unique) presentations, there can never be a generalized treatment. This applies particularly if treatment options are begun post-diagnosis. Effective treatments for neurological diseases, if they occur at all, can arise only from prophylaxis or the next-best option of extremely early-phase detection followed by strategic, targeted therapy. The only way to get to this stage is for governments and other entities to commit significant funds to providing a new perspective on such diseases. Essentially, this is a policy discussion, in which social priorities need to be carefully examined. Policy considerations are not the traditional role of scientists, but without the input of those doing the research, a policy re-evaluation will almost certainly not happen. Whether it does or does not is a choice. Needless to say, choices have consequences.

These last comments are really the focus of this book, and were fleshed out from some very preliminary thoughts as I walked the Camino Frances of the Camino de Santiago. For those who do not know it, the Camino actually describes a number of routes, mostly in Spain and France, which all end up in the Galician city of Santiago de Compostella. Even on a single route, although the conventional end point remains the same, the geography can vary from year to year, as a result of human activity and weather. How one actually walks the Camino varies with season, personal fitness, past or acquired injuries, frame of mind, companions, and so on. Not everyone finishes. For those who do complete the Camino, no two journeys are the same. Thus, one often hears the expression, "walking one's own Camino."

All of this leads to the point hinted at earlier: no two neurological disease manifestations, even in ostensibly the same disease, are actually the same, except perhaps at disease end state. Everyone walks their own Camino of neurological health. This metaphor, I think, has significant implications for neurological disease detection and treatment.

Four final points – caveats, really – need to be acknowledged, all of which will be discernible to readers in due course. First, just as neurological diseases are not linear in how they develop, progress, or complete, this book is not linear either. While there is a trajectory that leads from the first pages to the final conclusions, the book could not be written as if it were a simple story. Rather, it is recursive in fact and concept, with various themes being introduced and then reconsidered pages later as new information is added. Some readers may find that this makes parts of the book redundant. I hope, however, that such readers will see that any one such theme is expanded by the stage of the book and the discussions that have occurred since it was last raised.

Second, in some sections I describe the work of my laboratory and colleagues in more detail than I do the work of others. The reason is simple: I know my own work best – the valid parts as well as the invalid. I hope I have not done such self-selection too blatantly, or too often.

Third, in areas that are likely to prove particularly controversial, I err on the side of providing too many, rather than too few, primary literature references. This point ties in with the fourth caveat: The book is written mostly for my fellow neuroscientists and for those in the neurological disease world. This focus inevitably leads to some pretty dense – and reference-filled – expositions, which may be daunting for any nonspecialist scientists or the lay public. A glossary is provided at the end, which I hope will help.

That about sums it up.

Needless to say, in all of the following material, any errors in citation, content, or interpretation are purely my own.

Christopher A. Shaw
Victoria, BC, Canada

Endnotes

1 Scope Berdmore Davies (1782–1852) was a dandy and friend of Lord Byron.
2 Claude Jutra (1930–1986) was a Quebecois director, screenwriter, film editor, cinematographer, and actor. After being diagnosed with Alzheimer's and living with the condition for a time, Jutra committed suicide. In recent years, his reputation has been stained by allegations of pedophilia.

Acknowledgments

This book owes much to a number of individuals, for a great variety of reasons. First, I thank Justin Jeffryes of John Wiley & Sons for suggesting the project and for tolerating my numerous requests for extensions. The various support persons at Wiley were a pleasure to work with throughout the entire process and I am most grateful for their efforts on behalf of the book. Next, thanks are due to Claire Dwoskin for her financial support to my laboratory and her boundless encouragement in all things. Other supporters were the Luther Allyn Dean Shourds estate, the Kaitlin Fox Foundation, and various more official granting agencies, including the National Institutes of Health and the US Department of Defense.

My laboratory mates provided endless enthusiasm and cogent conversation, acted as sounding boards, and offered much other help as the project emerged. In no particular order, these were: Dr. Alice Li, Sneha Sheth, Jess Morrice, and others listed more specifically in the following.

Janice Yoo and Jessie Holbeck were most helpful in tracking down references and summarizing blocks of data for various chapters. In regard to the data summaries, Janice in particular was an amazing source, and her summaries enabled various sections to be completed. Indeed, without Janice, the book would not have been finished in anything like a timely manner. As the final deadline loomed, Janice took over all of the formatting and reference checking. For all of these reasons, my gratitude to her is boundless. Katie Blank did a fantastic job with the figures and tolerated my endless revisions. I also owe her a special debt of gratitude. Michael Kuo did final formatting, reference checks, and a huge range of jobs associated with getting this book through the copy editing and galley proof stages. I owe him a huge debt of gratitude as well.

Pierre Zweigers designed some figures for the ALS portion of the book and provided much useful discussion and commentary on several early drafts of some chapters. Bob Quellos provided valuable information on aspects of architecture. Dr. Thomas Marler of the University of Guam was kind enough to take pictures of cycads for the book. Dr. John Steele of Guam was most generous in allowing me access to some figures from his work and from the historical record on ALS-PDC. Dr. Greg Cox of Jackson Laboratories and Prof. Steven Hyman of the Broad Institute kindly provided copies of their Power-Point presentations on ALS animal models and the coming crisis in neurological disease research funding, respectively. Prof. Roger Berkowitz of the Hannah Arendt Center for Politics and Humanities of Bard College was kind enough to find the Hannah Arendt quote I use in Chapter 16. Prof. John Oller, Dr. Lucija Tomljenovic, Micheal Vonn, and Darcy Fysh provided extremely valuable critiques on drafts of part, or all, of the book. I owe much to those in the laboratory of Prof. Romain Gherardi for their kindness and guidance during my sabbatical in Paris. This includes not just Romain himself, but Profs. F.-J. Authier and Josette Cadusseau and various students and staff as well.

A posthumous thank you is due to my former PhD supervisor, Prof. Peter Hillman, who passed away while I was in the midst of writing the book. His influence has been felt throughout various stages of my career, particularly as they all coalesced in the following pages. My long-time friends and colleagues Dr. Denis Kay and Ken Cawkell provided many stimulating conversations related to topics in this book. My wife, Danika Surm, always found time in her incredibly busy schedule to allow me a few hours' work on this project here and there. My older children, Emma and Ariel, also helped in various ways, mostly serving as additional sounding boards for my endless babbling on the topics that follow. Joe's Café provided the caffeine that made it all feasible while I was writing in Vancouver.

Finally, I am most grateful to my department, Ophthalmology and Visual Sciences, and its various chairpersons over the years; to the Faculty of Medicine; and to the University of British Columbia itself. All have been supportive of my sometimes unconventional approaches to academic issues and all actually believe in that sometimes elusive application of the concept of academic freedom.

In this last year, as the book took shape in the various intellectual and geographically peripatetic ways in which it was written (Paris, Vancouver, Los Angeles, the Camino de Santiago, Lucy sur Yonne, and Victoria), my son Caius was born and my mother, Peggy O'Shea, and my father, Lou Shaw, died. This book is therefore dedicated to the future of my son and the memory of my parents. *Buen Camino* to my son as he travels through life and to my parents for lives well lived and long journeys well taken.

Christopher A. Shaw
Victoria, BC, Canada

Part I

The Dynamics of Neurological Disease

1

The Dynamics of Neurological Disease: Current Views and Key Issues

> *It was six men of Indostan*
> *To learning much inclined,*
> *Who went to see the Elephant*
> *(Though all of them were blind),*
> *That each by observation*
> *Might satisfy his mind.*
> *The First approach'd the Elephant,*
> *And happening to fall*
> *Against his broad and sturdy side,*
> *At once began to bawl:*
> *"God bless me! but the Elephant*
> *Is very like a wall!"*
> *The Second, feeling of the tusk,*
> *Cried, –"Ho! what have we here*
> *So very round and smooth and sharp?*
> *To me 'tis mighty clear*
> *This wonder of an Elephant*
> *Is very like a spear!"* [etc.[1]]
>
> John Godfrey Saxe

From the Preface

1) The human CNS is complex. It contains something on the order of 86 billion neurons, organized into multiple subsystems, surrounded by 85 billion supporting glial cells. Neurons are totally dependent on these support cells for their normal functions. Each neuron connects to multiple other neurons for an estimated 94 trillion synaptic connections. There should be nothing particularly controversial about anything in this paragraph for anyone in neuroscience/neurological disease research.

5) For all of these reasons, neurological diseases that are age-related (e.g., Parkinson's disease, ALS, Alzheimer's disease, and others) are going to be complex as well. The same applies to neuronal disorders at the other end of the age spectrum (e.g., autism spectrum disorder (ASD)).

1.1   Introduction

Certainly the first thing to consider when contemplating the human nervous system in health or disease is its overall complexity. In regard to the latter, the subject of this book, the sheer number of individual elements alone means that there are going to be multiple ways for any part of the system, any subsystem, or even individual cells such as the types of neurons and glia, to malfunction. Add to this the vast number of interconnections between neurons, circuits, and systems, and the potential for multiple forms of dysfunction grows greater still.

However, before considering how the human central nervous system (CNS) evolves into a disease state, it is important to appreciate just how utterly complex the system actually is.

1.2   The Complexity of Human Neurological Diseases

Few neuroscientists would disagree with the view that the human nervous system in general is quite complex. Indeed, some scholars and lay persons from various disciplines have opined that it is the most complex thing in the universe, or at least the most complex that humans know about. This last clause is essential given the robust hubris of *Homo sapiens*.

Regardless of just how complex the human nervous system is in the context of the rest of the universe, the questions which arise are these: First, how does such a complex system come into existence? Second, for the purposes of this book, how does it break down? It may be worth noting here that the nervous systems of most vertebrates are also relatively complex, particularly those of mammals. Largely for this reason, attempts to provide comprehensive and predictive animal models of neurological diseases are almost certain to run into many of the same problems as those associated with trying to understand the human CNS in the various states in which it may be, or become in the future.

The answer to the first question is the subject of developmental neurobiology, which examines the genetic and environmental factors underlying the formation of nervous system structure and function. In the latter regard, much has been learned about developmental features of the nervous system, the early and late forms of modifications, often termed "neuroplasticity," and the implications of the latter in particular for the remarkable capacity that any nervous system has to modify itself and thus alter behavioral responses to changing external circumstances (for a general review, see Shaw and McEachern, 2001).

The broad subject matter that comes under the rubric of neuroplasticity has been the focus of innumerable scientific research papers, reviews, and books. I was a co-editor of one of the latter, *Toward a Theory of Neuroplasticity* (Shaw and McEachern, 2001), which attempted to come to grips with the extensive subject matter at the time, a literature that will only have grown in the intervening years. The general topic of neuroplasticity will be considered here only in the context of the second question which is the focus of the chapters that follow.

Restating that question, can an admittedly complex structure/system be destroyed in a simple, perhaps unitary way, or must the innate complexity of the system in the first place make the dissolution of the system complex as well?

The answer is that both can occur, but with very different characteristics, depending on a spectrum of types of injury. For example, acute injury to the brain in the form of gunshot wounds or other major head trauma can certainly destroy the system rapidly. The myriad cellular chemicals and processes that are almost immediately released by macroscopic damage lead to the microscopic destruction of cells in a time frame of seconds to minutes. In the middle of the spectrum are traumatic injuries to the CNS that cause some level of destruction of neurons and glial cells, which may not be instantly fatal to the individual. In such cases, such as in cortical stroke or spinal cord damage, the initial trauma is often followed by secondary damage to surrounding neural cells and it is the latter that tends to exacerbate the initial injury. Indeed, such secondary damage may eventually be of larger scale and impact than the initial insult (Oyinbo, 2011).

At the other end of the spectrum are the so-called "progressive," age-related neurodegenerative diseases, which are neither acute in their initial stages, nor, as far as is known, of rapid onset. Rather, these "classical" neurological diseases (i.e., Parkinson's disease, amyotrophic lateral sclerosis (ALS), and Alzheimer's disease; Figure 1.1) appear in most cases to be more insidious in onset and progression. In general, there are few

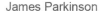
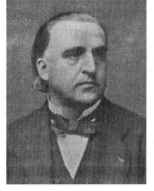
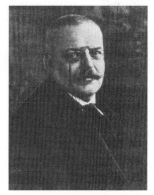

James Parkinson   Jean-Martin Charcot   Alois Alzheimer

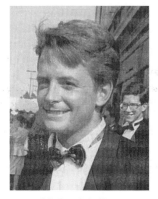
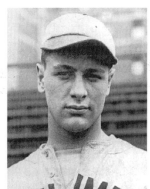
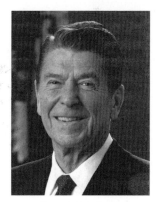

Michael J. Fox   Lou Gehrig   Ronald Reagan

Figure 1.1 Discoverers of the progressive, age-related neurological diseases and their famous victims (top to bottom): James Parkinson (Parkinson's disease was first described in his "Essay on the Shaking Palsy"; note that a verified picture of James Parkinson does not seem to be extant) and Michael J. Fox; Jean-Martin Charcot and Henry Louis ("Lou") Gehrig; Alois Alzheimer and Ronald Reagan.

reasons to believe that these diseases arise in a short time period. There may, however, be exceptions.

For example, forms of what look to be ALS-like motor neuron disorders have arisen relatively rapidly in some Gulf War Syndrome victims (Haley, 2003). Additionally, some ALS-like disorders in young women have been linked, at least temporally, to human papilloma virus (HPV) vaccine adverse reactions (Huang et al., 2009). In addition, there is a rapid-onset form of parkinsonism, now the basis of one of the major animal models of Parkinson's disease, that arises due to the direct action of the molecule 1-methyl-4-phenyl-1,2,3,6-tetrahydropyridine (MPTP). People afflicted with this form of parkinsonism had injected into their veins what they believed to be a synthetic opioid, 1-methyl-4-phenyl-4-propionoxypiperidine (MPPP), a street analogue of meperidine (Demerol). The inaccurate synthesis of MPPP gave MPTP instead (Langston et al., 1983). There are various other examples as well, which will be described in later chapters.

Parkinson's disease, ALS, and Alzheimer's disease typically develop slowly, and most evidence suggests that the pre-clinical stages of the diseases arise over the course of years to decades (Ben-Ari, 2008). One view is that some predisposing neuronal factors may arise *in utero*, similar to the "fetal basis of adult disease" (FeBAD) hypothesis proposed for cardiovascular disorders. This hypothesis and how it may apply to CNS diseases will be discussed in Chapter 10.

In what follows, it is important to stress that while traumatic acute brain injuries, stroke, and so on are the subjects of intensive research and are of clear medical and social importance, the focus of this book is really on the major neurological diseases, which occur progressively, meaning that the various signs and symptoms of any of these diseases will continue to worsen during the time course from clinical diagnosis until death.

It is at least a fair assumption that much the same progressive nature of such diseases occurs prior to the clinical stage, but the reality is that the field does not know much about this part of the progressive process. There are some hints from animal models of the various diseases, insofar as these accurately reflect the human condition (a point I will return to in Chapter 8), that pre-clinical stages actually resemble an early phase of what will become a "cascading failure" in the affected regions of the nervous system at a later time. The term "cascading failure" can be defined as the failure of one part in a system of interconnected parts that triggers the failure of other, successive parts (Bashan et al., 2013). During this cascade, the underlying biochemical and morphological processes build toward the general dysfunctions that begin to characterize the stage in which clinical diagnosis occurs. The point from clinical diagnosis onwards is, at this time, the point of no return for the neurological health of those regions of the nervous system affected, and indeed for the overall health of the patient. This latter point is well illustrated not only by the general lack of success in treating such diseases to date, but also through consideration of the numbers of molecules of all types that are found to be altered following post-mortem examination. The examples typically provided by various genomic, proteomic, and metabolomics arrays demonstrate huge differences between those with the disease state and those without (Figure 1.2).

If the end state of any of these diseases is cluttered with vast numbers of altered structures and molecular processes and thus not likely amenable to treatment, then it may be worthwhile at this juncture to consider the things that those attempting treatment would need to know in order to achieve success.

First, clinicians would need to know something about the actual etiology (or much more likely, etiologies) for that disease. As will be discussed in the following pages, apart from a few genetic mutations, which appear to be responsible for the "familial" forms of these diseases, we do not have much insight into that much larger fraction of neurological diseases that are termed "sporadic," or of unknown origin. It should also be stressed that just because some forms of neurological disease involve genetic changes, this should not be taken to imply that they are without anything apart from a genetic etiology or that they are completely separate from environmental factors. This point will be made clearer in the discussion of epigenetics in neurological diseases in Chapter 6.

In addition to having clearly demonstrated etiologies, the field would need a fairly accurate time course for the various pre- and post-clinical stages. Thus, if the diseases were of genetic origin, the time course would begin with that mutation; if it were due to a toxic molecule, the time course would begin with the introduction of that molecule.

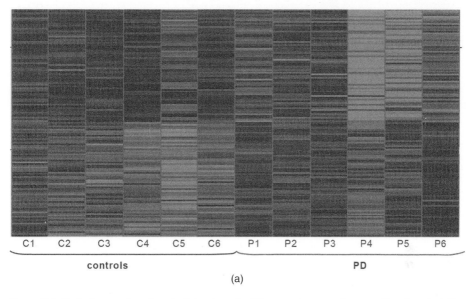

(a)

Figure 1.2 Typical examples of genomic/proteomic differences in neurodegenerative disease victims compared to control patients. (a) Relative expression levels of the 137 genes differentially expressed in Parkinson's disease (PD) samples relative to controls. Only genes that met the criterion of being altered by a factor of 1.5 relative to control and which passed the Wilcoxon test at the significant level of $p < 0.05$ were included. Genes are clustered by their relative expression levels over the 12 samples. Expression levels are color-coded relative to the mean: green for values less than the mean and red for values greater than it. *Source*: Grünblatt et al. (2004), used with permission from Springer Science and Business Media. (b) Genes differentially expressed in the motor cortex of sporadic ALS subjects: 57 of 19 431 quality-filtered genes (0.3%), represented by 61 probes, were differentially expressed (corrected $p < 0.05$), with each row in the matrix representing a single probe and each column a subject. Normalized expression levels are represented by the color of the corresponding cell, relative to the median abundance of each gene for each subject (see scale). Genes are named using their UniGene symbol and arranged in a hierarchical cluster (standard correlation) based on their expression patterns, combined with a dendrogram whose branch lengths reflect the relatedness of expression patterns. For each gene, the fold-change (diseased vs. control) and corrected p values are given. *Source*: Lederer et al. (2007), used under Creative Commons Attribution License. (See color plate section for the color representation of this figure.)

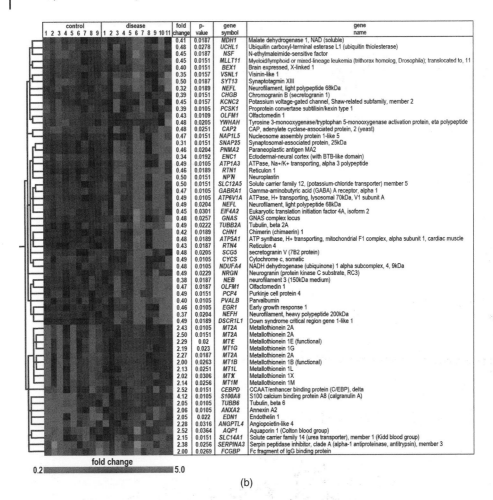

(b)

Figure 1.2 (*Continued*)

While there is now an existing literature describing "staging" for diseases such as Parkinson's and Alzheimer's, staging for ALS remains less defined (see Chapter 9). Regardless, the staging of the pre-clinical diseases is still largely unknown. To address this lack of information, the field would have to fill significant gaps in the basic knowledge of these diseases. For example, not much is known (yet) about risk factors, let alone causal factors. Worse, the likely additive – perhaps synergistic – actions of gene–gene, toxin–toxin, and gene–toxin interactions in neurological disease are only now, and quite slowly, emerging. The general absence of information on such interactions is very problematic for the attempt to understand disease origins since the great likelihood is that these are precisely the sorts of multiple events that are going to cause disease initiation and progression.

Delving downwards to more molecular levels, it would be crucial to have some idea about the activated genes and biochemical pathways at each of the still undefined pre-clinical disease stages. Achieving this level of pre-clinical analysis would be remarkably difficult, especially since the existing literature cannot do so very well even post-clinically. In particular, the field would need to identify abnormal biochemical processes that showed the propensity to cascade and thus trigger still further abnormal events.

Based on current genomic, proteomic, and metabolomic studies, such downstream events are likely to be huge in number, but of uncertain significance and time course. In the first case, the problem is one of separating putatively causal events that lead to stages of neurological disease from those that are merely bystander events, or even failed compensatory processes. To date, this goal has been difficult to achieve. At present, existing "biomarker" studies aimed at monitoring neurological disease onset and progression are still rudimentary in specificity, scope, and overall utility (for a review, see Shaw et al., 2007).

With every passing year, it becomes increasingly obvious that a great many genes, proteins, and other molecules are affected in Parkinson's disease, ALS, and Alzheimer's disease. The problem for potential therapeutics is not that the field has failed to identify a host of these, but rather the question of what to do with this burgeoning list of potential therapeutic targets. Thus, in cases where hundreds of molecules in the affected parts of the CNS are altered, it becomes quite hard to imagine – let alone achieve – any sort of realistic drug therapy that could deal with myriad downstream alterations in the CNS. Even if one could devise such therapeutics, it would be difficult to expect them to prevent disease progression without triggering nearly endless side effects that might prove equally deleterious to the CNS and to other organ systems.

1.3 The Nervous System as an Archetypical Complex System

The nervous system is a prime example of what is termed a "complex system" (Figure 1.3). This concept is not easily defined, but instead is described on the basis of the attributes any such system possesses.

Chapter 4 will delve into complex systems in more detail, but for now some of the key attributes to note are these: Complex systems have multiple, interconnected components, which, in response to an external stimulus, display "emergent properties." Emergent properties, in turn, lead to "complex adaptive behaviors" and at least one, if not many, changes in system output. A classic example of emergent properties comes from a consideration of social insects. A beehive is composed of many thousands of bees, whose cumulative complex behaviors are those of the colony as a unified entity, not

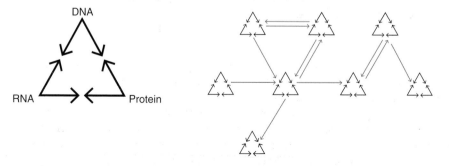

Figure 1.3 Schematic illustration of the complexity in DNA to protein interaction and in nervous system interactions.

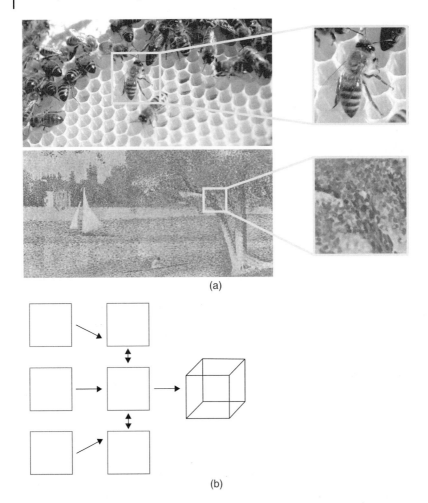

(a)

(b)

Figure 1.4 Emergent properties. (a) Top: an example of an emergent property, comparing an individual bee to a beehive. The properties of the hive are vastly more complex than those of the bee. Bottom: The "pointillist" paining, "A Sunday Afternoon on the Island of La Grande Jatte" (French: "Undimanche après-midi à l'Île de la Grande Jatte") by the post-impressionist French artist, Georges Seurat. (b) Schematic of emergent properties, showing individual elements of some systems (squares), an additional level of interaction between these elements, and a final emergent feature that is not necessarily predictable from the initial elements.

merely those of the individuals (Figure 1.4). Some other complex systems studied in detail in "complexity theory" include the stock market, political systems, ecosystems, and the weather. There are obviously many more.

Each of these complex systems can experience cascading failures due to the complex interconnections of the component parts. Thus, any failure of one circuit in an electrical device can lead to the destruction of other circuits and the overall failure of the device. Power grids that interconnect can experience cascading failures if one power plant in the network goes down. A more down-to-earth example comes from everyone's experience of how relationships and/or marriages implode.

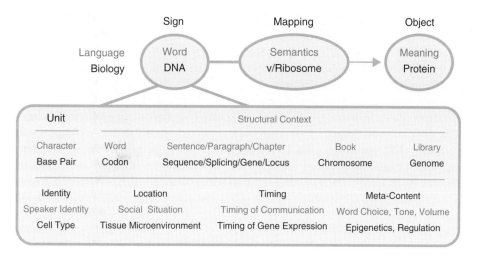

Figure 1.5 Basic concepts of biological signaling (biosemiosis) from DNA to cell function. *Source*: Gryder et al. (2013), used under Creative Commons Attribution License.

It may be instructive to view a common political situation as a metaphor for a declining nervous system. At first, a popular new government operates at high capacity and function, making few mistakes, and effectively coping with any challenges and minor upheavals. As time goes by, a cumulative deterioration begins to occur. The role of aberrant messaging (e.g., failed signaling – Signaling in biological systems has been termed "biosemiosis" or the biology of meaningful communication: Figure 1.5) leads to further signal disruptions. Bad messaging, lies, errors of judgment, and so on increasingly impact public confidence. The government becomes desperate and begins to make a series of even worse decisions. These decisions lead to further scandals. Government members begin to resign. And, in the end, a once-powerful political machine that a few months or years earlier seemed unassailable is brought down.

In the context of a neurodegenerative disease it is possible to postulate that the same general features of cascading failure occur. An initially highly functioning nervous system receives a limited number of insults which at first are coped with effectively by the various compensatory and redundancy features of the system. However, over time, the insults to the system become additive – or even synergistic – and the signaling becomes progressively degraded. Biological signaling in a biosemiotic sense begins to fail, creating additional incorrect messages and, hence, abnormal functions. The nervous system, once so adept at compensation, begins to miscompensate, exacerbating the overall dysfunction of the system. Eventually, the damage is too widespread to control and the overall decline is ensured.

In just such a way, Parkinson's disease, ALS, and Alzheimer's disease (and other neurological diseases) may occur. In such a context, neurological disease may represent just one example of the fate of any complex system in which a series of insults and increasingly failed signaling leads to system collapse.

System complexity is thus inevitably tied to the integrity of signaling and it is therefore the very aspect of complexity that needs to be understood first when dealing with human neurological diseases. In fact, it would be nearly impossible to argue that the nervous system of any animal is not at some level complex, at least in regard to function. As an example, some relatively simple nervous systems, such as that of *Caenorhabditis elegans*, a very primitive nematode (roundworm) used to model neuronal connectivity, can express rather complex behaviors, including learning and memory (Rankin, 2004; Sasakura and Mori, 2013). The level of interconnected elements even in such a simple nervous system clearly shows that emergent properties – in this case learning – can result from relatively simple neural activity.

At a more elaborate level of nervous system organization, social insects such as honey bees and ants can perform a great variety of extremely complex and purposeful behaviors (for bees, see Von Frisch, 1950). Vertebrate nervous systems are more complex still in the numbers of neurons, neuronal nuclei of specialized cells and functions, and interconnections within and between regions. And, of course, the emergent properties of vertebrates far exceed those of invertebrates. In the same manner, the complexity found in the nervous systems of mammals and the attendant emergent properties exceed those of other vertebrates.

Humans have the most complex nervous systems yet described. By adulthood, human brains have close to 86 billion neurons, at least 85 billion supporting glial cells, and upwards of 1 trillion synaptic connections (Murre and Sturdy, 1995; Azevedo et al., 2009; Walloe et al., 2014). The numbers in the overall human nervous system are without a doubt vastly larger, although those in the human spinal cord and peripheral nervous system, not to mention neural elements in other organ systems, do not yet appear to be known with any certainty. For the spinal cord, one estimate is 13 million neurons and twice that number of glial cells, but this may be at the low end (Glover, 2008).

By way of contrast, consider the common comparison of the human CNS to modern computers (Figure 1.6). Most current electronic devices, including computers, make use of transistors which are semiconductor devices used to amplify or switch electronic signals and electrical power. Microchips are composed of millions of integrated transistors. The transistor count is the most frequently used measure of integrated circuit complexity, and is roughly analogous to the synaptic connections between neurons.

In the world of personal computers, one of the fastest current processors is the Intel Core i7-4960X which is made for high-end desktop use. This processor contains

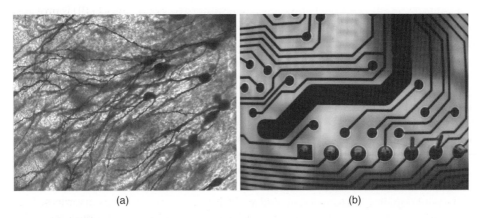

(a)   (b)

Figure 1.6 Microgram of a region of the human CNS compared to computer circuitry. (a) Golgi-stained neurons in the dentate gyrus of an epilepsy patient. 40× magnification. *Source*: MethoxyRoxy, used under Creative Commons Attribution License (https://commons.wikimedia.org/wiki/File:Gyrus_Dentatus_40x.jpg). (b) Computer circuit board. *Source*: Peter Shanks, used under Creative Commons Attribution License (https://www.flickr.com/photos/botheredbybees/2389301872).

1.86 billion transistors. In comparison, a mainframe computer such as IBM's zEnterprise EC12, released in 2012, has a processor containing 2.75 billion transistors. IBM recently launched a "neuromorphic" computer chip called TrueNorth, which is designed to work like a mammalian brain (Merolla et al., 2014; Service, 2014). It has 1 million digital "neurons" which connect to one another through 256 million "synapses." It contains 5.4 billion transistors. Even with this as a benchmark, the human brain has something like 10^5 more neurons and 10^4 more connections than any single computer.

The point of these comparisons is not to show that the human brain is superior in number of functioning elements (e.g., the numbers of neurons or synapses) given that one can envision future computers achieving comparable numbers. Indeed, a case could be made that the Internet, with its integrated web of computers, may have accomplished – if not exceeded – this level already. Rather, the point to be made is that computers, as complex systems, and the susceptibility of computer programs to signaling errors, may be quite analogous to the kind of susceptibility to failure seen in the human brain. In other words, the ways in which both computers and the human brain break down may be generally similar, as we will discuss later in this chapter.

This latter point returns to the initial question: Can a complex system such as the human nervous system break in a simple way? Obviously, as already discussed, in cases of acute trauma to the head or spinal cord, it can. However, if such trauma is not rapidly fatal, the nervous system of animals and humans shows a remarkable ability to compensate for the damage through the use of redundant neuronal circuits and by rewiring some brain areas.

The human literature is replete with just such examples. One of the more famous cases from the neurology literature is that of Phineas Gage. Gage was an American railway worker who had a large metal tamping rod blown through his head in an accidental explosion in 1848. The rod entered under his jaw and exited the top of his head, taking with it a considerable amount of cortical tissue. In spite of massive brain damage, Gage went on to recover and never lost most of his cognitive or motor abilities. He did suffer from epileptic seizures in later years, but in spite of these he managed to live on for 12 years after the initial injury.

A recent example of neural compensation for traumatic brain injury (TBI) is provided by the case of a Canadian army captain (now retired), Trevor Greene. Greene was struck on the head by an axe wielded by a Taliban insurgent in Afghanistan in 2006. His initial injuries appeared insurmountable. The axe blade had bisected the primary motor regions of the brain, and the overall damage was significant. Doctors at the Canadian Forces medical facility at Kandahar airbase, and later at a US military hospital in Germany, gave Greene's family little hope for his survival and believed there was virtually no chance of him ever recovering consciousness. In spite of this, Greene did regain consciousness and in the years since the injury he has progressed to the point where he can again talk. His cognitive abilities appear to be relatively intact, and he has regained considerable motor capabilities, the latter which seem to be improving gradually through the use of a form of imaging therapy.

These two cases point to the possibility of CNS recovery in various disorders. They will be addressed in more detail in Chapter 15. As a prelude to the later discussion, it is relevant to ask whether the Gage and Greene examples point to broader prospects for neural recovery from any brain injury. Both cases demonstrate the remarkable redundancy and plasticity of the nervous system, but do they have implications for age-related neurological diseases?

1.4   CNS Signaling Failures: Implications for Neurological Disease

Although an obvious truism, it is worthwhile in the context of the following chapters to remember that the nervous system is basically a signaling device. Information comes in from internal and external sources through various sensory receptors, is transduced into neural signals, and then undergoes multiple levels of processing within the CNS. Adaptive behaviors of the organism result. Just as with much simpler nervous systems, emergent properties also occur. For this reason, it is important at the outset to recognize the importance of the integrity of signaling between the nervous system's component parts for its successful functioning.

From this view, it follows that failures of signaling at any level are almost certain to have significantly negative consequences for neuronal function overall. At a macroscopic level, signaling errors can follow from events that impact the integrity of neuronal circuits and synapses within and between different regions of the brain. At a more microscopic cellular level, the levels of signaling include signals from DNA to protein and from protein to cell structure and function.

As will be considered in Chapter 5, the relatively small percentage of neurological diseases arising from the identified genetic mutations are in essence signaling errors in which the proteins necessary for normal neuronal function are not made or – often, worse – are made incorrectly. The resultant protein malfunction leads to cellular dysfunction, often eventually culminating in cellular (and, in this case, neuronal cell) death. Various toxins can impact signaling at various levels as well, including by altering gene expression, RNA transcription, the activity of intracellular organelles, and the cellular signals sent to other cells. Alternations at any of these levels will necessarily impact overall neuronal survival of the affected regions. Thus, however it is conceived, or regardless of the cause of the dysfunction, the breakdown of normal neuronal function leading to neurological diseases can ultimately be considered to arise from a type of signaling failure.

It is in this regard that the failure of the nervous system shares properties with the failures of other complex systems that depend on accurate signaling. Chapter 14 will address these concerns in more detail with a discussion of the biological meaning communicated between sending and receiving entities and the implications of such failure.

1.5   History and Key Characteristics of the Age-Dependent Neurological Diseases

Before considering the key age-related, progressive neurological diseases (Parkinson's disease, ALS, and Alzheimer's disease), it is perhaps worthwhile to put these into some sort of broad neurological disease perspective.

In general, neurological diseases/disorders are any that affect the nervous system, even if other organ systems are involved, and even if the primary disorder resides in these other organ systems, as in tuberculosis or diabetes.

To get a sense of the range of neurological disorders involved, I refer to those provided by a Canadian organization, Neurological Health Charities Canada (NHCC), an entity representing a range of nongovernmental organizations working on public awareness and fundraising for individual neurological disorders in Canada. NHCC, in partnership with the Public Health Agency of Canada (PHAC), devoted considerable effort, time, and money to cataloguing and describing incidence and prevalence levels for some 15 neurological disorders or disease conditions. It also provided some studies designed to look at risk factors and patient treatments. Although given in a specifically Canadian context, the list was thought by NHCC/PHAC to be broadly representative of those diseases arising in other countries in the industrialized Western world, and to some extent in the developing world as well. Overall, the final report included results from 18 separate projects (Neurological Health Charities Canada and Public Health Agency of Canada, 2014).

The neurological disorders included in the original mandate included, in alphabetical order: ALS, Alzheimer's disease and related dementias, brain injuries, brain tumors, cerebral palsy, dystonia, epilepsy, Huntington's disease, hydrocephalus, multiple sclerosis, muscular dystrophy, Parkinson's disease and parkinsonisms, spina bifida, spinal cord injury, and Tourette syndrome.

For a variety of reasons, a number of neurological disorders were not considered in the epidemiological surveys. These omissions, not trivial by any means, included some particularly important neurological disorders, such as autism spectrum disorder (ASD), macular degeneration, stroke, and schizophrenia and other mental disorders.

As the NHCC/PHAC studies began to sift through the initial epidemiological data, the overall range of neurological conditions, either included or not, resolved into particular categories: "developmental," "acute/traumatic," "age-related neurodegenerative," and "other." Some disorders can fit into various categories or subcategories, including:

- *Developmental*: Down's syndrome, cerebral palsy, spina bifida (ASD would have been in this category had it been in the initial project).
- *Acute/traumatic*: stroke, TBI (of which stroke can be one type), spinal cord injuries.
- *Age-related neurodegenerative*: ALS, Parkinson's disease and parkinsonisms, Alzheimer's disease and other dementias, Huntington's disease (macular degeneration, had it been included, would have been here).
- *Other*: schizophrenia and other so-called "mental disorders," neoplasms, Tourette syndrome, epilepsy.

Of these, Parkinson's disease, ALS, and Alzheimer's disease fit somewhere in the "age-related" general category, but are unique in that each is progressive and likely represents examples of "cascading failure" much like those cited earlier. This feature is typified by the spread from one part of the CNS to others after the initial onset. In ALS and Parkinson's disease, for example, cognitive decline may be a key sign of the latter stages of both diseases.

Further, as one of the disorders not considered by the NHCC, ASD may initially present as a developmental neurological disorder, but the underlying CNS abnormalities can create the eventual circumstances for later nervous system dysfunction with aging. This notion has not yet been explored, in part due to the simple fact that most of those currently diagnosed with ASD have not yet reached the age at which the age-related neurological diseases enter a clinical diagnosis stage. Nevertheless, Down's syndrome provides a clear precedent, with many of those with Down's developing Alzheimer's-like dementias in middle age (Zigman and Lott, 2007).

In the more acute neurological disorders (e.g., TBI and spinal cord injuries), the initial phases after injury are characterized by secondary damage to adjacent neurons and neural structures. Although often eventually stable after this secondary stage of damage, acute trauma may also have later neurological sequelae. One example involves the development of a "syrinx," or progressive cavitation of the central canal of the spinal cord, which may follow years after a spinal cord injury. As the syrinx grows, it creates pressure on various descending spinal cord nerve tracts and leads to degeneration of the axons in these tracts. The consequence, if left untreated, is a loss of motor and sensory functions below the syrinx.

1.6 The Fractal Nature of Complexity in the CNS

This chapter opened with a consideration of the dynamics of the nervous system, its overall complexity, and the inevitability of the complex interplay of factors that lead to neurological disease. It may be worthwhile here, at the outset, to consider some evolving concepts concerning cells and genes, as these will serve to inform some of that which follows.

The first point is that the standard cell "doctrine," in place for over 200 years, is likely to be, if not wrong, then quite incomplete. In brief, cell doctrine as applied to development has been seen as largely unidirectional. That is, dictated by the presumably one-way nature of genetic instructions. Emerging views in cell biology and genetics suggest that this view is not correct. Cells are not simply discrete entities, but rather, at a fractal level, composed of numerous organelles and molecules. They have, as Theise and others have described, a form of "quenched disorder" between being totally random and totally deterministic in their behaviors and interactions (Theise, 2005). Thus, at the nano level of the cell, cell doctrine breaks down as a concept. It also breaks down when considering macro level extracellular interactions. Conventional cell doctrine took the view that intracellular versus extracellular space is a rigid barrier, but this has increasingly been shown to be a limited concept. Similarly, cell lineages, far from being totally fixed, are affected by the same nano and macro considerations (Theise and Krause, 2002; Theise and d'Inverno, 2004; Kurakin, 2005).

The second "classic" notion is that gene transcription from DNA to RNA to cellular proteins is a one-way path. This view, promoted as the "Crick" doctrine, is also coming under scrutiny. In brief, recursive feedback at all levels appears to occur, making gene function highly modifiable (Pellionisz et al., 2013).

These newer conceptualizations of cells and of DNA signaling have clear implications for cell functions and lineages overall, as well as more particularly for the nervous system. If emergent properties can occur at the single-cell level, how much more likely are such properties to emerge in health and in disease in the vast complexity provided by multiple interactions within the human CNS?

To fully appreciate such considerations, it is necessary first to understand what the field of neurological disease research does – and does not – know about some of the diseases of the human nervous system, namely Parkinson's disease, ALS, and Alzheimer's disease. Details on this topic will be presented in the next chapter and will provide the basis for much of that which follows.

Endnotes

1 The Third approached the animal,
And happening to take
The squirming trunk within his hands,
Thus boldly up and spake:
"I see," quoth he, "the Elephant
Is very like a snake!"
The Fourth reached out his eager hand,
And felt about the knee.
"What most this wondrous beast is like
Is mighty plain," quoth he,
"'Tis clear enough the Elephant
Is very like a tree!"
The Fifth, who chanced to touch the ear,
Said: "E'en the blindest man
Can tell what this resembles most;
Deny the fact who can,
This marvel of an Elephant
Is very like a fan!"
The Sixth no sooner had begun
About the beast to grope,
Then, seizing on the swinging tail
That fell within his scope,
"I see," quoth he, "the Elephant
Is very like a rope!"
And so these men of Indostan
Disputed loud and long,
Each in his own opinion
Exceeding stiff and strong,
Though each was partly in the right,
And all were in the wrong!
MORAL.
So oft in theologic wars,
The disputants, I ween,
Rail on in utter ignorance
And prate about an Elephant
Not one of them has seen!
John Godfrey Saxe (1816–1887) and his version of the well-known Indian legend.

2

Clinical and Economic Features of Age-Related Neurological Diseases

"Science is built up with facts, as a house is with stones. But a collection of facts is no more a science than a heap of stones is a house."
Jules Henri Poincaré, *La Science et l'Hypotese*, 1908[1]

> **From the Preface**
>
> The same general considerations cited for Chapter 1 apply here.

2.1 Introduction

The diseases to be considered in this chapter – Parkinson's, ALS, and Alzheimer's – are the archetypical neurological diseases associated with middle and old age. There are, of course, exceptions to this statement, which will be addressed in subsequent chapters – particularly those that deal with the Guamanian forms of each of the diseases. One important notion to keep in mind is that Poincaré's comments are highly relevant when considering the details that currently exist concerning these neurological diseases, as well as others that will be considered later in brief.

At present, the field generally believes it knows a great deal about the basic features of each of these diseases, both behaviorally and in regard to the progressive pathological features within the central nervous system (CNS). There are some controversies regarding incidence and prevalence, precise numbers often being hard to come by as recently discovered by Neurological Health Charities Canada and Public Health Agency of Canada (2014). As well the costs – fiscal and emotional – to individuals and society can be uncertain. What is not yet available is a comprehensive structure into which to place the vast collection of facts and figures.

2.2 Parkinson's Disease

Of the three neurological disorders to be considered in this chapter, chronologically the first to be "discovered" was Parkinson's disease, originally termed the "shaking palsy."

Neural Dynamics of Neurological Disease, First Edition. Christopher A. Shaw.
© 2017 John Wiley & Sons, Inc. Published 2017 by John Wiley & Sons, Inc.

Parkinson's disease was named after its discoverer, the English surgeon, apothecary, and political reformer, James Parkinson. In 1817, in a now classic article, Parkinson described six patients he had examined, all with variations on the same mysterious illness (Parkinson, 1817).

Later characterizations of Parkinson's disease signs and symptoms included a variety of early features, often beginning on one side of the body before becoming bilateral in presentation. This now forms part of the staging of Parkinson's disease progression. It is also of some interest that the same sort of unilateral to bilateral presentation has recently been observed in an animal model of parkinsonism, as will be discussed in Chapter 14 (see Van Kampen et al., 2014b).

The symptoms of Parkinson's disease include stiffness of the extremities, clumsiness, slowness of movement, decreased arm swings when walking, decreased facial expression, and various dyskinesias, or movement disorders. Of the latter, tremors of the limbs at rest (resting tremor) and sometimes tremors associated with voluntary movement, such as reaching for an object (sustention tremor), are common. Another feature often observed is a characteristic "pill-rolling" behavior, which looks as if an imaginary pill is being rolled between the thumb and forefinger. Other signs of Parkinson's disease include a decrease in voice volume, a diminished capacity to distinguish odors, and decreased eye blinking. Depression often accompanies the disease, as does a decline in cognitive function, the latter in about 60% of cases (Muslimovic et al., 2009; Parkinson's Disease Foundation, 2015).

As Parkinson's disease progresses, a characteristically stooped posture emerges, along with akinesia, ataxia, bradykinesia, and festination. Additionally, the inability to control involuntary motion and the inability to voluntarily stop moving after being pushed (postural instability) occur. Patients in late stages of the disease can develop a fixed "reptilian" stare, a feature termed Parkinson's "facies." Many of these signs for "classical" Parkinson's disease closely resemble those of the Guamanian form of parkinsonism (Chapter 7), part of the overall ALS–parkinsonism dementia complex (ALS-PDC) collection of neurological disorders, which will be considered in more detail in Chapter 7.

2.2.1 Neuropathological Features

The *substantia nigra pars compacta* (SNpc; SN for short), part of the basal ganglia, is the largest nucleus in the midbrain (Figure 2.1a). It takes its name from a group of neurons that appear darkly colored (*substantia nigra* means "black body") because they contain the melanin-like pigment neuromelanin which arises from metabolism of the neurotransmitter dopamine. The primary pathological feature of Parkinson's disease is the loss of SN neurons. As these neurons degenerate and pigment is lost, the SN becomes paler in appearance (Figure 2.1b).

Numerous other changes precede the loss of neurons in the SN, and still further changes occur as the disease progresses (Braak and Braak, 1991; Braak et al., 2003; see also Chapter 9).

Neurons in the SN send axons to other areas of the brain, in particular to a region of the subcortical part of the forebrain, the striatum. This structure is composed of two interacting brain nuclei, the caudate and the putamen. In the striatum, dopamine released from neurons of the SN regulates the activity of striatal neurons which act to control many types of movement. The loss of the dopaminergic input to the striatum is thought to disturb the balance between neural excitation and inhibition. As dopamine levels in the striatum fall, there is an increase in inhibitory signals to motor regions of the brain. The disturbed inhibition/excitation balance is believed to be related to the emergence of some of the characteristic parkinsonism motor defects. In Parkinson's disease and

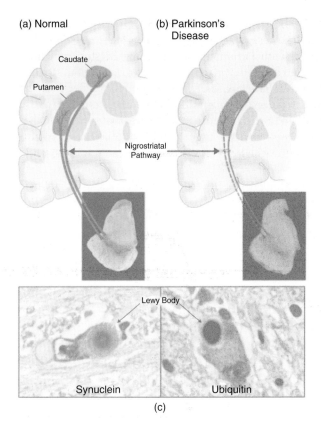

Figure 2.1 Key cellular features of Parkinson's disease. (a) Schematic representation of the normal nigrostriatal pathway, comprising dopaminergic neurons whose cell bodies are located in the SNpc (see arrows). These neurons project (thick solid lines) to the basal ganglia and synapse in the striatum (i.e., putamen and caudate nucleus). The micrograph demonstrates the normal pigmentation of the SNpc produced by neuromelanin within the dopaminergic neurons. (b) Schematic representation of the diseased nigrostriatal pathway. In Parkinson's disease, the nigrostriatal pathway degenerates. There is a marked loss of dopaminergic neurons that project to the putamen (dashed line), and a more modest loss of those that project to the caudate (thin solid line). The micrograph demonstrates depigmentation (arrows) of the SNpc due to the marked loss of dopaminergic neurons. (c) Immunohistochemical labeling of intraneuronal Lewy bodies in an SNpc dopaminergic neuron. Immunostaining with an antibody against α-synuclein reveals a Lewy body (arrow) with an intensely immunoreactive central zone surrounded by a faintly immunoreactive peripheral zone (left micrograph). Immunostaining with an antibody against ubiquitin yields more diffuse immunoreactivity within the Lewy body (right micrograph). *Source*: Dauer and Przedborski (2003), used with permission from Elsevier.

the other parkinsonisms discussed in this section, involuntary muscle contractions and uncontrolled movements result.

Some investigators believe that the initial anatomical lesion in Parkinson's disease is actually in the striatum, much as it is in Huntington's disease. In this view, the initial events involve the loss of the dopamine-containing terminals from SN neurons, followed by the death of the striatal neurons as a consequence of the loss of dopaminergic innervation. Lesions of the striatal terminals in various animal models produce a characteristic loss of SN neurons and the appearance of Parkinson's-like behavioral phenotypes. In these studies, chemically induced lesions in the striatum form the basis for the major *in vivo* animal models of Parkinson's disease, as discussed later.

Whichever stage comes first, the overall degenerative process appears to irreversibly damage both structures. In Parkinson's disease patients, brain imaging studies show that at the time of the onset of clinically defined symptoms, some 60% of SN dopamine neurons have already been destroyed and dopamine in the putamen segment of the striatum has been depleted by 80% or more (Rajput et al., 2008).

Advanced Parkinson's disease features degeneration of neurons outside of the nigro-striatal pathway, including neurons that use other neurotransmitters. Non-dopaminergic neurons that degenerate in other brain regions in Parkinson's disease include those containing noradrenaline (the *locus coeruleus*), serotonin (raphe nucleus), and acetylcholine (*nucleus basalis of Meynert* and the dorsal motor nucleus of the vagus nerve). The *nucleus basalis* is one of the primary loci for neural damage in Alzheimer's disease.

In addition, the olfactory regions of the brain, as well as regions of the cerebral cortex (cingulate and entorhinal) and parts of the autonomic nervous system, are also negatively affected. Abnormal cellular inclusions, termed "Lewy bodies," which are typical of Parkinson's disease SN and striatum, may be present in these areas as well (Figure 2.1c) (Hornykiewicz and Kish, 1987).

Additionally, non-neuronal cells in the periphery, such as blood platelets, show abnormal features, including damage to the mitochondria.

In spite of the fact that Parkinson's disease is widely considered to be largely a disorder of dopaminergic pathways, not all dopamine-containing cells are equally affected at the same time or to the same extent. For example, dopamine terminal loss occurs first in the dorsal and caudal putamen and only later in the ventral putamen and caudate nucleus; the mesolimbic dopaminergic neurons in the ventral tegmental area (VTA) adjacent to the SN are much less affected than the SN neurons themselves (Uhl et al., 1985; Kish et al., 1988). Consequently, there is significantly less depletion of dopamine in the nucleus accumbens (Price et al., 1978), one of the main sites of projection for these neurons (Uhl et al., 1985; Hornykiewicz and Kish, 1987).

In many cases of Parkinson's disease, and in many cases of the parkinsonism variants discussed later, post-mortem analysis reveals the presence of Lewy bodies in neurons of the SN and striatum, as well as various cellular projections of these neurons, forming what are termed "Lewy neurites." Lewy bodies and neurites appear to be mainly made up of an abnormally folded version of the protein α-synuclein, but they include other proteins as well, such as ubiquitin.

Whether Lewy bodies are causal to neurodegeneration or merely a downstream by-product of a system in distress is still unclear, but a prevalent view is that their formation is, at least in part, the former (Goedert et al., 2013). From this view emerges the perspective that the abnormal proteins, especially α-synuclein, are a key pathological marker of the disease and one of the early, if not initiating, disease-state events. Largely for this reason, one of the most widely used *in vivo* models of Parkinson's disease is a transgenic model in which human mutant α-synuclein is overexpressed (Recchia et al., 2008). Adding some weight to the notion that α-synuclein is indeed a fundamental part of the overall emerging state in Parkinson's disease is the observation that α-synuclein pathology is also found in peripheral cutaneous nerves, the autonomic nervous system, the enteric nervous system, the spinal cord, the lower brainstem, some limbic structures, and the neocortex (Iwanaga et al., 1999; Fumimura et al., 2007; Ikemura et al., 2008; Del Tredici et al., 2010).

Mechanistically, Parkinson's disease SN neuron loss appears to involve dysfunctions in mitochondrial complex 1 (Banerjee et al., 2009). Additionally, as in the other neurological diseases discussed in this chapter, neuroinflammatory processes appear to be active and to involve both astrocytes and microglia within areas undergoing degeneration (Tansey and Goldberg, 2010).

Finally, the blood–brain barrier appears to be compromised in Parkinson's disease (Gray and Woulfe, 2015), which may explain (in part) disease progression.

2.2.2 The Parkinsonisms

Overall, Parkinson's disease as a distinct neurological disease entity is one of a number of disorders of the so-called parkinsonisms. Each of the parkinsonisms shares some of the characteristic behavioral signs and symptoms, as well as some of the same underlying anatomical lesions, primarily those involving the degeneration of neurons in the SN.

Examples of these Parkinson's-like diseases include the following: "manganese madness," found historically in some manganese miners (Cotzias et al., 1971, 1974); dementia pugilistica, in certain high-contact sports involving head injuries, including boxing (Saing et al., 2012); parkinsonism following encephalitis (*encephalitis lethargica*) (Bojinov, 1971; Ogata et al., 1997; Sacks, 1999); and a further type induced by injection of the street drug MPTP (see Chapter 1). In addition, there are several parkinsonisms that combine features of other neurological diseases, especially the various forms of dementia.

One of the latter disorders is progressive supranuclear palsy (PSP), which features widespread neuronal death outside of areas usually found in idiopathic Parkinson's disease (Steele et al., 1964, 2014). In addition, PSP shows a widespread distribution of tau neurofibrillary tangles (NFTs), a hallmark feature of Alzheimer's disease (see Section 2.4). In many ways, PSP resembles ALS-PDC of Guam, perhaps the most studied of the parkinsonisms (see Chapter 7). It also resembles the form of parkinsonism that is found on the French Caribbean island of Guadeloupe (Guadeloupe PDC, or G-PDC) (Caparros-Lefebvre et al, 2002; Shaw and Höglinger, 2008).

2.2.3 Rating Schemes

An emerging view of Parkinson's disease is that the neurological features and time lines that fall under the conventional Parkinson's disease rubric actually describe a spectrum of related neurological disease manifestations that share a final end state but not necessarily the same rate of progression or all the same signs and symptoms (Sherer and Mari, 2014). The spectrum nature of Parkinson's disease as one of the parkinsonisms is quite apart from the even more obvious variations found within the more general class of "parkinsonisms." This point will become clearer in Chapter 9 when I describe the categorization schemes for the disease in the context of potential underlying and perhaps common disease etiologies.

The characteristic staging of Parkinson's disease after clinically-defined onset follows one or more of the following classification schemes which refer to the stages of the disease.

2.2.3.1 Hoehn and Yahr Scale

This is a commonly used clinical rating method that defines broad categories of motor function (Hoehn and Yahr, 1967):

- *Stage 1*: Unilateral involvement only, usually with minimal or no functional disability.
- *Stage 2*: Bilateral or midline involvement without impairment of balance.
- *Stage 3*: Bilateral disease, mild to moderate disability with impaired postural reflexes. The patient remains physically independent.
- *Stage 4*: Severely disabling disease, but the patient is still able to walk or stand unassisted.
- *Stage 5*: Confinement to bed or wheelchair, unless aided.

2.2.3.2   Modified Hoehn and Yahr Scale

This has the following stages (Goetz et al., 2004):

- *Stage 1*: Unilateral involvement only.
- *Stage 1.5*: Unilateral and axial involvement.
- *Stage 2*: Bilateral involvement without impairment of balance.
- *Stage 2.5*: Mild bilateral disease with recovery on the pull test.
- *Stage 3*: Mild to moderate bilateral disease, some postural instability. Patient remains physically independent.
- *Stage 4*: Severe disability, but the patient is still able to walk or stand unassisted.
- *Stage 5*: Wheelchair bound or bedridden, unless aided.

2.2.3.3   Schwab and England Activities of Daily Living Scale

This scheme is designed to estimate the abilities of Parkinson's patients relative to unaffected persons. It can be assessed by the medical caregiver or by the patient as follows (Schwab and England, 1969):

- *100% – Completely independent*: Able to do all chores without slowness, difficulty, or impairment.
- *90% – Completely independent*: Able to do all chores with some slowness, difficulty, or impairment, but may take twice as long to perform them.
- *80% – Independent on most chores*: Takes twice as long to perform chores. The patient is conscious of difficulty and slowing of movement.
- *70% – Not completely independent*: Finds it three or four times more difficult to do chores. Chores thus take up a large part of the day.
- *60% – Some dependency*: Can do most chores, but very slowly and with much effort and many errors. Some chores are impossible to perform.
- *50% – More dependent*: Needs help with approximately half of all chores. Experiences difficulty with everything.
- *40% – Very dependent*: Can assist with all chores, but can do few alone.
- *30% – More dependent*: Operates with considerable effort. Can do a few chores alone now and then, but generally much help is needed.
- *20% – Dependent*: Can do nothing alone, but can do some chores with help. The patient is now a severe invalid.
- *10% – Totally dependent*: Helpless without assistance.
- *0% – Vegetative*: Basic functions alone remain (swallowing, bladder, and bowel function are compromised). The patient is bed-ridden.

2.2.3.4   Unified Parkinson's Disease Rating Scale

This is currently the most commonly used method of categorizing Parkinson's disease in a clinical setting. The Unified Parkinson's Disease Rating Scale (UPDRS) was first developed in the 1980s, and in the original version it included the Hoehn and Yahr Scale and Schwab and England Scale (Fahn et al., 1987). In 2007, the Movement Disorder Society (MDS) published a revision of the UPDRS, known as the MDS-UPDRS, which has four sections (Goetz et al., 2007b; Movement Disorder Society, 2014):

- *Part 1*: Non-motor aspects of experiences of daily living (13 items).
- *Part 2*: Motor aspects of experiences of daily living (13 items).
- *Part 3*: Motor examination (18 items).
- *Part 4*: Motor complications (6 items).

2.2.4   Progression

These ratings schemes are provided to show the aspects of the progression of the disease post-diagnosis. Parkinson's disease typically evolves from symptom onset to end stage (or, more correctly, end state) within 8–10 years in the *relatively* well-defined patterns described earlier. But, as noted, there are significant variations (Sherer and Mari, 2014). Generally, however, the severity of motor symptoms progresses steadily, with dementia often appearing in the later phases of the disease.

Although the severity of signs and symptoms is thought to correspond directly to the level of damage inside the nervous system, the precise relationship between behavioral changes and cell loss is unclear, since most measurements of the latter are only made after death.

2.2.5   Other Organ System Involvement

In Parkinson's disease, in addition to the changes in neural systems already cited, there are changes in both the size and the biochemistry of blood platelets (Ferrarese et al., 1999; Behari and Shrivastava, 2013; Koçer et al., 2013). What this means is not clear, other the notion that Parkinson's disease, like the other neurological diseases discussed in this chapter, is likely to be a multisystem disorder.

2.2.6   Parkinson's Disease Clusters

The general nature of neurological disease clusters will be discussed in the next chapter. Here, it will suffice to note that there are only two actual clusters of the so-called "parkinsonisms" that are not the classical presentation of the original disease described by James Parkinson. These are ALS-PDC of Guam and the Western Pacific and G-PDC.

2.2.7   Risk Factors

Parkinson's/parkinsonism risk factors include rural living (possibly associated with greater exposure to toxic agricultural chemicals), head trauma, increasing age, and male sex. In regard to agricultural chemicals, a large-scale risk-factor study under the auspices of the NHCC/PHAC showed pesticide/herbicide exposure of various kinds to be a key risk factor for the disease (Public Health Agency of Canada, 2015).

Negative correlations include smoking: the risk of Parkinson's disease amongst smokers is 60% lower than amongst nonsmokers for reasons that remain quite unclear. Speculation in this regard has focused on the role of nicotinic acetylcholine receptors in the brain (James and Nordberg, 1995; Fujita et al., 2006).

The different subtypes of parkinsonism, the two clusters of ALS-PDC and G-PDC, and the risk associated with agricultural chemicals highlight that most forms of parkinsonism are likely to arise primarily from environmental, rather than purely genetic factors. Although genetic forms of early-onset Parkinson's disease do occur (see Chapter 5), it is worth noting here that these mutations comprise only a small fraction of all cases of the disease – certainly under 10%, and possibly even less, of the total.

The mutations identified to date include genes coding for the proteins parkin, ubiquitin, α-synuclein, and LRRK2 (to name only the major ones). Other very rare mutations, usually affecting single families, have been described as well. In relation to parkin, ubiquitin, and α-synuclein, the normal functions of these proteins are not known in any great detail. What the abnormal forms do to advance the disease is even less clear.

While the debate surrounding the potential genetic factors in Parkinson's disease has been taking place since the late 1800s, the question was thought to have been resolved in 1999 with the publication of an epidemiological study based on identical and fraternal twins (Tanner et al., 1999). In this study, almost 200 male twins with Parkinson's disease were identified in data from the US Veterans Administration based on an initial prospective group of nearly 20 000 twins. The study reported that the concordance rate for Parkinson's disease in monozygotic twins was not significantly greater than for dizygotic twins. This outcome suggested that genetic factors were *not* causal in most cases, the exception being for the early-onset forms of the disease (i.e., beginning before age 50).

These results are not without controversy and at least one study has suggested a stronger genetic role for Parkinson's disease amongst identical twins (Wirdefeldt et al., 2011). In addition, a genome screen for sibling pairs suggested a genetic linkage on chromosomes 1, 9, 10, and 16 for the sporadic form of the disease as well (DeStefano et al., 2001).

2.2.8 Current Treatment Options

There are various treatment options for Parkinson's disease and other of the parkinsonisms, some relatively efficacious, some much less so. These will be addressed in more detail in Chapters 13 and 14, but as a prelude, the following applies: Replacing dopamine by giving patients the dopamine precursor molecule L-3,4-dihydroxyphenylalanine (L-DOPA) can provide relatively long reversals of Parkinson's disease paralysis. One particular parkinsonism case caused by an encephalitis infection and treated by L-DOPA was the basis of a best-selling novel, and later movie, *Awakenings* (Sacks, 1999).

The success of L-DOPA treatment is rarely permanent, however, and in more advanced stages of the disease, L-DOPA can induce severe movement dyskinesias that are, in many cases, almost as debilitating as the disease itself. Direct brain injections of fetal SN cells have given mixed results, with the duration of benefits being variable in length. The success rate appears to vary considerably between treatment centers. Stem-cell therapies have not been successful to date.

2.2.9 Animal Models

Numerous attempts have been made to create animal models of Parkinson's disease, with most focused on inducing the rapid degeneration of dopaminergic neurons of axons from neurons in the SN (Blesa et al., 2010). This strategy arises from the view that this loss is the crucial and perhaps initial feature of the disease in human patients. While such means of inducing parkinsonism outcomes are typically highly artificial, it is notable that Parkinson's/parkinsonism-like symptoms can also more naturally develop in animals upon the ingestion of various neurotoxins (e.g., the seeds of the cycad *Cycas micronesica* (Van Kampen et al., 2014b; see Chapter 7), yellow star thistle (Mettler and Stern, 1963), and other plants).

A number of genetic models using transgenic animals expressing various mutant proteins have also been created and tested. These models sometimes fail to produce neuron death in the SN, but this remains a highly active area of current research. The use of genetic models in general, and in relation to the mutant superoxide dismutase 1 (mSOD1) model for ALS more specifically, will be addressed in Chapter 5.

2.2.10 Parkinson's Disease in Relation to Other Neurological Diseases

Parkinson's disease has typically been viewed as a completely distinct neurological entity, separate from other neurological diseases. This view largely prevails in spite of the fact that the variant forms of parkinsonism often display clear signs of dementia, many with features practically identical to those of Alzheimer's disease. Notable examples are some of those neurological disease variants already mentioned. For example, ALS-PDC, G-PDC, and PSP all share the expression of an Alzheimer's-like dementia. In addition, some 60% of patients diagnosed with classical Parkinson's disease go on to show signs of dementia and damage to other parts of the brain. Further, Lewy bodies, which are so characteristic of many cases of Parkinson's disease, can show up in the SN of Alzheimer's disease patients. Similarly, NFTs and senile plaques, characteristics of Alzheimer's disease, can be found in some Parkinson's cases (Braak and Braak, 1990). Non-neural systems, notably blood platelets, can also be affected in Parkinson's disease.

2.2.11 Demographics

Parkinson's disease occurs more often in men than in women, with a ratio that ranges from 1.5 to 1 to almost 4 to 1 (Gillies et al., 2014). In terms of overall prevalence and incidence, the numbers cited in Section 2.2.12, however determined, make Parkinson's disease the second most common age-related, progressive neurological disease after Alzheimer's disease.

2.2.12 Incidence and Prevalence

2.2.12.1 United States and Canada

Most of the following data are derived from the Parkinson's Disease Foundation (US), Parkinson Society Canada, and Health Canada (all as of 2010).

In the United States, approximately 1 million people have Parkinson's disease. Incidence is approximately 60 000 per year in a population of over 319 million. In Canada, prevalence is approximately 100 000. In population terms, this is comparable to the United States, which has a roughly 10 times larger population. Incidence in Canada is given as 10–20 per 100 000, which again is comparable to the United States.

In North America overall, the prevalence data can be broken down by age cohort: 113/100 000 amongst those aged 50–59 years; 540/100 000 amongst those aged 60–69 years; 1602/100 000 amongst those aged 70–79 years; and 2953/100 000 amongst those aged over 80 years (Ross and Abbott, 2014).

2.2.12.2 Worldwide

While incidence levels in the rest of the world vary, there appears to be a trend to higher levels in countries of the Northern Hemisphere. In the industrialized Western countries, some evidence suggests increased incidence levels for various movement disorders, including Parkinson's, with an overall change of between two and fourfold from the late 1970s to the late 1990s (Pritchard et al., 2004). Age, sex, and location appear to affect the rate of change.

Incidence levels increase with age, but the average age of onset for both sexes is about 65 years, although an estimated 15% of people with Parkinson's are diagnosed before the age of 50.

2.2.13 Changes in Incidence/Prevalence over the Last 30 Years

2.2.13.1 United States and Canada

Changes in incidence/prevalence were reported to be stable in Minnesota from 1976 to 1990 (Rocca et al., 2001). This is only one state amongst 50, so the accuracy of these data are not certain for the United States overall. In Canada, the data do not seem to be reliable, although one report for the province of Manitoba showed no increase from 1980 to 2006 (Lix et al., 2010), mirroring the US study. Concerning the latter data, a recently released document prepared for the NHCC/PHAC gives similar outcomes (Public Health Agency of Canada, 2015).

2.2.14 Costs

2.2.14.1 Cost Per Patient

2.2.14.1.1 United States
- *Total costs*: $6000/year for medications, plus $25 000 for surgical treatments. Assisted-living facilities or nursing homes can cost upwards of $100 000/year (The Michael Stern Parkinson's Research Foundation, 2013).

2.2.14.1.2 Canada
- *Total costs*: $12 000 per year for medications, plus $15 000–20 000 per procedure for surgery (Parkinson Society Canada and Health Canada, 2003).

2.2.14.2 Societal Costs

2.2.14.2.1 United States
- *Total costs (including treatments, social security payments, and lost income)*: $25 billion/year (Parkinson's Disease Foundation, 2010).
  There are variant cost estimates from other sources:

- *Total costs*: $14.4 billion/year (Kowal et al., 2013):
  - *Direct costs*: $8 billion/year.
  - *Indirect costs*: $6.3 billion/year.

2.2.14.2.2 Canada
- *Total costs*: $446.8 million/year (Canadian Institute for Health Information, 2007):
  - *Direct costs*: $201.9 million/year.
  - *Indirect costs*: $244.9 million/year.

There are variant cost estimates from other sources:

- *Total costs*: $558.1 million/year (Parkinson Society Canada and Health Canada, 2003):
  - *Direct costs*: 87.8 million/year.
  - *Indirect costs*: 470.3 million/year.

2.2.14.3 Projected Cost Increases

The prevalence and economic burden of Parkinson's disease are projected to grow substantially over the next few decades due to the aging Baby Boomer population if prevalence ratios remain constant. Nursing home care will be a major contributor to medical costs and reduced employment will be a major indirect cost (Kowal et al., 2013). If Parkinson's incidence also increases, however, then the numbers listed in this section will be on the low side.

2.3 Amyotrophic Lateral Sclerosis

ALS, a type of motor neuron disease (MND), was "discovered" almost 50 years after the first descriptions of Parkinson's disease in 1817. Its formal debut was given in 1865 by Jean Martin Charcot, a French neurologist (Charcot, 1865). ALS later got its more common name from baseball's Lou Gehrig, who died of the disease in 1941.

The formal name of ALS describes its basic features: "amyotrophic," for the typical atrophy and loss of tone of the affected muscles; "lateral," for the degeneration of fibers in the lateral columns of the spinal cord; and "sclerosis," for the actual lesions in these same columns.

2.3.1 Loci of Onset

In ALS, motor weakness and deficits are commonly first observed in the legs or arms, a sign indicating the loss of lower motor neurons. ALS may also begin in the brain ("bulbar" onset), with early symptoms including dysarthria and dysphagia. These features also eventually occur when disease onset begins in the spinal cord and spreads rostrally.

The initial site of onset appears to influence disease severity and progression. Most of those with ALS (65%) initially show unilateral limb onset, presenting in either the legs or arms as a muscle weakness with fasciculations. These patients progress to end-state disease in 3–5 years. Some 30% present with bulbar onset, with initial symptoms including dysarthria and dysphagia (Hardiman et al., 2011; Ravits et al., 2013; Swinnen and Robberecht, 2014). These patients are typically older and have a much more rapid development of the disease end state (2 years) (Chiò et al., 2011).

As above, disease onset may often start on one side, much as in Parkinson's disease, before becoming bilateral. Again, as with Parkinson's disease, some animal models of ALS mimic this feature (see Chapter 11). Unlike Parkinson's or Alzheimer's, in which patients can live with the disease for decades, death in ALS usually occurs rapidly, typically due to respiratory failure caused by the loss of innervation of the diaphragm due to the loss of motor neurons of the C3, 4, and 5 levels of the spinal cord.

The underlying pathological process in ALS is typically one in which upper and/or lower motor neurons controlling the muscles of the limbs and respiration degenerate and the muscles they innervate subsequently atrophy. The upper motor neurons controlling voluntary movement are those arising from the motor cortex or brain stem which carry motor information by way of spinal tracts to the lower motor neurons. These upper motor neurons are the large pyramidal cells (termed "Betz cells") found in layer V of the primary motor cortex. Lower motor neurons are found in the gray matter of the spinal cord (termed "anterior horn cells"), in the anterior nerve roots, or within the cranial nerve nuclei in the brain stem. Lower motor neurons innervate the skeletal muscles.

ALS is itself subdivided into a variety of early-onset forms of a primarily genetic origin, termed "familial ALS" (fALS). The later-onset forms, termed "sporadic ALS" (sALS), are of still unknown origin. The vast majority of cases are of the sporadic form. fALS presents with an age of onset that is 10 years earlier than sALS.

ALS is the most common disease type in a spectrum of other MNDs. These others include primary lateral sclerosis, which affects upper motor neurons alone, and progressive muscular atrophy, which affects only lower motor neurons. Another MND is progressive bulbar palsy, which impacts the lowest motor neurons of the brain stem.

2.3.2 Neuropathological Features

The lower motor neurons are subdivided into α-motor and γ-motor neuron subtypes. The former innervate the extrafusal muscle fibers of skeletal muscles to initiate muscle contractions. The latter innervate the intrafusal muscle fibers of muscle spindles. The main neuronal lesions of ALS in the spinal cord primarily affect α-motor neurons, but here again there are differences between sALS and fALS. In the latter, most cases show signs of limb onset without bulbar involvement, and less than 20% of fALS cases show signs of both lower motor neuron dysfunction and upper motor neuron degeneration.

At disease end state in sALS, surviving motor neurons typically show the presence of ubiquitin-positive cytoplasmic aggregates, which suggest proteosomal involvement in the disease (Al-Chalabi et al., 2012). Another main pathology involves shrunken anterior nerve roots (Yachnis and Riviera-Zengotita, 2014), likely a consequence of motor neuron loss. Evidence for increased astrocytic and microglial proliferation suggests inflammatory processes during the disease time course.

In regard to neuronal pathology, there are several characteristic intracytoplasmic pathological features in sALS. These include: "Bunina bodies" which are small granular inclusions, usually found only in the cytoplasm and in dendrites which are ubiquitin–negative (Figure 2.2); skein-like inclusions of thread-like structures in the cytoplasm; and round hyaline inclusions in the cytoplasm. The latter two inclusions stain positively for ubiquitin (Kato, 2008; Yachnis and Rivera-Zengotita, 2014). Cytoplasmic TDP-43-positive inclusions are also common in sALS, but are a scarce finding in the mutant *SOD1*-linked familial form of the disease (Mackenzie et al., 2007).

In fALS, two major forms have been identified: those with neuronal changes similar to sALS and those that show posterior column involvement and lack skein-like inclusions (Kato, 2008). There are, however, a considerable range of variations.

fALS can also be subdivided based on some of the typical sALS proteins associated with ubiquitin-positive inclusions. Other distinguishing features of sALS compared to fALS include abnormal translocation of TDP-43 with the formation of cytoplasmic inclusions. The latter occurs in sALS and the non-m*SOD1* forms of fALS, such as *TARDBP* and *C9orf72* (Mackenzie et al., 2007; Al-Chalabi et al., 2012), as will be described in Chapter 5.

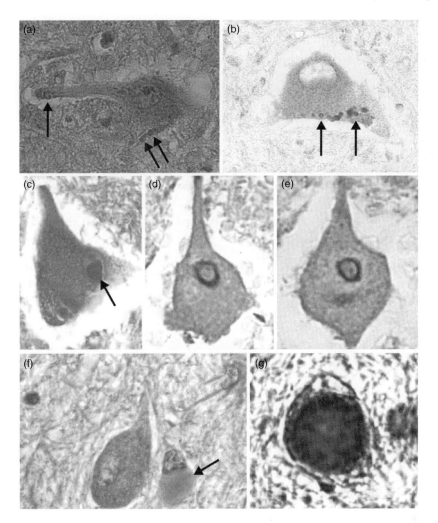

Figure 2.2 Key cellular features of ALS. (a,b) Light micrographs of Bunina bodies. (a) Bunina bodies in an anterior horn cell of an sALS patient. Bunina bodies are small eosinophilic inclusions (approximately 1–3 μm in diameter) that stain bright red with hematoxylin–eosin (H-E). They are observed within the cytoplasm (double arrows), arranged in a chain-like formation, and within dendrites (arrow), appearing as a cluster. (b) Cystatin C immunostaining. Bunina bodies are positive for cystatin C (double arrows). A Bunina body (indicated by the center arrow) appears as a round structure with a central-lucent core, which corresponds to a cytoplasmic island containing neurofilaments and other micro-organelles at the ultrastructural level. (c–e) Light micrographs of neuronal Lewy body-like hyaline inclusions (LBHIs). (c) A round LBHI (arrow) is observed in the cytoplasm of the anterior horn cell, composed of an eosinophilic core with a paler peripheral halo. A small, ill-defined LBHI (arrowhead) is also seen in the cytoplasm of the anterior horn cell, consisting of obscure, slightly eosinophilic materials. H-E staining was used. (d,e) Serial sections of a neuronal LBHI in a spinal anterior horn cell immunostained with antibodies against (d) m*SOD1* and (e) ubiquitin. An intraneuronal LBHI is clearly labeled by the antibodies to *SOD1* and ubiquitin. The immunoreactivity for both *SOD1* and ubiquitin is almost restricted to the halo of the LBHI. (f) Light micrograph of an astrocytic hyaline inclusion (Ast-HI) in the spinal-cord anterior horn. The Ast-HI (arrow) is round and eosinophilic. The astrocyte bearing the Ast-HI is morphologically different from the adjacent neuron. The nucleus of the cell bearing the Ast-HI resembles that of a reactive astrocyte (double arrowheads), and not that of an oligodendrocyte (arrowhead). H-E staining was used. (g) A neurofilamentous conglomerate inclusion, showing intense immunohistochemical positivity for phosphorylated neurofilament protein. Scale bar: (a–e,g) 30 μm; (f) 10 μm. *Source*: Kato (2008), used with permission from Springer Science and Business Media. (See color plate section for the color representation of this figure.)

fALS typically shows misfolded SOD1 proteins, a finding not usually seen in sALS cases. This conclusion remains controversial and appears to strongly depend on the antibody being used to label the misfolded protein (Liu et al., 2009; Pokrishevsky et al., 2012; Rotunno and Bosco, 2013).

2.3.3 Rating Schemes

2.3.3.1 El Escorial Diagnostic Criteria

The characterization of ALS clinically typically involves the use of one of several schemes. The El Escorial diagnostic criteria were first developed in 1994 by the World Federation of Neurology (WFN) Research Group on Motor Neuron Diseases (Brooks, 1994), and later revised in 2000 (Brooks et al., 2000). El Escorial was designed to aid in diagnosing and classifying patients for clinical studies, therapeutic trials, and molecular genetics research.

According to these criteria, the diagnosis of ALS requires symptoms of both lower and upper motor neuron degeneration and the progressive spread of symptoms or signs, together with the absence of electrophysiological or pathological and neuroimaging evidence for other disease processes (Brooks et al., 2000). These criteria categorize patients into "clinically definite," "clinically probable," "clinically probable – laboratory supported," and "clinically possible" groups. However, the sensitivity of the criteria has been found to be low in clinical practice and early diagnosis (Traynor et al., 2000).

In 2006, clinical researchers proposed a modification to the existing criteria to increase sensitivity without losing specificity (de Carvalho et al., 2008). The new Awaji–Shima criteria allow electromyographic evidence of denervation, including fasciculations, to carry equal weight to clinical evidence. The modified criteria have been shown to significantly increase sensitivity, resulting in earlier diagnosis and thus earlier potential entry into clinical drug trials (Douglass et al., 2010; Costa et al., 2012).

2.3.3.2 ALS Functional Rating Scale

A second scheme (see Table 2.1), the ALS Functional Rating Scale (Revised) (ALSFRS-R), is a validated rating procedure designed to monitor the progression of disability in patients with ALS (Cedarbaum et al., 1999). The ALSFRS-R was developed to provide better coverage of respiratory difficulties than the original ALSFRS. It does not take into account the effects of symptom duration. However, expressing an ALSFRS-R score as a function of disease duration does provide a clinically relevant measure of disease progression (ΔFS) that can be employed to stratify patient cohorts (Kimura et al., 2006; Labra et al., 2016) and which provides predictors of overall survival.

2.3.3.3 Forced Vital Capacity

Forced vital capacity (FVC) is a measurement used as an index of respiratory function, particularly in relation to potential respiratory compromise in ALS patients (Brinkmann et al., 1997). FVC measures the volume change of the lungs between a full inspiration to total lung capacity and a maximal expiration to a residual volume. The use of FVC has some clear advantages and disadvantages. For example, it is easy to perform and can be used to measure progression and predicted survival times (Czaplinski et al., 2006), and is the best indicator of impending respiratory failure (Fallat et al., 1987). On the other hand, it may lack sensitivity as an early indicator of the disease.

Table 2.1 The ALSFRS scaling system for ALS.

Measure	Score	Finding
1. Speech	4	Normal speech process
	3	Detectable speech disturbance
	2	Intelligible with repeating
	1	Speech combined with non-vocal communication
	0	Loss of useful speech
2. Salivation	4	Normal
	3	Slight but definite excess of saliva in mouth; may have night-time drooling
	2	Moderately excessive saliva; may have minimal drooling
	1	Marked excess of saliva with some drooling
	0	Marked drooling; requires constant tissue or handkerchief
3. Swallowing	4	Normal eating habits
	3	Early eating problems; occasional choking
	2	Dietary consistency changes
	1	Needs supplemental tube feeding
	0	NPO (exclusively parenteral or enteral feeding)
4. Handwriting	4	Normal
	3	Slow or sloppy; all words are legible
	2	Not all words are legible
	1	Able to grip pen, but unable to write
	0	Unable to grip pen
5a. Cutting food and handling utensils (patients without gastrostomy)	4	Normal
	3	Somewhat slow and clumsy, but no help needed
	2	Can cut most foods, although clumsy and slow; some help needed
	1	Food must be cut by someone, but can still feed slowly
	0	Needs to be fed

(Continued)

Table 2.1 (Continued)

Measure	Score	Finding
5b. Cutting food and handling utensils (alternate scale for patients without gastrostomy)	4	Normal
	3	Clumsy, but able to perform all manipulations independently
	2	Some help needed with closures and fasteners
	1	Provides minimal assistance to caregiver
	0	Unable to perform any aspect of task
6. Dressing and hygiene	4	Normal function
	3	Independent and complete self-care with effort or decreased efficiency
	2	Intermittent assistance or substitute methods
	1	Needs attendant for self-care
	0	Total dependence
7. Turning in bed and adjusting bed clothes	4	Normal
	3	Somewhat slow and clumsy, but no help needed
	2	Can turn alone or adjust sheets, but with great difficulty
	1	Can initiate, but not turn or adjust sheets alone
	0	Helpless
8. Walking	4	Normal
	3	Early ambulation difficulties
	2	Walks with assistance
	1	Non-ambulatory functional movement
	0	No purposeful leg movement
9. Climbing stairs	4	Normal
	3	Slow
	2	Mild unsteadiness or fatigue
	1	Needs assistance
	0	Cannot climb stairs

10. Dyspnea (new)	4	None
	3	Occurs when walking
	2	Occurs with one or more of the following: eating, bathing, dressing (ADL)
	1	Occurs at rest; difficulty breathing when either sitting or lying
	0	Significant difficulty; considering using mechanical respiratory support
11. Orthopnea (new)	4	None
	3	Some difficulty sleeping at night due to shortness of breath; does not routinely use more than two pillows
	2	Needs extra pillow in order to sleep (more than two)
	1	Can only sleep sitting up
	0	Unable to sleep
12. Respiratory insufficiency (new)	4	None
	3	Intermittent use of BiPAP
	2	Continuous use of BiPAP during the night
	1	Continuous use of BiPAP during the night and day
	0	Invasive mechanical ventilation by intubation or tracheostomy

NPO, nil per os; ADL, activities of daily living; BiPAP, bilevel positive airway pressure.
Source: Cedarbaum et al. (1999).

2.3.4 Progression

As in Parkinson's disease, the progressive nature of ALS is a key feature in that regardless of which group of motor neurons is initially affected, the pathological process typically spreads to other groups, ultimately destroying α-motor neurons in the ventral spinal cord and upper motor neurons in the motor cortex and brain stem. Patients eventually suffer from partial or complete paralysis of the limbs.

Although the loss of motor function leading to death definitely involves the motor neuron cell bodies, their axons, and the muscles they innervate, it is not yet clear which of these might be the initial locus of degeneration. One view holds that the motor neurons are the proximal site of the disease and thus are primarily affected. In this view, as the motor neurons degenerate, their axons and eventually the neuromuscular junction degenerate as well, to be followed by muscle atrophy. This view is supported by several animal models of the disease (Blizzard et al., 2015), including one for the Guamanian variant (Lee et al., 2009). An alternative view, largely derived from the animal model of m*SOD1*, is that the process starts at the muscle end plate and works its way in a retrograde direction back to the motor neurons (Fischer et al., 2004). The correct sequence is not known in human patients and it seems likely there is considerable variation.

2.3.5 Rates of Disease Progression

As already noted, those ALS patients with bulbar-onset forms of the disease reach the end state more rapidly than those with lower motor neuron onset. Some ALS patients in the latter case survive for a decade or longer (Pupillo et al., 2014). Factors associated with longer disease duration include age at onset and sex.

2.3.6 Age of Onset and Sex Distribution

The usual age of onset for sALS in North America is in the 5th to 6th decade of life, with a decade earlier onset for fALS. Male victims of the disease exceed females by about 50% (Mehta et al., 2014).

2.3.7 Other Organ System Involvement

In addition to the loss of motor neurons in the disease, various changes in skin structure have been noted from the time of Charcot (1880) to the present. A series of papers by various investigators, mostly from Japan, have described a change in collagen that occurs coincidentally with the loss of motor neurons (Ono et al., 1999). The fact that both neurons and skin are of ectodermal origin may be an important clue to disease origin, although this point has not been widely investigated. It does highlight, however, that in ALS, as well as the other neurological diseases considered in this chapter, other organ systems are somehow involved, even if only secondarily.

2.3.8 ALS Clusters

There is at least one ALS cluster. There may be a second. The first is the form of ALS on Guam and elsewhere in the Western Pacific, which will be described in detail in Chapter 7. The second is a subgroup of patients with Gulf War Syndrome (Haley et al., 1997; Haley, 2003). Epidemiological studies for the latter suggest a roughly twofold increase in ALS levels in US military personnel during the 1991 Gulf War compared to the civilian population. While the incidence is not as extreme as that for ALS-PDC on Guam and elsewhere, the age of onset is considerably younger than in classical ALS. This age feature is also a major characteristic of ALS-PDC on both Guam and Irian Jaya (Galasko et al., 2002; Spencer et al., 2005a).

2.3.9 Risk Factors

Risk factors for ALS include exposure to various agricultural chemicals and heavy metals. Smoking is also a risk factor (Weisskopf et al., 2004; de Jong et al., 2012), unlike for Parkinson's disease. A potential link to pesticides/herbicides as a key risk factor was identified by epidemiological studies by the Public Health Agency of Canada, as mentioned in Section 2.2.

As with Parkinson's disease, most cases of ALS are sporadic. This observation suggests an environmental etiology, rather than one of genetic origin. A fraction of fALS is caused by mutations in a gene that codes for the antioxidant protein SOD. As cited previously, the generation of transgenic mice carrying various copies of the mutant human gene has been a key focus of animal studies of the disease since the early 1990s.

SOD1 mutations are expressed in about 25% of patients with fALS. However, fALS only makes up 5–10% of all ALS cases. m*SOD1* thus accounts for no more than 2% of all cases of ALS. Unlike familial Parkinson's disease in which the mutation deletes the protein or makes it ineffective, m*SOD1* is described as a "toxic gain of function" mutation, meaning that it adds some still unknown fatal factor that initiates or propagates the processes leading to neuronal degeneration.

In addition to m*SOD1*, a dozen or more extremely rare mutations leading to forms of MND have been studied. Other mutations are constantly being discovered, as will be described in Chapter 5.

A genetic susceptibility factor has been identified in the form of variant genes coding for different forms of the cholesterol transport protein, apolipoprotein E (APOE). The same gene-variant protein is associated with a greater risk for Alzheimer's disease (Raber et al., 2004).

In spite of the limited evidence for genetic causality factors in the vast majority of ALS cases, until fairly recently the field has focused almost entirely on the *SOD1* mutation in humans, or in transgenic animals expressing the human mutation. Newer studies have begun to focus on mutations involving *TARDBP*, *FUS*, and *C9orf72*, among others (see Chapter 5).

2.3.10 Current Treatment Options

At present, no treatment regime works well in relieving the signs, symptoms, progression, or in ensuring survival, amongst those afflicted with ALS. The available treatments will be discussed at length in Chapters 13 and 14.

2.3.11 ALS in Relation to Other Neurological Diseases and Disorders: Cognitive Impairment

For years, ALS was considered a completely distinct entity with no crossover to either Parkinson's or Alzheimer's disease. It is now known that this view is, in large measure, incorrect. As in Parkinson's disease, a form of dementia affecting the frontal lobes of the brain occurs in at least 20% of all ALS patients. This is termed "frontotemporal dementia"

(FTD) (ALS-FTD) and it induces profound personality changes and cognitive impairment in all cases. It shows up neuropathologically as deposits of tau protein in the frontal cortex (Irwin et al., 2007). Other ALS patients show little loss of cognitive function prior to end-state disease. These distinctions highlight, yet again, that there is a wide spectrum of presentation of ALS with dementia. In regard to FTD itself, some 50% of cases have motor neuron involvement (Swinnen and Robberecht, 2014).

Another link between sALS and FTD is the presence of ubiquitinated inclusions that are positive for TDP-43 translocations (Neumann et al., 2006). To add to the spectrum nature of these disorders, the intronic hexanucleotide repeat expansion found in another genetic mutation leading to ALS, *C9orf72*, shows up in almost 25% of FTD cases (DeJesus-Hernandez et al., 2011; Renton et al., 2014). This repeat expansion is also present in about 40% of fALS cases (Renton et al., 2014). The nature of these mutations in ALS and FTD will be discussed in greater detail in Chapter 5.

Finally, as in Alzheimer's disease, as well as ALS-PDC and PSP, classical ALS occasionally shows deposits of abnormal tau protein in various regions of the nervous system (Strong et al., 2005).

2.3.12   ALS and Other CNS Regions

Although ALS has usually been considered to involve only motor neurons, there is an older, lesser-known scientific literature demonstrating that this view is not correct. Anatomical evidence for widespread cortical and SN damage has been in the literature since the 1980s (Hughes, 1982; Lowe, 1994), with some indication that it may date back much further (Holmes, 1909).

Finally, in ALS, other organ systems are affected as well. For example, patients' skin collagen seems to be altered, as mentioned earlier.

2.3.13   Animal Models

Most animal studies of ALS over the last 20 years have focused on exploring features and mechanisms in animals with the inserted mutant human form of the *SOD1* gene, but always at much higher copy numbers than are found in human fALS patients who express only one such copy (see Zwiegers et al., 2014). Although the model is considered to reflect the underlying pathological processes in human ALS without the involvement of other neural areas, there is increasing evidence that it is far from specific (Petrik et al., 2007a). The latter may more accurately reflect the human disease. Currently, there are few good environmental models of ALS, although some have recently been followed up (Wilson et al., 2002; Andersson et al., 2005; Tabata et al., 2008).

2.3.14   Incidence and Prevalence

The following mostly concerns sALS, the dominant type of ALS. A smaller fraction of what follows includes fALS.

2.3.14.1   United States and Canada
In the United States, the prevalence of ALS is estimated at 30 000 people; in Canada the number is 2500–3000. Incidence is approximately 2–3/100 000 per year in both countries.

2.3.15 Changes in Incidence/Prevalence over the Last 30 Years

2.3.15.1 United States
A small overall increase in disease death rate was noted between 1979 and 1983, with a subsequent plateau until 1998 (Sejvar et al., 2005). From 1999 to 2009, there was no definitive trend in the annual ALS-associated death rate, and some studies suggested a possible decrease. However, these numbers were age- and group-specific (Mehal et al., 2013).

2.3.15.2 Canada
In the province of Nova Scotia, there has apparently been a stable incidence of ALS since 1984 (Bonaparte et al., 2007). However, it is difficult to assess a country's overall incidence-level changes over time from data from one province alone.

2.3.15.3 Worldwide
There seems to be a trend toward a gradual increase in incidence and prevalence (Chiò et al., 2013). However, those countries/regions with formerly extremely high ALS rates (ALS-PDC-like disorders; see Chapter 7) show a significant decline in the incidence and prevalence of ALS-like disorders (Plato et al., 2003; Spencer et al., 2005a).

Worldwide prevalence has been estimated at 500 000 (Chiò et al., 2013). This is an important number to keep in mind during later discussion of the main model of ALS to date (i.e., m*SOD1*, which has dominated the field for a generation). Given current estimates of the impact of *SOD1* mutations, this equates to no more than 5000 persons worldwide.

Finally, in regard to overall ALS incidence levels, one study has estimated a two- to four-fold increase since the 1970s and has linked this to the probability of increasing environmental factors (Pritchard et al., 2004).

2.3.16 Costs

2.3.16.1 Cost Per Patient

2.3.16.1.1 United States
- *Total costs*: $63 693/year (Larkindale et al., 2014):
  - *Direct costs*: $49 010.
  - *Medical costs*: $31 121/year (including both out-of-pocket cost and insurance-paid amounts).
  - *Nonmedical costs*: $17 889/year.
  - *Indirect costs*: $14 682/year.

2.3.16.1.2 Canada
- *Total costs*: Over $150 000 per patient over the course of the disease (ALS Canada, 2013):
  - *Direct costs for the average course of the disease*: $49 108/3.4 years.
  - *Indirect costs annually*: $36 467/year.
- *Total costs*: $89 158/year (Gladman et al., 2014):
  - *Direct costs*: $32 337/year.
  - *Out-of-pocket*: $19 574/year.
  - *Government/nonprofit organization supported*: $12 763/year.
  - *Indirect costs*: $56 820/year.

2.3.16.2   Societal Costs

2.3.16.2.1   United States
- *Total costs*: $1.023 billion (Larkindale et al., 2014):
  - *Direct costs*: $786.9 million.
  - *Indirect costs*: $235.7 million.

2.3.16.2.2   Canada
- *Total costs*: $182.4 million (Canadian Institute for Health Information, 2007):
  - *Direct costs*: $13.79 million.
  - *Indirect costs*: $168.57 million.

2.4   Alzheimer's Disease

Chronologically, Alzheimer's disease was the last of the major age-dependent, progressive neurological diseases to be described clinically and anatomically. It was named after the German neuropathologist and psychiatrist Alois Alzheimer. In a paper published in 1906, Alzheimer described the characteristic behavioral features of the disease, including the selective loss of memory and the inability to learn new tasks (Alzheimer, 1906).

Pathologically, Alzheimer's disease features damage to the parts of the brain primarily involved in memory and learning, notably regions of the neocortex and hippocampus. It also involves neurons that make the neurotransmitter acetylcholine in the *nucleus basalis* of Meynert. The damage to the brain in Alzheimer's disease involves the loss of neurons and the overall shrinkage of the cortex, concomitant to a continued loss of function (Alzheimer's Association, 2015b).

Alzheimer's disease makes up some 60% of all dementia cases (Alzheimer's Society of Canada, 2010). Dementia itself is generally defined as a loss in cognitive abilities. For example, decreases in memory, language skills, judgment, and visual–spatial performance all qualify as indices of dementia. Altogether, dementias of all types represent the most common form of intellectual impairment in those over 60 years of age. Dementia can be the consequence of stroke, head trauma, alcoholism, drug intoxication, infectious diseases of the brain, or exposure to toxic molecules such as aluminum (see Chapter 6). An earlier form of mental impairment is termed "mild cognitive impairment" (MCI) and is thought to be a precursor to more severe dementia (Authier et al., 2001).

There are also forms of dementia that arise from the so-called "prion" diseases, such as inheritable Creutzfeld–Jabob disease (CJD) and foodborne prion disease (variant CJD). Prions are self-replicating protein particles (Prusiner, 2001). The diseases they induce can be confused with Alzheimer's disease based solely on behavioral effects and psychological tests, but the underlying neuropathology is quite different, necessitating post-mortem examination of the brain. Another type of Alzheimer's-like dementia is an early-onset form associated with Down's syndrome, as cited earlier.

In general, distinguishing non-Alzheimer's dementias from Alzheimer's disease by behavioral measures alone is difficult. In fact, the only definitive diagnosis of the disease is made following post-mortem histological examination of the brain.

As also mentioned earlier, Alzheimer's-like dementias can combine features of other neurological diseases, including some of the parkinsonisms (e.g., ALS-PDC of the various locations in the Western Pacific, PSP, G-PDC) and disorders such as FTD. The latter can coexist with ALS.

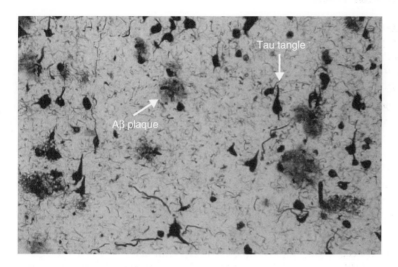

Figure 2.3 Pathological hallmarks of Alzheimer's disease. Post-mortem tissue sample from an Alzheimer's-disease patient brain showing typical neuropathology, including Aβ plaques and tau NFTs. *Source*: O'Brien (2015, http://sage.buckinstitute.org/amyloid-beta-and-alzheimers-disease/).

2.4.1 Neuropathological Features

Alzheimer's-disease brains display two characteristic "hallmark" anatomical features that set this disease apart from other dementias (Figure 2.3). First, an Alzheimer's brain typically shows the presence of sheets of misfolded, insoluble amyloid beta (Aβ), which surround and sometimes encompass neurons and other cells in the cortex and hippocampus. These deposits form dense structures, termed "plaques." Amyloid protein arises from the cleavage of Aβ precursor protein (APP). APP is normally produced in the brain and is not pathological, although its exact role is not fully understood. The pathological metabolism of APP produces Aβ.

Although Aβ has long considered a key causal factor in Alzheimer's disease, this conclusion is not necessarily correct. A countervailing view has gained widespread acceptance, bolstered by the older literature, which shows that the forms of Alzheimer's disease on Guam (PDC and Marianas dementia) are essentially identical in behavioral and pathological features to classical Alzheimer's disease, except in the relative absence of amyloid plaques (Kurland, 1972, 1988). For this reason, it may be that Aβ is not required in order to express the behavioral and pathological events of the Alzheimer's-disease state, although it likely contributes to the overall toxic cellular environment in the diseased brain.

A second key morphological feature of Alzheimer's disease is the presence of NFTs, comprising clumps of an abnormally phosphorylated form of tau protein. Tau protein is normally associated with neuronal microtubules and their function. Abnormal tau accumulates inside the damaged cells and is thought to disrupt normal transport adding to the overall pathology, including synaptic and neuronal losses during the course of the disease (The National Institute on Aging and Reagan Institute Working Group on Diagnostic Criteria for the Neuropathological Assessment of Alzheimer's Disease, 1997).

While NFTs are a hallmark sign of Alzheimer's disease, there are some interesting variations. For example, abnormal tau presentation has been found in Parkinson's patients, in various of the parkinsonisms (including PSP, ALS-PDC, and G-PDC), in FTD, and even in conventional ALS. Each of these cases could fall into an emerging disease categorization of "tauopathies," in which the proposed underlying theme is a crucial involvement of abnormal tau (Bayer, 2015).

This interpretation may not be correct. The reason is again linked to ALS-PDC on Guam. There, many otherwise neurologically normal people seem to express Alzheimer's-like tangles of tau protein (Kurland, 1988). One interpretation of this outcome is that tau does not induce the disease state itself, but is rather a consequence of, or response to, it. Support for this view comes from studies in cell culture, in which tau appears following various toxic insults (Kisby et al., 1999). In this interpretation, abnormal tau is a "downstream" event; that is, one that is less important in the early stages compared to the final stages of the disease.

Similarly, the aggregations of mutant proteins in Parkinson's disease in Lewy bodies may also be a late-stage event. Even in Huntington's disease, the inclusions of the mutant protein huntingtin are not clearly related to disease progression and hence are perhaps a by-product of the overall disease state, rather than the proximal cause of neuronal death.

As in Parkinson's disease and ALS, a neuroinflammatory process involving both astrocytes and microglia is present (Heneka et al., 2015). As also in Parkinson's disease, mitochondrial morphology and function are compromised (Wang et al., 2009) and there is evidence of cerebrovascular dysfunction in terms of decreased cerebral blood flow (Bell and Zlokovic, 2009).

The commonality of protein "opathies" in each of the considered diseases (sometimes different proteins, but sometimes not) and the evidence for neuroinflammation and mitochondrial dysfunctions suggest that these sorts of event are not unique features of any of the diseases, but rather "downstream" consequences at a near end state for a range of neurological diseases.

2.4.2 Rating Schemes

Alzheimer's disease staging is performed using the following measurements.

2.4.2.1 Global Deterioration Scale

Also known as the Reisberg Scale, this divides the disease into six stages of ability (Reisberg et al., 1982):

- *Stage 1*: No dementia, with no cognitive decline and no memory problems.
- *Stage 2*: No dementia, with a very mild cognitive decline, including memory lapses and forgetting of familiar names and locations of objects; neither lapse is obvious to others.
- *Stage 3*: No dementia, with mild cognitive decline, including mild forgetfulness, difficulty in learning new things, difficulty concentrating or a limited attention span, problems with orientation (such as getting lost), communication difficulties (such as finding the right word), loss or misplacing of objects, and difficulties handling problems at work. These changes are noticeable to family, friends, and coworkers.
- *Stage 4*: Early-stage dementia, with moderate cognitive decline, including some memory loss regarding personal history, difficulty with complex tasks (finances, shopping, planning dinner for guests, etc.), decreased knowledge of current and recent events, and impaired ability to perform challenging mental arithmetic.
- *Stage 5*: Mid-stage dementia with moderately severe cognitive decline, including major gaps in memory and the need for help with day-to-day tasks.

- *Stage 6*: Mid-stage dementia with severe cognitive decline, including continued memory loss and loss of awareness of recent events and experiences; the need for assistance with bathing or a fear of bathing; difficulty counting; personality and emotional changes, such as confusion, anxiety, suspiciousness, anger, sadness/depression, hostility, apprehension, delusions, and agitation; disruption of normal sleep/waking cycle; obsessions, such as repetition of simple activities; decreased ability to use the toilet or incontinence.

2.4.2.2 Functional Assessment Staging

Functional Assessment Staging (FAST) focuses more on an individual's level of functioning in daily living activities, rather than on cognitive decline as per the Reisberg Scale.

- *Stage 1*: Normal adult, no functional decline.
- *Stage 2*: Normal older adult, personal awareness of some functional decline.
- *Stage 3*: Early (putative) Alzheimer's disease, noticeable deficits in demanding job situations.
- *Stage 4*: Mild Alzheimer's disease, requiring assistance in complicated tasks.
- *Stage 5*: Moderate Alzheimer's disease, requiring assistance in choosing proper attire.
- *Stage 6*: Moderately severe Alzheimer's disease, requiring assistance in dressing, bathing, and toileting; experiences urinary and fecal incontinence.
- *Stage 7*: Severe Alzheimer's disease, with a decline in speech ability to about a half-dozen intelligible words and progressive loss of the ability to walk, sit up, smile, and hold the head up.

2.4.2.3 Clinical Dementia Rating

The Clinical Dementia Rating (CDR) is a semi-structured, clinician-rated interview based on ratings of a patient's functioning in six domains commonly affected in Alzheimer's disease: memory, orientation, judgment and problem solving, community affairs, home and hobbies, and personal care (Hughes et al., 1982). Its stages are:

- *CDR-0*: No dementia. No symptoms.
- *CDR-0.5*: Mild. Memory problems are slight, but consistent. Some difficulties with time and problem solving. Daily life slightly impaired.
- *CDR-1*: Mild. Memory loss moderate, especially for recent events. This loss interferes with daily activities. Moderate difficulty with problem solving. Cannot function independently at community affairs. Difficulty with daily activities and hobbies, especially complex ones.
- *CDR-2*: Moderate. More profound memory loss, retaining only highly learned material. Disorientation with respect to time and place. Lack of good judgment and difficulty handling problems. Little or no independent function at home. Can only do simple chores and has few interests.
- *CDR-3*: Severe. Severe memory loss. Lack of orientation with respect to time or place. No judgment or problem-solving abilities. Cannot participate in community affairs outside the home. Requires help with all tasks of daily living and with most personal care. Often incontinent.

2.4.3 Other Organ System Involvement

As with Parkinson's disease and ALS, Alzheimer's patients may show other system involvement as the disease progresses. Specifically, a link to insulin-3 deficiencies has been reported (Steen et al., 2005; Craft et al., 2013). The importance of this observation, apart from once again reinforcing the notion of Alzheimer's disease as a multisystem disorder, is not known.

2.4.4 Alzheimer's Disease Clusters

There are only two Alzheimer's-like disorders currently considered to form clusters: ALS-PDC and, perhaps, G-PDC (Caparros-Lefebvre et al., 2002; Shaw and Höglinger, 2008). The latter exhibits strong cognitive dysfunctions, much like various of the other parkinsonisms.

As with Parkinson's disease and ALS, the vast majority of cases of Alzheimer's – some 90% – are sporadic. Of the remainder, only 50% have a familial component, which seems to be due to four dominant genes: presenilin 1 (*PSEN1*), presenilin 2 (*PSEN2*), *APP*, and *APOE*, located on chromosomes 14, 1, 21, and 19, respectively (Schellenberg et al., 1992; Levy-Lahad et al., 1995; Rogaev et al., 1995).

Notably, *APOE* is considered a susceptibility gene for the disease, rather than a causal one. Other genetic susceptibility factors have been identified, including genes coding for structural proteins of the neuronal cytoskeleton and proteins involved in neurotransmission (Woodhouse et al., 2009).

The fact that most cases of Alzheimer's disease cases are sporadic – just like Parkinson's disease and ALS – should lead to a more rigorous evaluation of possible environmental causal factors. In spite of this, there are no definitive links to any environmental toxins, although there is some highly suggestive evidence concerning some forms of aluminum (Exley and Esiri, 2006; Walton and Wang, 2009; Tomljenovic, 2011). Most of the focus in animal models of Alzheimer's disease has been on transgenic mice expressing human genes for abnormal APP or presenilin (as discussed in more detail in Chapter 5).

2.4.5 Risk Factors

Agricultural chemicals have been listed as potential risk factors for Alzheimer's disease (Krewski 2014a,b; Public Health Agency of Canada, 2015).

2.4.6 Current Treatment Options

At present, no pharmaceutical treatment has any significant effect on the progression of Alzheimer's disease. The available treatments – most completely ineffective – will be discussed at length in Chapters 13 and 14. Some newer perspectives on Alzheimer's disease may be more promising.

2.4.7 Demographics

Alzheimer's disease is highly age-dependent in that it affects only 2.4 per 100 000 people aged 40–60, but 127 per 100 000 people older than 60 in the United States. Increasing age is thus the greatest risk factor for Alzheimer's disease, with disease onset much broader than for Parkinson's disease or ALS. Overall, 1 in 10 individuals over 65 and nearly half of those over 85 are affected (Bowler et al., 1998). Total Alzheimer's disease numbers are estimated at 5 million in the United States, making it the number one major age-dependent neurological disease, and the one with the greatest prevalence after epilepsy. Proportional levels occur in Canada (Public Health Agency of Canada, 2015).

The relatively small percentage of inherited forms of Alzheimer's disease are of earlier onset than sporadic forms and can strike individuals as early as the 3rd or 4th decade of life. As noted, these make up only a small fraction of the overall number of cases. A recent study by Pritchard and Rosenorm-Lanng (2015) suggests a general downward trend in age of onset, however, even in the sporadic forms. These data are of interest in the context of observations of ALS-PDC, which suggest that its age of onset is inversely linked to incidence. In other words, as incidence increases, age of onset decreases, and *vice versa*.

Sex plays a role in Alzheimer's disease: the ratio of males to females is nearly equal before age 75, but females are favored by a ratio of 2.5 : 1 after age 85 (Hebert et al., 2013; Alzheimer's Association, 2015a), perhaps suggesting that gonadal hormone deficiency following menopause contributes to disease onset and/or progression.

Besides sex and old age, other risk factors for Alzheimer's disease include head trauma and lack of education (Alzheimer's Association, 2015a).

2.4.8 Incidence and Prevalence

2.4.8.1 United States

- *Prevalence*: In 2014, an estimated 5.2 million Americans of all ages had Alzheimer's disease. This included an estimated 5 million aged 65 and older and approximately 200 000 under age 65. One in nine people aged 65 and older (11%) had the disease (Alzheimer's Association, 2014) – a number similar to that reported by Bowler (1998).
- *Incidence*: In 2014, 469 000 people aged 65 or older were projected to develop Alzheimer's disease (Alzheimer's Association, 2014).

2.4.8.2 Canada

- *Prevalence*: In 2011, 747 000 Canadians had dementia of various types. Accurate specific prevalence and incidence data for Alzheimer's disease are not available.
- *Incidence*: According to an older study by McDowell et al. (2000), the overall age-standardized incidence rates are 21.8/1000 for women and 19.1/1000 men aged 65 or older, giving 60 150 new cases of Alzheimer's per year in Canada.

Much of the confusion in both countries stems from the difficulty in distinguishing Alzheimer's disease pre mortem from other forms of dementia.

2.4.9 Changes in Incidence/Prevalence over the Last 30 Years

2.4.9.1 United States

An increase of incidence of 3.96% between 1992 and 2005 was reported by Akushevich et al. (2013). The reasons for this are not clear. Other studies have not shown any increases in Alzheimer's disease incidence (Rocca et al., 2011).

2.4.10 Costs

2.4.10.1 Costs Per Patient

2.4.10.1.1 United States

- *Total costs*: $46 669 per person annual payment for those aged 65 and older (versus $14 772 per person annual health care costs for those without Alzheimer's disease) (Alzheimer's Association, 2014).

- *Total costs when care purchased in the marketplace*: $56 290/person (Hurd et al., 2013):
  - *Direct costs (out-of-pocket spending, Medicare, formal home care)*: $28 501.
  - *Indirect costs (caregiving time valued according to replacement cost)*: $27 789.

2.4.10.2   Societal Costs

2.4.10.2.1   United States
- *Total costs*: $214 billion/year in 2014 (Alzheimer's Association, 2014). Medicare and Medicaid are expected to cover $150 billion (70%) and out-of-pocket spending is expected to be about $36 billion (17%). Where the rest of the funds will come from is not clear.

2.4.10.2.2   Canada
The values for Canada are quite variable by agency and year. Perhaps the most detailed are those provided by Alzheimer's Canada in their document, *Rising Tide* (Alzheimer's Society of Canada, 2010).

- *Total costs (2008)*: approx. $15 billion:
  - *Direct costs*: approx. $8 billion.
  - *Lost opportunity costs (unpaid caregiver's lost income)*: approx. $5 billion.
  - *Indirect costs*: approx. $2 billion.
- *Projected costs for the near term (2018)*: $36.7 billion:
  - *Direct costs*: $19.6 billion.
  - *Lost opportunity costs*: $12.3 billion.
  - *Indirect cost*: $4.8 billion.

2.4.10.3   Projected Cost Increases

2.4.10.3.1   United States
The segment of the US population aged 65 and older is expected to grow dramatically in the next decades, and total annual payments for people with Alzheimer's disease are projected to increase from $214 billion in 2014 to $1.2 trillion in 2050 (Alzheimer's Association, 2014). This dramatic rise includes a sixfold increase in government spending under Medicare and Medicaid and a fivefold increase in out-of-pocket spending. One study has projected that intolerable financial burdens will impact the viability of the American medical system (Hyman, 2012). Similar considerations likely apply to other countries as well.

2.4.10.3.2   Canada
The number of Canadians living with cognitive impairment, including the various dementias (with Alzheimer's disease as a key fraction of the total), will double to 1.4 million by 2031. The costs will climb to $293 billion a year by 2040 (Alzheimer's Society of Canada, 2012).

2.4.10.3.3   Worldwide
The costs are estimated at US$604 billion per year at present, and are set to increase even more quickly than the projected increase in prevalence (World Health Organization and Alzheimer's Disease International, 2012).

2.5   Summary of the Data on the Progressive, Age-Related Neurological Diseases

The preceding summaries for Parkinson's disease, ALS, and Alzheimer's disease are intended merely to provide brief synopses of the extensive, complicated, and sometimes contradictory sets of data within and between the different diseases. In regard to the epidemiological data, it is perhaps noteworthy how much is not known about diseases that are so well established and that have been so widely studied for well over a century – or, in the case of Parkinson's disease, for almost 200 years.

In regard to the prevalence and incidence data for these diseases, some confusion arises due to the inability of some epidemiological studies to separate classical Parkinson's disease from the other parkinsonisms and movement disorders; this problem becomes more acute in regard to Alzheimer's disease, which epidemiology is often not able to distinguish from other dementias. Such problems have plagued a recent effort in Canada to come up with accurate national figures for both diseases (Public Health Agency of Canada, 2015).

As will be discussed in detail in later chapters, each of these diseases is truly complex and almost surely involves multiple crucial phases between onset and CNS subsystem collapse. To truly understand the progression of any of these diseases, these multiple levels of pathology would have to be considered. Such levels would range from observations and measurements on altered behavior to detailed analyses of changes at both the systems and cellular levels. Cellular-level analysis would have to consider the underlying pathological events in cellular biochemistry and gene expression.

Even if the field had all of this information, this alone would not be sufficient to allow the field to understand these diseases or their pathological evolution. Simply put, studying a process as complex as the cell death pathways in neurological disease by examining only those events seen at some end state can never put all the elements into the correct temporal order. Thus, the sequence of events, or "time line," is absolutely crucial (Figure 2.4). In spite of this, almost nothing is known about pre-clinical disease time lines. Most behavioral or *in vivo* work on humans is done after clinical diagnosis, or

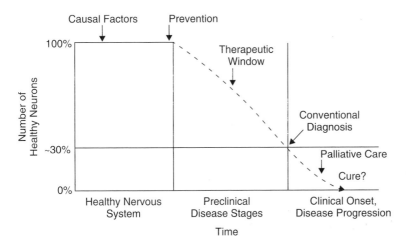

Figure 2.4 Simplified schematic of a proposed timeline of neurological diseases.

even later (see Chapter 9). Virtually all anatomical and biochemical studies on humans are done post mortem. The majority of animal models for each disease are designed to get to an equivalent to the human clinical state as rapidly as possible, and thus suffer from the same difficulties.

2.6   Neural Loci and Mechanisms of Action

Beyond the issues posed by the rather diffuse nature of neurological disease epidemiology which has largely failed to provide definitive answers to questions about risk factors, lie additional problems of a crucial nature: In which neural compartments do the diseases originate? What are the likely mechanisms underlying neuronal degeneration? Answering the former should, in principle, provide clues to the latter.

As will be discussed in the various chapters that follow, in terms of the primary locus of degeneration, the field does not yet know to what extent the initial damage is cell-autonomous (i.e., originating in the neurons most affected) or non-cell-autonomous (i.e., originating in other cell types). This is extremely problematic, since without this information, assigning mechanisms of action is pretty close to impossible.

Some of this problem may be the reason that for all of the diseases in question, numerous cell-autonomous and non-cell-autonomous actions have been proposed, each with a variety of potential sites whose dysfunction is considered to be primary to cell death. These have included various organelles in neurons or glial cells, including the endoplasmic reticulum, mitochondrion, the proteasome, and others. Altered cell membranes and receptors and the neurotransmitters/neuromodulators for the same have all been implicated in the different regions of neurons, including the soma, dendrites, and axons. The transport mechanisms of various molecules, both anterograde and retrograde, have been cited for both neurons and glial cells. DNA/RNA transcriptional errors have been proposed, not to mention a host of mutant gene effects. Concerning the latter, both those that are deletions of crucial function and those that are described as a "toxic gain of function" mutation are possible.

In terms of underlying cellular mechanisms, oxidant stress, excitotoxicity, and the full range of those aspects of cellular functioning that would be disrupted by any malfunction of the various organelles have also been proposed.

In regard to the very nature of neuronal degeneration, I have so far failed to distinguish between two key types of cell death that can occur in the neurological diseases: apoptosis (programmed cell death) and necrosis (cell death following injury). In fact, evidence for both types has been noted in the neurological disease literature for all of the diseases discussed here (Hyman and Yuan, 2012; Mattson, 2000). A more recently described form of cell death pathway, termed "necroptosis," has been considered for ALS (Re et al., 2014). Necroptosis contains features of both necrosis and apoptosis.

All of these events – and certainly there are more – are not only plausible, but are likely to occur at some stage in the sequence leading to cellular degeneration and culminating in the disease end state. These features of neurological diseases and models are not referenced here, as all will appear later in the book. All have been therapeutic targets at one time or another, with, in hindsight, quite predictably null results. The situation overall is reminiscent of the John Godfrey Saxe quote that opens Chapter 1.

Determining which of these elements/events is involved is likely not possible in human studies. Given this, the alternative that has been widely used in the field is to turn to various model systems in order to gain some traction on questions about causality, progression, and cascading events.

Therefore, it is to these models that I will turn in Chapters 14 and 15 in order to consider the promise they have offered for understanding neurological diseases. Before this, however, it is important to consider the spectrum nature of neurological diseases.

Endnote

1 Jules Henri Poincaré (1854–1912) was a French mathematician, theoretical physicist, and philosopher of science.

3

Spectrums of Neurological Disease, Clusters, and Ubiquity

> *Just the place for a Snark! I have said it twice:*
> *That alone should encourage the crew.*
> *Just the place for a Snark! I have said it thrice:*
> *What I tell you three times is true*
> Lewis Caroll, "The Hunting of the Snark,"
> 1874

And in regard to the same:

> *"His crew are simply Tom, Dick and Harry, with the Baker as Everyman. We are*
> *all there, all in the same boat, all heading in the wrong direction, going the wrong*
> *way."*
> Alexander L. Taylor, *The White Knight*, 1952

From the Preface

The same general considerations cited for Chapter 1 apply here.

3.1 Introduction

As mentioned in the previous chapters, an emerging view that is beginning to take hold amongst those studying Parkinson's disease and ALS is that these diseases are not unitary entities, but are better described as spectrum diseases. If they are indeed parts of their own spectrums, then a safe bet would be that Alzheimer's disease is as well. These notions will be explored in this chapter and later in the book.

3.2 Spectrums of Neurological Disease

It is increasingly clear that most of the neurological diseases considered here fit into their own disease spectrums: a clear example of "nested complex systems," or a complex system within a larger complex system (Figure 3.1). For example, Parkinson's disease, ALS, and Alzheimer's disease are all encompassed within a larger schema of related

Neural Dynamics of Neurological Disease, First Edition. Christopher A. Shaw.
© 2017 John Wiley & Sons, Inc. Published 2017 by John Wiley & Sons, Inc.

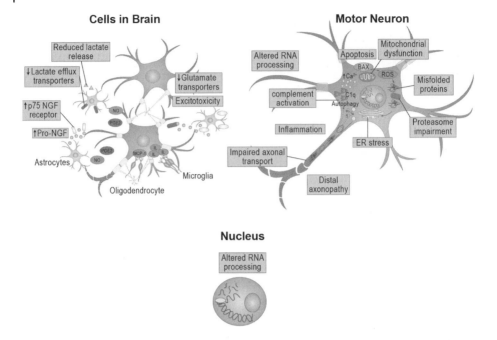

Figure 3.1 Examples given are those of neurons in the brain in context to the various glial cell types (astrocytes, microglia, and oligodendrocytes) and some of the changes seen in neurological diseases (left figure). A motor neuron with some of the identified cellular changes is also shown (right figure). *Source*: Modified from Ferraiuolo et al. (2011), with permission from Macmillan Publishers Ltd.: [*Nature Reviews Neurology*].

neurological disorders such as ALS-PDC (see Chapter 7) and others in which features of two or more of these diseases are simultaneously present. In ALS-PDC, the spectrum includes a form of ALS that appears to be virtually identical to classical ALS, a form of parkinsonism with a dementia component, and a more Alzheimer's-like dementia. Not everyone afflicted by ALS-PDC has all of the features of each disease subset, but a considerable number do, at least as expressed over time. In PSP, parkinsonism is combined with a clear dementia that may not present in conventional Parkinson's disease until later in the time line of the disease. Guadeloupe PDC in many regards resembles both PDC on Guam and PSP, as noted previously.

A similar realization has begun to emerge even within a conventionally "pure" disease such as conventional Parkinson's disease (Sherer and Mari, 2014).

In much the same way, ALS is only one type of motor neuron disease (MND). Even within traditional ALS, there are forms that appear to originate with the loss of either upper or lower motor neurons, as cited previously, and additional subgroups according to how the disease spreads within the neuraxis, its rate of progression, the presence or absence of changes in other neural systems, and so forth (Strong and Rosenfeld, 2003).

As for Alzheimer's disease, it is abundantly clear that not only is Alzheimer's only one sort of age-related dementia (Hebert et al., 2013), but that even within Alzheimer's disease itself a spectrum of subtypes occurs. The latter is true not only in regard to so-called "typical" Alzheimer's disease in comparison to the Alzheimer's-like form of ALS-PDC, but also within the classical Western form (Mega et al., 1996; Perl et al., 1998).

In addition, as an older scientific literature amply demonstrates, the so-called "conventional" neurological diseases are not really completely unique in the nature of their neurological lesions (Figure 3.2). ALS can show damage to other central

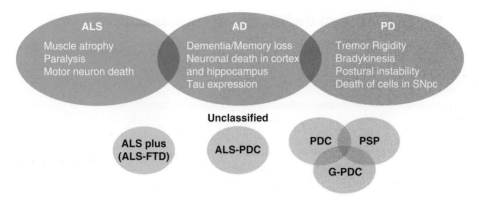

Figure 3.2 Overlapping features of the age-related neurological diseases, and a fractal version of the same.

nervous system (CNS) regions (e.g., the nigro-striatal system), as cited previously – an observation mirrored in animal models of the disease (Andersson et al., 2005; Petrik et al., 2007a; Tabata et al., 2008). The same is true in Parkinson's disease, as cited already, and in parkinsonism disease models (Wilson et al., 2002).

In regard to the preceding, it is not the case that these observations in humans and animals are unknown, but rather that they are often simply ignored, perhaps as inconveniences to the presumed purer forms of the diseases. This view may arise from a perspective that since ALS is primarily an MND, and since the proximal cause of death is the loss of motor neurons leading to muscle atrophy, any other neural subsystems affected are incidental and thus of lesser importance. The same applies in Parkinson's disease, primarily a movement disorder, in which the cognitive deficits are sometimes seen to be relatively less important than the loss of SN neurons and the attendant motor dysfunctions.

The reasons for this perspective are likely complicated and range from the understandable desire by many in the field to have the different diseases seem simple in their presentation to the sometimes outright antipathy in grant review panels toward anything that seems to be a messy, boundary-crossing disorder. How likely would it be, for example, for an ALS grant panel to fund a study that showed Parkinson's disease features as well? It is not that such grants never get funded; it just does not happen often. The outcome thus becomes a self-censoring exercise in which known observations from the scientific literature – moreover, ones that might contribute essential clues to disease etiology and progression – are downplayed and thus effectively minimized. This is not always the case, and some neurological diseases have been linked through the notion that all are, in part, "proteinopathies" (Calne and Eisen, 1989 and the subsequent literature).

Larger numbers of cases of these various diseases overall simply make clear the relative heterogeneity of each and the extent of the overlap between them. Unfortunately, even increasing the numbers does not necessarily tell researchers much about the causal or contributory susceptibility factors that underlie any such disease. For example, the total number of cases of ALS across North America, separated as they are geographically and temporally, has not told the field anything definitive about etiologies in spite of dedicated epidemiological efforts to do so. The same situation applies to Parkinson's and Alzheimer's diseases as well. There is, however, a solution, albeit a fairly rare one.

Before I address this, however, it is important to consider what might be termed the "dimension of the problem" problem.

3.3   The Dimension of the Problem when Assessing Potential Causal Factors in Neurological Diseases

Trying to zero in on the etiological factors leading to the age-related neurological diseases has proven to be an empirically daunting task, and one that, viewed from a distance, seems more of a random walk than a targeted strategic means leading to their identification.

The following are some of the constraints that nature has imposed on the search. First, if taking a genomics approach, with all the caveats that go with this (see Chapter 5, there are something like 23 000 human genes to examine. Amongst these, many of the induced proteins (estimated to be about 100 000) are expressed in the CNS, at least at various stages of neurodevelopment. Given the complexity of CNS biochemical and signaling pathways, the alteration or deletion of any one such protein could negatively impact critical aspects of normal neural metabolism, signaling, or other functions. The protein kinase family and its multifaceted interactions in neurological disease serve to illustrate this point (Krieger et al., 2003) (Figure 3.3). It would be surprising if altering gene function through mutation did not also do so at multiple levels.

Much the same applies to gene polymorphisms, in which the protein products can have altered efficacies (e.g., with apolipoprotein E (*APOE*)) (Raber et al., 2004).

Chapter 5 will consider the genes that have so far been shown to be involved in some familial forms of the various neurological diseases. These are limited in number and cannot actually tell the field much about the sporadic forms of the diseases, but a currently dominant perspective holds that particular genetic abnormalities will universally equate to the expression of a particular neurological disease. From this viewpoint, it follows for some researchers that mutant genes will point the way to common biochemical pathways that are also triggered by one or many of the putative environmental neurotoxins. Some of the latter will be discussed in Chapter 6.

This "gene-centric" perspective appears to be shared by a considerable number of scientists in the field, and it has clearly dominated research in Parkinson's disease, ALS, and Alzheimer's disease for decades. The power of the "genetics equals disease state" viewpoint has, to no great surprise, also spilled over into research funding, with a significant fraction of basic research dollars aimed at related areas, including: the seemingly endless hunt for mutant genes; the identification of gene-induced biochemical pathways and the interactions they trigger; the modeling of these genes and pathways; and the search for therapeutics to combat the resulting aberrant proteins.

The notion that a single gene can cause a single disease outcome also illustrates the power of reductionist models of neurological disease. There are examples in which such views are clearly warranted, such as in Huntington's disease. However, they also arise incorrectly as a derivative form of Koch's postulates about infectious disease etiologies.

An overwhelming problem for those trying to apply a similar perspective to neurological diseases – or at least the sporadic forms of Parkinson's disease, ALS, and Alzheimer's disease – is that, to date, the total number of genes involved in any of the familial forms has not risen much above about 10%. That number could change, of course, with more detailed searches through the genomes of the emerging familial cases, including more detailed analyses of various single-nucleotide polymorphisms (SNPs). However, it might also demonstrate that such research is beginning to asymptote out to a ceiling on just how many causal gene-based cases of neurological diseases actually exist. At least for some in the ALS research community, this statement will

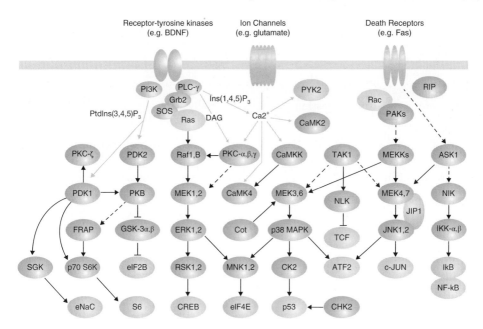

Figure 3.3 Protein kinase pathways activated in ALS and animal models (m*SOD1*) of ALS. In this example, activation of receptor tyrosine kinases can occur via an increased release of growth factors from neurons and non-neuronal cells produced as a regenerative response in ALS (Wagey et al., 1998). Tyrosine-specific protein kinases are shown in pink and serine/threonine-specific protein kinases and mitogen-activated protein kinase (MEK) isoforms are shown in blue. Transcription factors are shown in green, monomeric GTPases in yellow, and other in brown. Direct activation is indicated with solid black arrows, whereas indirect activation is indicated by dashed arrows. Actions of second messengers are shown by green arrows. ATF2, activation transcription factor 2; BDNF, brain-derived neurotrophic factor; CHK2, checkpoint kinase 2; CK2, casein kinase 2; Cot, cancer Osaka thyroid; DAG, diacylglycerol; eIF, eukaryotic initiation factor; eNaC, epithelial Naϸ channel; FKBP, FK506 binding protein; FRAP, FKBP-rapamycin-associated protein; Grb2, growth factor receptor-bound protein 2; GSK-3a, glycogen synthase kinase 3a; IKKa, IKB kinase a; Ins(1,4,5)P3, inositol (1,4,5)-trisphosphate; JIP1, JNK-interacting protein 1; JNK1, c-JUN N-terminal kinase 1; p38 MAPK, p38 mitogen-activated protein kinase; MEKK, MEK kinase; MNK, MAPK-interacting kinase (MAPK signal integrating kinase); NIK, NF-kB-inducing kinase; NLK, Nemo-like kinase; PAK, p21-activated kinase; PDK, 3-phosphoinositide-dependent kinase; PI3K, phosphatidylinositol 3-kinase; PdtIns(3,4,5)P3, s phosphatidylinositol (3,4,5)-trisphosphate; PKB, protein kinase B; PLC-g, phospholipase Cg; PYK2, proline-rich tyrosine kinase 2 (phosphotyrosine kinase 2). *Source*: Krieger et al. (2003), used with permission from Elsevier. (See color plate section for the color representation of this figure.)

be viewed with concern, particularly in light of the newer genetic mutations linked to fALS, which have been greeted with great fanfare (e.g., *C9orf72*, *FUS*, and *TARDBP*). A response to such possible concern, along with a more detailed discussion of the genetic bases for some neurological diseases, will be given in Chapter 5.

The next set of factors that can trigger or exacerbate neurological diseases is those found in the environment, whether produced by nature or by human activity. The story of ALS-PDC and related disorders linked to environmental toxins (see Chapter 7) clearly establishes the potential role of such toxins, but leaves open the related question of how many there might be in the human environment. The list is likely to be experimentally endless. Human activity adds a thousand new molecules to the environment each year (Glover and Rhoads 2006). This additional toxic burden is carried by each person currently alive in North America, and is placed atop the already huge numbers added over the last few generations, let alone since the beginning of the Industrial Revolution. How many of these molecules are neurotoxic on their own? The answer is likely, "many." And, while it is perhaps also likely that most will not cross the blood–brain barrier directly, many others will.

The more complicated question – one not usually explored in any depth in the scientific literature – is what happens when these potential toxins combine temporally or sequentially and at different stages of neuronal development or in different periods of life. Indeed, the likelihood that toxin additive effects (let alone synergistic effects) exist is high, and thus the number of things that can contribute to disease etiology is larger still.

The problem gets worse when one considers gene–toxin interactions (Figures 3.4 and 3.5). While those genes found directly to induce neurodegeneration are limited (as discussed earlier and in Chapter 5), gene polymorphisms, and thus potential susceptibilities to toxins, on their own or in combination, are going to be much more common.

Several simple examples from human genetics and variant biochemistry illustrate this point very well. In brief, one concerns the genetic polymorphism that fails to make the correct form of the enzyme that cleaves ethanol, alcohol dehydrogenase. Those who carry its variations fail to adequately or rapidly detoxify alcohol and are thus more

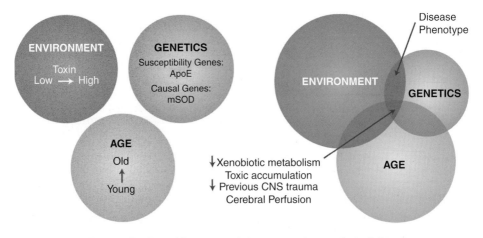

Figure 3.4 Simple example of possible gene–toxin interactions in neurological disease.

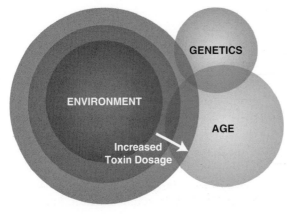

Figure 3.5 More complex example of possible gene–toxin interactions in neurological disease.

likely to experience what are termed "alcohol use disorders" (AUDs) than are those with different forms of the enzyme. In the absence of alcohol, however, such individuals have no negative effects of the variant protein expression. Similar circumstances and outcomes apply also to those with genetic polymorphisms for the enzymes that degrade lactose or gluten. These examples are examined in greater detail in Chapter 12.

There is no simple answer to the question of how to simplify this situation, but there is one partial solution, albeit with caveats. That is to seek clusters of neurological diseases that are sporadic – for which no clearly dominant genetic etiology exists.

3.4 Neurological Disease Clusters

For ALS, or any other neurological disease where the etiology/ies remain unknown, the best approach to the myriad subtypes and vast potential number of factors, both genetic and environmental, is to identify a disease "cluster." This is basically a large number of individuals in a relatively constrained geographical space and period of time who appear to have the same disease (Figure 3.6). However, the subject of what precisely defines a cluster appears to be contentious for those in the neurosciences, and even amongst epidemiologists (Sabel, 2014).

Nevertheless, finding neurological disease clusters offers one approach to coping with the huge range of variables imposed by time and geography. It thus serves as an acknowledged means of reducing the potential causal factors, interactions, and so forth to a much more manageable number of possibilities. This does not mean, as I will show, that the identification of a neurological disease cluster will necessarily lead to a clear identification of those same putative factors.

While finding such neurological disease clusters would be helpful, there are actually very few real examples of the same. Those historical clusters that seem generally agreed on are the following. The first concerns instances of lathyrism expressed in prisoners of war during World War II, but described far back in history as well. The second is the adult-onset and developmental neurological disorders associated with methyl mercury toxicity exposure at Minimata Bay, Japan. The third is the neurological deficits

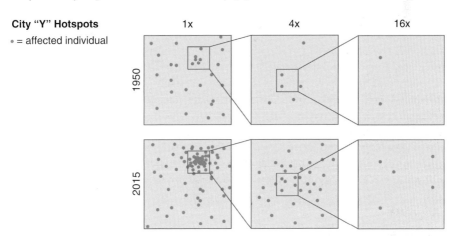

Figure 3.6 In this scheme, two imaginary years are shown (1950 and 2015) showing increasing numbers of disease victims in the time period. Different scales are shown showing how the distributions might appear at various magnifications.

found in some individuals who consumed domoic acid-contaminated mussels in Eastern and Central Canada. All of these real clusters are discussed in this section to place the presentation of ALS-PDC as a true neurological disease cluster and "geographical isolate" in a clearer context.

3.4.1 Lathyrism

Lathyrism is a muscle-wasting disorder associated with the consumption of the chickling pea, *Lathyrus sativus*. Lathyrism's symptoms have been known in conjunction with chickling peas, grass peas, vetch, and other legumes for over 2000 years, and came to the attention of neurologists at the end of World War II (see Kisby, 2000, who cites Hippocrates referring to lathyrism in ancient Greece). Lathyrism outbreaks at that time were associated with wartime conditions in prison camps: in one particular case, a German Army-controlled forced-labor camp in the Ukraine. The prisoners had largely subsisted over a long period on a diet of grass peas. The outcome was a neurological disorder characterized by muscle spasms and weakness in the legs. Other studies showed that the toxicity from members of the *Lathyrus* genus was not restricted to humans: animals, particularly adult male horses, that consumed the peas showed similar hind-limb weakness or even paralysis. Once a normal diet was restored, most human and animal victims of chronic lathyrism showed partial recovery, but muscle weakness, stiffness, cramps, and other pathological features could persist for life. Of note to some of the material that follows in regard to ALS-PDC is that lathyrism in humans was more common in males than females by a ratio of almost three to one.

L. sativus contains the plant amino acid, β-N-oxalylamino-l alanine (BOAA), first isolated from the grass pea by Bell and O'Donovan (1966). BOAA appears to be a signaling molecule in some plants, possibly involved in the uptake and transport of zinc. Although it is not normally found in the diet of humans, when it occurs at high doses it can overactivate neurons through its action as a glutamate agonist at the α-amino-3-hydroxy-5-methyl-4-isoxazolepropionic acid (AMPA) receptor, one of three main ionotropic glutamate receptors in the CNS (Weiss et al., 1989). When stimulated by glutamate, or by BOAA acting as a glutamate agonist, BOAA causes a high flux of calcium to enter neurons. In lathyrism, the neurons affected are typically motor neurons, and the action of BOAA causes action potentials to propagate uncontrollably.

In general, persistently high levels of BOAA can kill or damage motor neurons in the spinal cord, thereby affecting the control of skeletal muscles. As the motor neurons weaken or die, muscle atrophy occurs. In regard to the last point, much the same general process appears to occur in ALS, albeit not likely for the same reason. The difference between lathyrism and ALS, however, is one of the degree of neuronal dysfunction in that with lathyrism, most of the motor neurons are not destroyed during the course of the disease, whereas with ALS they are.

Lathyrism bears some similarities to the highly unusual neurological disease spectrum ALS-PDC of Guam and the Western Pacific. This is of particular interest given that BOAA was once considered a potential causal factor for the Guamanian disorder.

3.4.2 Minimata

One of the better-known cases of a neurological disease cluster involved a severe case of industrial pollution at Minimata Bay, Japan, in the late 1950s. Some inhabitants of Minimata showed a range of neurological signs, including seizures, intermittent loss of consciousness, and repeated periods of perturbed mental state. Many of those affected progressed into a permanent comatose condition. Birth defects, including severe mental retardation, rose to epidemic levels.

The impact on so many people in such a relatively short period of time led to the identification of the causal factor: methyl mercury, long known to be a neurotoxin, had made its way from a nearby chemical facility into the fish in the bay, then into the people who consumed them (for a summary, see Risher et al., 2002).

3.4.3 Domoic Acid

Another cluster of neurological disease was identified in the eastern provinces of Canada in the late 1980s (Perl et al., 1990). Over a period of days, a relatively large number of people became severely ill with early symptoms of diarrhea and vomiting. A number of those afflicted appeared to have neurological consequences, including severe and often permanent short-term memory loss. Some of those who became ill died, and post-mortem analyses revealed damage to the hippocampus, one region of the CNS involved in learning and memory.

Given the numbers involved and the time and space constraints, public health officials and epidemiologists were able to trace the illness to the consumption of cultivated mussels from the province of Prince Edward Island. Toxicology studies of the mussels showed high levels of the neurotoxin domoic acid. Eventually, the entire path of the disease was understood: Mussels, as filter feeders, eat various sorts of plankton. During plankton blooms, some species of plankton synthesize domoic acid. As the mussels feed, they accumulate domoic acid. When humans eat the contaminated mussels, the toxin makes its way into the brain where it stimulates kainate receptors, a subtype of the ionotropic glutamate receptor family. The neurons thus activated succumb to overstimulation by excitotoxic cell death.

3.4.4 Summary

The neurological disease clusters discussed in this section are relatively well known – and very unusual – since, with the exception of ALS-PDC and Guadeloupe PDC (G-PDC), they represent acute, rapidly or relatively rapidly occurring geographical and temporal concentrations of neurological disease victims.

Acute cases in which some toxin is present at high enough levels to impact large numbers of people, such as with the methyl mercury at Minimata or the domoic acid poisonings in Eastern Canada, may be easy to solve based on geography and time frame. Most neurological diseases, however – including the progressive, sporadic, age-dependent examples highlighted in this book – have not proven to be so simple. In fact, with the exception of these cases and a few others, when seeking etiological factors for most neurological diseases – especially in regard to toxins – it appears far more likely that toxin exposure occurs at a low but chronic level. This appears to fit the epidemiology of neurological diseases in that if the level of the toxin(s) is typically low few people will show neurological disease outcomes over short periods of time. Further, this observation is in accord with the notion that, whatever the cause of a neurological disease, it may take years or decades for the cumulative damage to become clinically obvious.

The impact of low-level toxicity affects the speed at which population effects can emerge. In consequence, neurological disease clusters do not form around low-level chronic toxins. Add to this the additional variables of age, sex, other trauma to the nervous system, and variations in genetic susceptibility, and the likely reason that neurological disease clusters are the exception rather than the rule becomes clearer.

Another complication is that modern Western society, perhaps particularly in North America, is largely mobile – vastly more so than that of anyone's immediate ancestors. One grows up in one part of the country – or even a different country – goes to school somewhere else altogether, follows a career or spouse/partner still elsewhere, and finally retires in yet another place. The lack of geographical consistency and our lack of understanding of when the disease process begins vastly complicate the enormous problems of sifting risk factors against a backdrop of what may be ubiquitous low-level toxin exposure.

3.5   Ubiquity

As already noted, there are few clusters of neurological disease that satisfy the conditions of numbers as well as of geography and time considerations. Neurological diseases, in general, occur in most places within most industrialized countries in relatively uniform distributions.

What both these observations suggest is the following: except in rare circumstances, where the causal toxin is at a high concentration and/or interacts with genetic suscepti-bility factors present in a large part of the population (as perhaps on Guam), those who succumb to a diseases represent a small part of the overall population. A larger fraction of the same part is not affected until toxin exposure increases.

What makes those who succumb different than those who do not is thus likely the relative impacts of toxin dose and genetic background and the presence of other toxin synergies or other comorbid conditions, along with sex and age. Any or all of these factors can shift a conceptual bell curve to the right, thereby increasing the numbers of those who will express the disease.

3.6   Nested Complex Systems: Proximal versus Distal Events as They May Relate to Neurological Diseases

As an example of complexity, consider the following from the perspective of geography rather than from that of neurological disease. If one is trying to get to the center of Washington, DC, specifically somewhere near the White House, from somewhere outside the city, here are the options: From the areas surrounding the city, the choice of routes is large. Basically, one can head for the White House from any direction and eventually get into the general vicinity. Some routes are fairly direct, others more circuitous. At a macro scale the number of routes, if coming by car, shrinks as one gets closer and closer to the destination. By the time one can see the structure, there are only a few ways to get there. Closer still, one has one or two routes to the front door. If we scale the journey to one on foot, the range of options increases dramatically for both distal and proximal approaches. The options only become constrained at the last stages.

Taking this as general example, now imagine the destination is not a geographical one like the White House, but rather a pathological one such as the last step leading to the death of any particular type of neuron in the CNS (Figure 3.7). There are, for example,

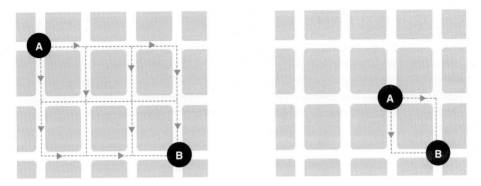

Figure 3.7 Convergence of proximal and distal events in neurological diseases.

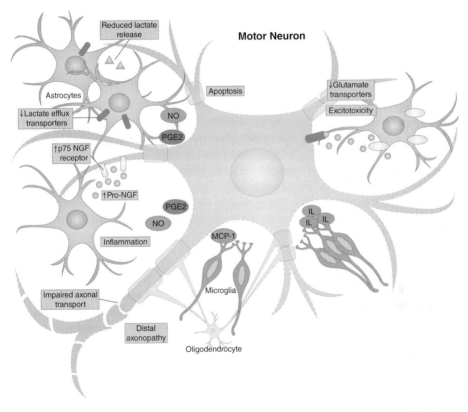

Figure 3.8 Cell- versus non-cell-autonomous mechanisms of neuronal degeneration in ALS. *Source*: Modified from Ferraiuolo et al. (2011) with permission from Macmillan Publishers Ltd.: [*Nature Reviews Neurology*].

a vast number of cell-autonomous or non-cell-autonomous ways to kill a motor neuron in ALS, or at least to render it dysfunctional. The first term, "cell-autonomous," refers to the myriad interacting events that occur within one cell type; the second, "non-cell-autonomous," refers to the interactions between various cell types that can impact events in an individual cell (Figure 3.8).

If one now changes the scale from major events such as glial dysfunction or a failure in axonal transport to the myriad changes in either of these events (or in any of the other degenerative cascades) that move that particular cascade forward, one is left with a subset of complex interactions. For example, at the glial cell level, there will be literally hundreds, if not thousands of crucial glial and neuronal factors that contribute to the successful interactions between both types of cell, the failure of any one of which might be a key part of the degenerative cascade.

The point of all of this is that just as there is a vast range of possibilities in how one gets from destination A to Z, there are a very large number of ways to accomplish the destruction of neurons in the CNS, either individually or as part of circuits and systems.

The implications of such a view are that we are unlikely ever to find totally unique ways to kill neurons at any level. The number of such ways may be limited, but they will not likely be singular. Indeed, at this stage, ALS researchers cannot define with any precision whether motor neurons die by an apoptotic process or by necrosis, or by a newly defined process termed necroptosis (or even other cell death mechanisms). The actuality is that these all occur (Mattson, 2000; Hyman and Yuan, 2012; Re et al., 2014), likely with very different antecedents and thus pathways leading to whichever form of cell death.

Of course, neurological diseases might still turn out to be relatively simple, "single"-pathway types of events in that various differing initial factors converge on a common cell-death pathway. Many researchers in the various subfields of neurological disease research hope that this view is correct.

As a prime example of this sort of hope, consider the ongoing search for aberrant genes – in terms of mutations, deletions, or "toxic gains of function" – in any of the neurodegenerative disorders ranging from autism to Alzheimer's disease.

A recent very illustrative example concerns the *UBQLN2* gene identified from a number of families in which ALS is relatively prevalent. The gene codes for a protein involved in proteasome function, the ubiquitin-like protein ubiquilin 2. The dysfunction of this protein has been linked by researchers to forms of fALS and to ALS with dementia/frontotemporal dementia (FTD) (Deng et al., 2011). These researchers contend that the mutation evokes a cascade of degenerative events leading to motor neuron and hippocampal cell death, and that ultimately this putative pathway involving ubiquilin 2 malfunction will turn out to be a common one for other neurodegenerative diseases. (It is worth mentioning here, and repeating later in the book, that similar views are common, from an environmental perspective, to those seeking so-called "universal toxins" in neurological diseases.)

Excitement over the Human Genome Project has led to the widely held view that most diseases are the result of particular gene mutations. Hence, if a gene is abnormal, an abnormal outcome (the disease) will arise. The analogy is often made to Huntington's disease, where this belief largely holds true. From this perspective, if science screens enough genes and gene segments, then eventually it will find the master genetic defect that is the basis of all forms of any particular neurological disease. This notion is common in ALS, where studies of mutant superoxide dismutase 1 (mSOD1) have led the field for over 20 years. It is backed up by the position that even if mSOD1 or the newer genetic players such as *C9orf2* are not the key, then at least they lead to neurodegeneration pathways that are common to both the genetic/familial and the sporadic forms of the disease. In this view, if one understands the mSOD1 pathway to lead to motor neuron death, then this is a fundamental piece of the puzzle leading to the overall disease manifestations in ALS, both familial and sporadic.

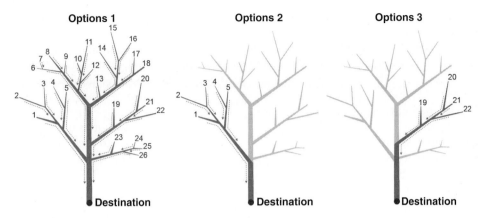

Figure 3.9 Branches on a tree as a schematic depiction of converging pathways in neurological disease. In Option 2 (and 3), only some branches will lead to the roots.

This notion is illustrated in a simple schematic manner in Figure 3.9, which shows a tree with many branches, each leading to a common trunk. If the roots are the ultimate goal, then the trunk will reach them regardless of which branch was initially used to get to get there.

What if, however, the genetic forms have radically different pathways from one another, let alone from environmental causes? In other words, what if there is not one tree with one main trunk leading to the roots, but multiple trees with multiple branches leading to multiple trunks?

The literature remains conflicted on this issue, but it might be safe to say that there are more researchers, at least in ALS, who favor the single tree/single trunk model of neurological disease.

Much the same perspective dominates Parkinson's and Alzheimer's disease research, where it is just as likely to be incorrect, for the same reasons as discussed for ALS.

3.7 The Path to "Curing" Neurological Diseases

The mission statements of most governmental and nongovernmental organizations that are concerned with patient advocacy and research into the various neurological diseases speak of finding "cures" to any particular disease state. It may be useful, at the outset of this section, to consider what is meant by "cure," both in general, and more specifically in terms of neurological diseases such as Parkinson's disease, ALS, and Alzheimer's disease.

Various definitions of "cure" exist, including the following: to remove an ailment or disorder; to restore to good health; and a course of medical treatment effective in combating a disease. There are others, but these give the general idea. Basically, they all posit a return to some pre-existing condition of health that existed before the onset of disease.

To some extent, cures can occur, even for serious illnesses such as cancers, when they go into long-term remission. Likewise, in most non-life-threatening infectious diseases, various medical and nonmedical treatments can restore a person to their prior condition of health. For more serious diseases, this may not happen. Similarly, cardiovascular diseases can be cured by drugs or various surgical interventions, although whether or not the cure is actually to a pre-existing state of cardiovascular health is debatable. The same holds true for most organ transplants and for replacement of original body parts by mechanical devices (e.g., hip replacements).

All of this illustrates that a cure in such cases is not necessarily a complete return to the state of health that existed before the onset of the disease, but rather to something in between. In many cases, such an outcome could legitimately be considered a cure from the perspective of both the patient and the medical community.

How does this apply to neurological diseases? The first thing to realize is that with very few exceptions, medicine has not cured any neurological disease. It may in part control them, as in epilepsy and some forms of mental illness, but it does not cure them, since the underlying problems do not get resolved and the effectiveness of any drug regimen is often transitory.

The situation is vastly more complicated for the age-related, progressive neurological diseases. First, by the time of clinical diagnosis, a large percentage of neurons in the affected brain or spinal cord have died. Notwithstanding the hopes laid on stem cell research, therapies capable of replacing dead neurons are not yet a reality (indeed, they may never be, for reasons to be discussed in Chapters 13 and 14). Second, neurons in the brain do not exist in isolation, but rather in coordinated circuits. Even were stem cell therapies capable of putting *de novo* immature neurons into the affected regions of the CNS, getting them to connect properly would still be a major challenge, and one that is not yet routinely accomplished.

Consider, for example, what would have to be achieved in ALS. Many motor neurons have been destroyed by the time of clinical diagnosis. If they were somehow replaced, the new naïve motor neurons would still need to integrate into functional circuits within the appropriate spinal cord segment, and they would also have to sprout axons that could correctly innervate muscles located up to 1 m away. Since the latter cannot currently be achieved for spinal cord injuries in general, any assertion that such replacement of functional neurons can be carried out in ALS is, at least at this time, unlikely in the extreme. This statement is made in the context of some recent, albeit preliminary, advances in spinal cord repair surgeries (Tabakow et al., 2013, 2014), but it should be noted that the overall complexity of motor neuron loss in ALS is certainly greater than that of traumatic spinal cord injury. Further, the progressive nature of ALS adds an additional level of complexity since the factors that initiated the disease state are still likely to be operating in the system. Many of these same constraints apply to Parkinson's disease and Alzheimer's disease, as well.

For these reasons, what is really being discussed when we talk about "curing" neurological diseases is not a restoration of a pre-existing state of health, but rather a halting of disease progression before a stage that is even worse, namely late-stage dysfunction and death.

This more modest aim sounds as if it should be relatively feasible. At present, however, it is not. The reason for this state of affairs has three parts: Part one is that in order to prevent a disease process from progressing, one would have to know the causal agent(s) and the stages of disease progression. For the diseases under discussion, this information simply does not exist at present. Part two, which will be explored in more detail in Section 6.4, is that there is not likely to be one single causal factor, or even a few causal factors, to contend with. Part three is that at clinical diagnosis, many more than the initial neuronal insults are extant, leading the overall system rapidly toward a point of cascading failure.

There may be solutions to some of this, but they will not come by trying to force the disparate manifestations of any one neurological disease into a single model, or into a single treatment modality.

Rather than "atomizing" the problem by being overly reductionistic in our approach (as noted by Gould and Lewontin, 1979), the likely solution is going to arise from learning to look at these diseases across their respective spectrums of presentation. In this view, the goal will be to come up with a means of addressing multiple risk and causality factors, numerous interactions between genes and toxins, and multiple "other" biochemical and physiological variations across the human population.

In other words, in place of atomizing neurological diseases and thereby treating them as simple entities in health and illness, treatments will have to acknowledge their overall complexity and thus deal with the reality that complex systems are prone to complex dysfunctional states.

It is thus to a discussion of complex systems in general, and of the nervous system in particular, that I turn in the next chapter.

4

Complexity, Cascading Failures, and Neurological Diseases

> *"An organism is atomized into 'traits' and these traits are explained by natural selection for their functions...[in contrast,] organisms are integrated entities, not collections of discrete objects. Evolutionists have often been led astray by inappropriate atomization"*
>
> Gould and Lewontin (1979, p. 585)

From the Preface

9) Because of the complexity and interconnectedness of the CNS, damage at any level must necessarily cascade to other levels (e.g., cell to circuit, circuit to a particular region, etc.). So-called "cascading failures" will, at some point, trigger a total system collapse. Thus, after such a critical stage is reached, no effective therapy will be possible. For this reason, therapies designed to target late stages of disease, namely most at the "clinical" diagnosis stage, will inevitably fail and may simply exacerbate rather than relieve underlying pathological processes. The concepts from biosemiosis of the "true narrative representation" (TNR) apply here.

4.1 Introduction

As the quote which opens this chapter indicates, those working in the neurological disease world are often inclined, as in various disparate fields, to atomize problems. This may especially occur when considering central nervous system (CNS) dysfunctions given the complexity of the nervous system. The extent to which it occurs will be apparent from the discussion of model systems in Chapter 8. Before that, however, I want to step back and consider the nature of complex systems in general.

4.2 Introduction to Complexity Theory and Complex Systems

The following discussion can only serve to put the nervous system into the broadest context of complex systems. It is not capable of doing more than this given the massive amounts of information available on complex systems and their behaviors. Readers

Neural Dynamics of Neurological Disease, First Edition. Christopher A. Shaw.
© 2017 John Wiley & Sons, Inc. Published 2017 by John Wiley & Sons, Inc.

interested in pursuing any of the subfields of complexity theory will find a wealth of available literature, only some of which is cited here.

Complex systems are often hard to define precisely, but they share common characteristics. As cited by various authors, complex systems have multiple, interconnected elements and, crucially, the whole system has properties not derivable from the individual parts (Gilli and Rossier, 1981). Further, the interactions are nonlinear in that they are not simply the sum or multiples of the individual parts. Complexity in such systems may be disorganized, with a very large number of parts, or organized, with a more limited number. Organized complexity exhibits so-called "emergent" properties: properties of the entire system, rather than of any single element. Common examples include the behaviors of solitary ants or bees versus those of the colony, or the activities of a single neuron compared to neurons in a circuit or larger neural region of the CNS.

Numerous complex systems have been studied and modeled. These include the nervous systems of animals and humans, the colony behaviors of social insects, various political and social structures, the functioning of stock markets and economies, and the climate.

A complex system may be a "nested" part of larger complex systems. Conversely, it may also be composed of numerous smaller complex systems. For example, within the nervous system are numerous neural subsystems (e.g., the cerebellum, the cortex, etc.).

The aspect of nonlinearity that is typical of complex systems has generated some of what is termed "chaos theory," a discipline that has found a great deal of resonance in various fields over the last 20 years, including in the neurosciences. The property of a dynamical system that changes over time includes chaotic behaviors and "sensitivity to initial conditions." The latter term means that small perturbations at different points in the system can lead to significantly different future outcomes. This notion is sometimes referred to colloquially as the "butterfly effect."

Complex systems are usually open systems that operate far from equilibrium but retain, at least for part of their existence, stability. They always contain both positive and negative feedback loops.

A special type of complex system is termed a "complex adaptive system." As with other complex systems, these are composed of multiple, interconnected elements. They are considered adaptive in that they can change and learn from experience. Many of the types of complex system just listed qualify as complex adaptive systems. The nervous and immune systems, with their capacity to learn, remember, and change behavior, are perhaps the most striking examples.

One key feature of complex systems and complex adaptive systems that arises as a result of the strong coupling between components is that a failure in one or more components can lead to a cascading failure in which the entire system is catastrophically compromised. Numerous examples exist in the material and biological world, ranging from the collapse of computers and power grids to neurological diseases.

How things fail in networks has been a subject of much recent speculation and theorizing. One fairly recent example was considered in an article that attempted to model the collapse of the Italian power grid which used interconnected national networks (Buldyrev et al., 2010) (Figure 4.1). In this incident in 2003, a power failure at one location led to the loss of telecommunications and thus stopped instructions being sent to other locations, rapidly triggering further local collapses which cumulatively plunged much of Italy into darkness. Overall, the model of the collapse of the power grid in this case shows that isolated clusters of surviving stations remained as the overall network between clusters was erased. Scaling downwards, it is likely that such clusters would themselves collapse, being individually composed of interacting subnetworks of critical elements.

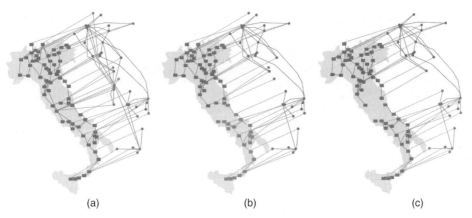

(a)   (b)   (c)

Figure 4.1 Example of a cascading failure: Italian power grid collapse. Illustration of an iterative process of a cascade of failures using real-world data from a power network (located on the map of Italy) and an Internet network (shifted above the map) that were implicated in an electrical blackout in Italy in September 2003. The networks are drawn using the real geographical locations, and every Internet server is connected to the geographically nearest power station. (a) One power station is removed (red node on map) from the power network, and as a result the Internet nodes that depend on it are removed from the Internet network (red nodes above the map). The nodes that will be disconnected from the giant cluster (a cluster that spans the entire network) at the next step are marked in green. (b) Additional nodes that were disconnected from the Internet communication network giant component are removed (red nodes above map). As a result, the power stations depending on them are removed from the power network (red nodes on map). Again, the nodes that will be disconnected from the giant cluster at the next step are marked in green. (c) Additional nodes that were disconnected from the giant component of the power network are removed (red nodes on map), as are the nodes in the Internet network that depend on them (red nodes above map). *Source*: Redrawn from Buldyrev et al. (2010), used with permission from Macmillan Publishers Ltd: [*Nature*]. (See color plate section for the color representation of this figure.)

4.3   Computer Programs and Computer Crashes

It is an obvious truism that scholars (and others) tend to compare human systems of different types to various technological features in their own time and place. Currently, in regard to nervous system function and dysfunction, comparisons to computers, and particularly computer failures, are common (and have been for a number of years) (Gigerenzer and Goldstein, 1996).

Computers do not, of course, equal human nervous systems, neither in their overall complexity, nor in the number of possible interconnections, nor in the emergent properties that are the hallmark of human brain functions. Analogies have also been drawn to the Internet, which comprises an interconnected series of computers (Leiser, 2011). This comparison may not be particularly accurate in terms of function, but in dysfunction it may be more analogous. As the overall topic itself would suffice for a full book, or series of books, I will confine myself here to some considerations involving the general impact of signaling errors.

In brief, a number of events can interfere with the proper functioning of a computer. These include intrinsic hardware and software issues, user errors, and malicious interference in the form of viruses and worms. One might imagine similar levels of problems in the CNS; for example, hardware and software problems might be considered to be similar to genetic, epigenetic, or environmental issues that impact CNS development; user errors could equate to exposure to environmental toxins, causing deleterious gene–toxin

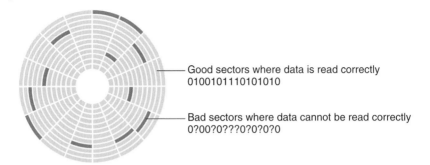

Good sectors where data is read correctly
0100101110101010

Bad sectors where data cannot be read correctly
0?00?0???0?0?0?0

Figure 4.2 How computer hard drives fail.

interactions and the like; and malicious interference might be compared with a range of pathological insults, including injuries and various infectious pathogens.

Another aspect, which may seem more mundane, yet could in fact be crucial, is the very nature of the signals being sent between different programs and between different cell types or sub-CNS regions. Corrupted or incomplete signals in computers can degrade the integrity of the programs, causing them to become less efficient and slower, eventually leading to the complete, catastrophic failure of the system (e.g., the dreaded "blue screen of death").

Modern computers have extensive validation/"defragging" programs to try to ensure that this does not happen. But, of course, it does (see Figure 4.2). Validation is an intrinsic part of a computer program, and seeks to prevent incorrect input messages from generating incorrect outcomes (but, of course, junk messages do get through). Defragging cleans up the hard drive. A lot of the problem has to do with how computer programs are produced. Most are developed by a number of different teams who are responsible for different elements. These program elements may be further broken down and worked on by other teams, and so on. At some point in the development of a final program, the disparate elements are put together. This is typically where problems arise. The challenge is that the program is now likely larger than the sum of its parts and it becomes virtually impossible for any one person to know what is happening in regard to errors and thus in regard to solving them.

The paradox is that the more complex a brain system or computer program gets, the closer it is to potential failure. The balance to be struck in computing – not always successfully – is to have the computer carry out as many functions as possible without doing any that could lead to failure. This might be one reason why computers may never have truly emergent properties (Bhalla and Iyengar, 1999), although this remains a point of contention in the field.

In terms of human brains, it is likely that as valuable as the emergent properties of CNS function are for human consciousness and cognition, the price to be paid at an individual, rather than population, level may include neurological failures in the form of neurological diseases.

4.4 Biosemiosis in the CNS (Part 1)

Biosemiosis is a relatively new field, combining, as the name suggests, aspects of biological systems and semantics (i.e., meaning). In other words, it broadly refers to biological system signaling, either internally or externally. To be more specific, Oller (2014) uses the term "pragmatics," noting that while semantics is abstract, pragmatics is concrete. Oller further notes that, "in between there is a mapping relation that takes some surface expression of the conceptual meaning (semantic) and makes it perceivable (pragmatically)" (pers. comm.).

The use of semantics in the current context refers specifically to the signals sent between biological entities at any level. For example, at a cellular level it includes the messages encoded in DNA, which lead to the synthesis of particular proteins, as well as the interactions of various cellular molecules and organelles, which lead to the appropriate cellular functions. At higher levels, it can refer to cell-to-cell communication, to the signals sent between various nervous system subsystems, and eventually to messages sent between individuals (e.g., in spoken human language).

Various events can prevent accurate – and, thus, effective – signal transmission. For example, mutations in DNA or transcriptional errors by RNA in nervous system cells (or any other cells) can lead to incorrect proteins being made. Crucially, in neurological disease, such errors can lead to misfolded proteins that lack appropriate biological functions. Further, the interference of such proteins and/or the impacts of various kinds on cell organelle can lead to cellular failure.

The list of such potential signaling failures is large. It will be addressed in more detail in later chapters in the context of cell-autonomous loci in neurological diseases. For example, failures in signal transmission between cells in the nervous system can arise from anything that acts to diminish neurotransmitter release or that alters receptor or second messenger proteins. It can also include disruptions in the effective actions of other nearby cells in the nervous system, as with the various types of glial cell. Specifically, these latter functions include the various neuronal supporting roles played by astrocytes, the protective/scavenger cell functions of microglia, and the enhanced cell conduction properties (and tropic support) provided by the oligodendrocytes. Disturbances involving such supporting cells are non-cell-autonomous (see Chapter 3), in that they arise initially from outside of any individual neuron.

4.4.1 Degraded Biological Signals in CNS Pathology

There are various examples from the literature where degraded biological signals impact the ability of CNS subsystems to respond to, or to compensate for, an injury. Several examples of blocked "pathological plasticity" are worth considering.

The first involves "denervation supersensitivity," a phenomenon that arises following the loss of the connections between motor neurons and the muscle fibers they innervate. The observation, in what is now an older literature, is that denervated muscle fibers show a redistribution of nicotinic acetylcholine receptors away from the neuromuscular junction (the end plate) and toward the extrajunctional regions of the muscle fiber. The normal response at the muscle end plate to acetylcholine released by the motor neuron is an action potential followed by individual muscle fiber contractions. This no longer occurs in denervated muscle fibers. Instead, the fibers in the denervated muscle responds with twitches when they receive stray acetylcholine released elsewhere. These fibers are said to have undergone denervation supersensitivity (Cannon, 1939; Cannon and Rosenblueth 1949; Thesleff and Sellin, 1980) (Figure 4.3).

Denervation supersensitivity can be blocked by providing gross electrical stimulation to the affected muscle. The electrical signal in this case is not the normal signal that would be discretely provided by the appropriate motor neuron axon acting on its target end plate, but rather a nonsense signal whose impact is to prevent the attempted reorganization of the end plate. The noise in the system (i.e., the failed normal signal – or failed

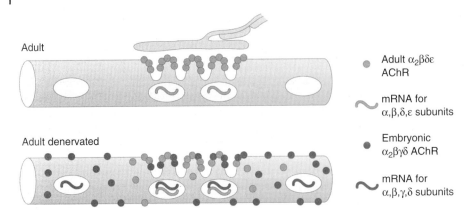

Figure 4.3 Denervation supersensitivity. *Source*: Redrawn from Nicholls et al. (2012).

biosemiosis) is such that no correct response is achieved (Kim et al., 1984; Wærhaug and Lømo, 1994; Andreose et al., 1995; Lain et al., 2009).

A second example comes from some earlier work my colleagues and I conducted on visual cortex plasticity in kittens. One form of neuronal plasticity in higher mammals is called "ocular dominance plasticity," which is observed when one eye is occluded for a period of time in early postnatal life. This period, in which plastic modifications of morphology and function can occur, is termed the "critical period." Cats, as an example of animals with frontal-facing eyes and stereoscopic vision, tend to have each eye dominate some portion of visual cortex input layer 4. During development, input fibers from the lateral geniculate nucleus segregate into ocular dominance bands within layer 4. Layer 4 neurons then project – usually in equal measure – to neurons in the other layers of the visual cortex, such that most neurons in these layers are equally responsive to stimulation of either eye (Hubel and Wiesel, 1962). Kittens deprived of form vision, usually by eyelid suture or other forms of occlusion during the critical period, will show a resulting dominance of cells in layer 4 and other layers of cortex that favors the open eye over the occluded eye (Wiesel and Hubel, 1963). This ocular dominance shift is one of the best studied forms of neuroplasticity in mammals.

My colleagues and I wondered if the same sort of biological noise as in denervation supersensitivity could block ocular dominance shifts. That is, if the visual cortex were provided with increased neural firing due to either abnormal electrical or chemical stimuli, would this prevent an ocular dominance shift from occurring? To answer this question, kittens in their critical periods had one eye occluded by eyelid suture while one hemisphere was either implanted with stimulating electrodes or had infusions of glutamate, the universal CNS excitatory neurotransmitter. In both cases, the outcome was that the region of cortex that received treatment did not undergo an ocular dominance shift, while surrounding regions of the visual cortex and all regions in the contralateral visual cortex with no implant did (Shaw and Cynader, 1984). As with the example of denervation supersensitivity, our interpretation was that the "noise" provided by the increased neuronal activation had drowned out the correct signal coming from the open eye and prevented the visual cortex from making its appropriate adaptive change.

Although these examples, and others, reflect the blocking of a form of adaptive plasticity, they nevertheless illustrate the power that incorrect signals, as forms of misinterpreted biosemiosis, can have for neuronal modification.

Another example, also from the visual plasticity field, was an experiment in which we tested the impact of neural noise on the orientation selectivity of visual cortical neurons. In adult cats, individual neurons in the visual cortex tend to favor a particular orientation of line segment within a region of visual space. This region is termed the "receptive field" and is that region of the visual field to which individual visual cortex neurons maximally respond when provided with the most appropriate stimulus (Hubel and Wiesel, 1962). In the visual cortex cumulatively, all orientations are represented. Most neurons favor not only particularly oriented line segments, but also those segments that move in particular directions orthogonally to the orientation of the line. Both of these features, orientation and direction selectivity, are under the control of regions of the receptive field that contribute inhibitory input to the overall structure. Both features can be modified by early experience. Animals reared in their critical periods looking at only one orientation of line or at objects that move in only one direction have modified neuronal responses in the visual cortex in which neurons favor only those visual features the animals experienced (see, e.g., Spinelli and Jensen, 1979).

To probe the impact of noise on these features in adult cats, we infused the $GABA_A$ antagonist bicuculline to block inhibitory activity in a small region of visual cortex in order to increase overall neuronal activity. After several weeks of such treatment, the regions of cortex close to the infusion sites showed that most neurons had lost either orientation selectivity, direction selectivity, or both. Other regions of the visual cortex away from the infusion sites were unaffected and showed normal adult neuronal properties. The effect seemed to be permanent, as even up to a year after the infusions had ended, the loss of orientation/direction selectivity remained. These results demonstrate that even in adult animals outside of the critical period, abnormal signaling in the form of noise can deprogram a previously correctly wired neuron. The caveat to these results is that they were not published in the peer-reviewed literature and thus need to be considered as unsubstantiated. However, they are a good fit to those cited earlier concerning the impact of noise on ocular dominance shifts.

Such results, and others, clearly point to the crucial nature of correct biological signaling for either establishing or maintaining normal neuronal functions. These outcomes are, in general, important for any consideration of therapeutic approaches to neurodegenerative diseases, as well as for such firmly established procedures as vaccination. These aspects will be considered in more detail in Chapter 14.

4.5 Complexity in the CNS and the Impact of Genetic and Environmental Insults

In advance of the next chapters, which will explore in detail particular examples of genetic mutations and toxins putatively involved in neurological diseases, the following question can be posed: How exactly does any given genetic mutation or alteration, any toxin, or any interaction of genes and toxins impact the CNS, leading to neurodegeneration?

In the following, I will use ALS as the example, although many of the points to be discussed apply equally to Parkinson's or Alzheimer's diseases, and to other neurological disorders as well.

In ALS, motor neurons die, leading to loss of innervation of particular muscles, a resultant loss of function, and, eventually, death, as the muscles of respiration are affected. In how many different ways could this happen? The answer is that there are numerous

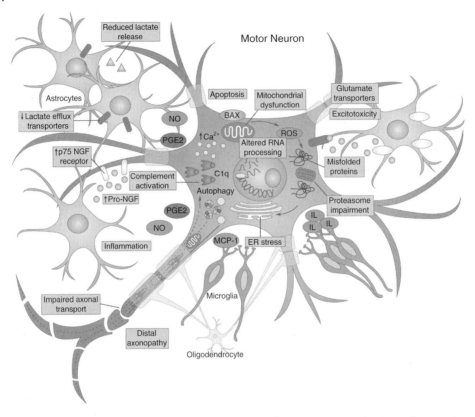

Figure 4.4 More complete example of cell- versus non-cell-autonomous mechanisms of neuronal degeneration (see Figure 3.8). *Source*: Modified from Ferraiuolo et al. (2011) with permission from Macmillan Publishers Ltd: [*Nature Reviews Neurology*].

ways to kill motor neurons, or to render them dysfunctional, and these involve both cell-autonomous and non-cell-autonomous events (Clement et al., 2003) (Figure 4.4).

At the cell-autonomous level, an aberrant gene or toxin can have a deleterious impact on a range of cellular structures or functions. A very short list of cellular structures considered in the literature includes: the neuronal membrane; various ionotrophic and G-protein receptors; organelles such as the mitochondrion, endoplasmic reticulum, and proteasome; molecular chaperones such as the various heat-shock proteins; transport structures inside the soma or axon; and the axon terminal/neuromuscular junction/end plate. Genetically, DNA alterations may encode nonsense messages to the RNA. In turn, altered RNA function may lead to transcriptional mistakes in protein synthesis, leading, for example, to alterations in protein structure. Biochemically, there can be changes in antioxidant molecules which increase oxidant stress by increasing free radical production and causing further alterations in energy metabolism through impacts on mitochondrial electron transport chain molecules. Alterations in the transport proteins needed for adequate axonal functioning can occur. Malfunctions in proteasome protein subunits or the molecular chaperones cited earlier can lead to the build-up of aberrant and/or misfolded proteins, which can in turn impact the actions of other cellular processes, either chemically or mechanically.

It should be borne in mind that such changes are not likely to be "one-hit" sorts of processes, but instead are highly interactive. At a cellular level, two of the most commonly considered putative mechanisms for neuronal death are excitotoxity and mitochondrial dysfunction, often cited as alternatives to each other. However, the two are *not* independent events at all, and indeed separating them either temporally or structurally is close to impossible: Excitotoxic molecules such as glutamate or the various glutamate agonists can induce prolonged cellular depolarization, thereby acting to increase calcium influx into a neuron. The latter flux triggers the activation of proteolytic enzymes, amongst other things. The changes in ionic currents across the cell membrane can induce corresponding changes in mitochondrial membranes, leading in turn to the collapse of mitochondrial activity. In its absence, the cell's energy stores are rapidly depleted, leading to a loss of cellular ionic integrity and loss of the cellular and mitochondrial membrane potentials. Because these two factors – and many others – are so dynamically interconnected, it is almost meaningless to speak of one occurring without the other. Thus, excitotoxicity will lead to mitochondrial collapse; and mitochondrial collapse will lead to cell membrane dysfunction, the functional equivalent to excitotoxicity. Without some means of looking at the two types of event in model systems in real time, one cannot realistically separate the temporal sequence of events, which likely occurs in a time frame of seconds to minutes. Such a resolution has not been achieved to date; it seems increasingly likely that it may never be.

In a real sense, this does not matter. The net result, regardless of what comes first, is system collapse at the cellular level. In terms of potential therapeutics, one can perhaps imagine (and writers of various grants and articles often *do* imagine) that various prophylactic neuroprotective agents will act to prevent either excitotoxicity or mitochondrial damage. How any such drug might do both is an open question, especially when the sequence of events is not likely to be known with any precision in model systems, let alone in human neurological diseases.

Overall, the great likelihood is that all of these events occur, but the precise sequence is not known. Indeed, such a sequence is not known for human neurological diseases and has not been established with any certainty even in *in vitro* or *in vivo* animal models.

None of the attendant difficulties improves as one scales upward to the non-cell-autonomous level. Instead, the situation becomes vastly more complex. Consider the minimal number of potential cellular players in ALS: the motor neurons (particularly α-motor neurons, but also γ-motor neurons), sensory neurons, astrocytes, microglia (in their various functional roles as either neuroprotectors or neuroscavengers), and oligodendrocytes (acting in either or both of their signal propagation and trophic roles), as well as the target muscle fibers. The latter send trophic signals back to the motor neurons, and one study using the often problematic mutant superoxide dismutase 1 (m*SOD1*) model of ALS (or at least fALS) posited that the loss of motor neurons originated at the level of the muscle end plate, with motor neuron degeneration being retrograde in direction (Fischer et al., 2004).

The situation is further complicated by being fractal as each of the cell types is subject to the cell-autonomous alterations already cited. Beyond this lie the potential impacts of non-neural cells, including cells of the vasculature and various immune system cells, each with its own signaling molecules.

Thus, if one asks the apparently simple experimental question of why motor neurons die in ALS, any of these factors will probably be involved at some stage. This contrasts with motor neuron loss in polio (poliomyelitis), a viral infection of motor neurons that is self-limiting and does not spread to other motor neurons not initially affected by the virus. This characteristic difference between ALS and polio and its implications will be addressed in more detail in Chapter 15.

The actual question here is not one of cell-autonomous versus non-cell-autonomous actions, but is more likely to do with the different sorts of non-cell-autonomous actions. In ALS, immune function seems to be compromised either as a primary or a secondary characteristic of the disease. In contrast, in polio, an effective immune response is largely responsible for the cessation of motor neuron loss.

Sorting any of this out in human patients, especially by the time they are normally diagnosed with ALS, is virtually hopeless as a future goal. Model systems, either *in vivo* or, even more so, *in vitro*, are not able to provide more than snapshots of the myriad processes at play. All of this has major implications for the success of the various therapeutic approaches that will be detailed in Chapters 13 and 14.

One obvious consequence of the potential interactions cited here is that the cumulative weight of these forms of cellular dysfunction must almost inevitably lead to a form of cascading failure, when some "tipping point," or point of no return, has been reached. This is obvious from the rapid decline of ALS patients and the precipitous rate of decline in at least the m*SOD1* animal model of fALS. What the various m*SOD1* studies show, depending in great measure on the type of mutation, the species background strain, the sex, and any drug treatments, is variable periods leading to disease initiation and, thus, long-term survival. Strikingly, the data do not show much variance in the rate of decline once the onset of dysfunction has begun, at least not as measured by the apparent rate of behavioral decline or survival as plotted on standard Kaplan–Meier curves. What these curves in fact look like is fairly straight lines from birth to the beginning of the decline, then a precipitous drop that seems relatively invariant in slope regardless of the other circumstances of the experiment (Figure 4.5). Such a curve certainly has the appearance of being consistent with the nervous system of the affected animals having hit a tipping

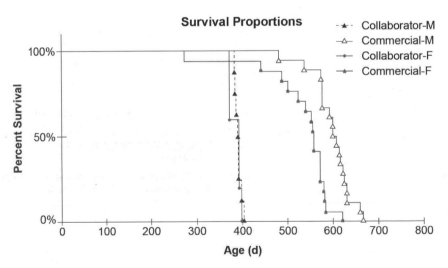

Figure 4.5 Kaplan–Meier curves for an m*SOD* model of ALS. Transgenic animals with a lower cycle threshold (CT) value exhibited an increased survival time. Bonferroni correction for multiple comparisons indicated a significant difference between animal supplier and life span. Inter-sex comparisons showed that collaborator-derived progeny reached the end point earlier, while commercially derived progeny with a lower CT value reached it much later, beyond 1.5 years of age. ***$p < 0.001$. Collaborator male n = 8; collaborator female n = 5; commercial male n = 18; commercial female n = 17. *Source*: Zwiegers et al. (2014), used under Creative Commons Attribution License.

point and triggered a cascading failure beyond recovery, or at least beyond self-recovery by any form of neuronal compensation, sprouting, neurogenesis, or plasticity.

The experimental outcomes from which this conclusion derives may reflect some of the more artificial aspects of the model, notably the multiple copy number of the mutant gene expression needed to induce motor neuron death (Zwiegers et al., 2014). But these outcomes may also reflect a very real aspect of cascading failure, not only in animal models of ALS, but in the disease itself.

There is currently no way of directly observing such an effect in the human disease. The absence of this information is of more than trivial academic interest, since without it there is no way to know at what stage therapeutics could be successfully used to intervene in the disease process, which drugs might work in such interventions, or even whether treatment regimens need to vary from individual to individual. This last point will be discussed in Chapter 15 in the context of the notion that each instance of neurological disease is, to a great extent, unique to the individual.

Therapeutics is further compromised by the fact that the field does not know much about disease etiologies for sporadic age-related neurological diseases. Combining these concerns, one begins to get a sense of the dimension of the problem that must be solved before effective therapeutics can be developed. In this sense, it is not at all surprising that treatments started post clinical diagnosis routinely fail. Indeed, such treatments, of whatever variety (drugs, stem or fetal cells, gene transplants, etc.), are likely to continue to fail well into the future, as will be discussed throughout the last section of the book.

As discussed earlier, cascading failures are typical of complex systems, regardless of origin: interpersonal relationships, political processes, the stock market, and the human nervous system. Perhaps especially in the latter case, it is difficult to imagine that any one part of the system can cease to function without eventually impacting all the others. I will explore this notion in other chapters on various neurological diseases and, later, in a discussion of various animal models of ALS.

4.6 Tipping Points and Time Lines of Disease Progression

The concept of a tipping point in a cascading failure is very relevant to discussions of the collapse of any complex system, obviously including the nervous system in neurological diseases (Rouse, 2006) (Figure 4.6). In such a state, it is as if the system has reached a point of transition, or "percolation," to use a term from complexity theory. The question in relation to the nervous system is at what stage the pathological events (of whatever nature) will reach the point of no return, after which the deterioration of the nervous system becomes virtually impossible to either halt or reverse.

Such data have not yet entered the literature on human neurological diseases. In part, this is because no one knows when the diseases begin because pre-clinical stages are

Figure 4.6 Illustration of a tipping point.

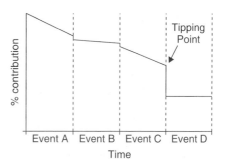

currently undetectable and thus merely the territory of speculation. The field does, however, know something about the stages of some neurological diseases after they have been diagnosed (see Chapter 9).

This lack of information might be alleviated by effective biomarkers of disease onset and progression and there is some indication that useful tools may be forthcoming. Indeed, the search for such biomarkers continues to occupy the efforts of various scientists. However, no effective biomarkers for the early stages of any of the age-related neurological diseases have yet been identified.

One can imagine the creation of the neurological equivalent of the Framingham study on cardiovascular disease. However, the numbers that would have to be screened to accomplish such an analysis would be astronomical. For example, to pull out those who might end up with ALS, the field would have to screen 100 000 people in order to get 3 or 4 future victims, given current incidence levels; for Parkinson's and Alzheimer's the number of potential victims would be higher, maybe on average up to about 20 per 100 000, but this is still far too low to draw much inference about disease staging and progression without screening millions of individuals over prolonged periods. This leaves animal models, each of which has various caveats, as will be discussed in Chapter 8.

Before that, however, it is important to consider the nature of the evidence for either genetic or environmental (toxin) etiologies in neurological diseases because the literature for both is firmly based on model system approaches.

5

Genetic Determinants of Neurological Disease

"Monogenic diseases result from modifications in a single gene occurring in all cells of the body. Though relatively rare, they affect millions of people worldwide. Scientists currently estimate that over 10 000 of human diseases are known to be monogenic. Pure genetic diseases are caused by a single error in a single gene in the human DNA. The nature of disease depends on the functions performed by the modified gene. The single-gene or monogenic diseases can be classified into three main categories: dominant, recessive, [and] X-linked."

World Health Organization

From the Preface

2) The complexity of the nervous system arises due to the interplay between genetic programs and environmental influences. This complexity includes the interactions that lead to neurodegeneration. Gene defects in the germ cell line and in the early developing CNS are likely to be fatal or result in profoundly disturbed neuronal functions. Environmental impacts on the CNS depend crucially on the stage of development: prenatal ones are likely to be of greater impact than those occurring in postnatal life, while early postnatal ones will be more impactful than those later in life. The concept of the "fetal basis of adult disease" used in other fields of study likely applies to neurological disease just as strongly (or even more so) to those disorders with which it is more conventionally associated. Environmental impacts also crucially depend on the number of CNS levels impacted (e.g., from genome to the whole CNS).

3) It is almost certain that gene defects/mutations alone will not explain most types of age-related neurological disease. Nor, for that matter, will obvious environmental stressors/toxins be found to be solely responsible in most cases. Hence, gene–toxin interactions are the likely source of most such diseases, acted upon by a number of other variables across the lifespan.

Neural Dynamics of Neurological Disease, First Edition. Christopher A. Shaw.
© 2017 John Wiley & Sons, Inc. Published 2017 by John Wiley & Sons, Inc.

5.1   Introduction

In much of the neurological disease literature, strong claims are often made that some genetic mutation or particular toxin exposure is the sole cause of one or more neurological diseases. Usually, the authors of these articles are very careful in how the issue is framed, given that working scientists typically try not to go beyond their data. The mainstream media, however, often overstate the importance of the work for curing or preventing the diseases in question. Sometimes, this is done with the collaboration of the researchers and/or the university where the work was done. There are numerous reasons for such a state of affairs, but these are beyond the scope of this book.

The quote at the start of this chapter is from the current World Health Organization (WHO) website (www.who.int). Of the examples given for monogenetic disorders, only three are actually primarily neurological: Tay Sachs, Fragile X, and Huntington's disease. It is important to keep this in mind when considering the following material.

5.2   Causality versus Coincidence

A key issue for some of the claims made about disease etiology lies in confusing correlation with causality. The problem is obviously not solely one confined to neurological disease research, but rather permeates much of the biomedical literature of various subspecialties, as well as other scientific (and social and political) disciplines. For example, in the often highly contentious subject of vaccine effectiveness, one finds those on both sides of the issue inferring causality, or denying the same, where none has actually been clearly established or rejected. A number of humorous examples can also be found that demonstrate how obviously absurd correlations can be found for virtually any two events that appear to be temporally linked.

As well-known as this basic problem generally is, many researchers occasionally, or sometimes frequently, fail to distinguish correlation from causality in whole, or in part. This problem tends to occur more in observational studies than in experimental ones, and it crops up frequently in epidemiological studies where various risk factors are considered to be associated with some disease state.

Experimental studies are not immune, however. For example, a related manifestation can occur when a researcher observes a change in some biochemical pathway associated with a disease state and infers from this that the altered molecule is causal to the disease. The altered pathway is often associated with a demonstrated mutant gene or the effect(s) of a toxin. The implicated molecule could, of course, be the cause. However, it is equally likely that the molecule is either a "bystander" molecule secondarily affected by something else, or even a compensatory molecule that the system has increased (or decreased) in an effort to fend off the emerging pathology.

Broadly speaking, there are several ways to address the problem of confusing correlation with causality. The first is through a longitudinal approach: one establishes a baseline of some state, introduces one variable amongst potentially many in question, and watches the hoped for process(es) emerge. This is hard to do in practice in *in vivo* animal models, harder still in human populations, and virtually impossible in the context of neurological diseases in humans. These problems will be addressed in more detail in Chapter 8.

The other way to approach the causality issue is to apply the so-called "Hill criteria," first described by British statistician A.B. Hill (Hill, 1965). Hill described nine features that should be met in an attempt to assign causation to any association. Broadly, these include situations where the following conditions are found to apply in disease states:

1) The strength of the association is strong (as measured by appropriate statistical tests that also achieve statistical significance).
2) There is broad consistency of the observed association (i.e., the association has been repeatedly observed by different researchers and/or in different places, circumstances, and times).
3) The specificity of the association is established (i.e., a single putative causal factor produces a specific effect – but see later).
4) A temporal relationship of the association is clear in that exposure precedes outcome.
5) A biological gradient or dose–response function exists such that increasing the amount of exposure in dose or time to the putative factor increases the risk.
6) Biological plausibility is likely (i.e., the mechanisms of action generally agree with a currently accepted understanding of the pathological processes at work in the disease in question).
7) Coherence exists between the current data and existing knowledge, such that data appear to be congruent with generally known facts of the natural history and biology of the disease.
8) Experimental or semi-experimental evidence exist for causality.
9) An analogy with similar evidence exists (e.g., different toxins may result in similar disease outcomes because they adversely affect the same underlying processes linked to a specific disease).

In neuropsychiatry, four of Hill's nine criteria are usually considered critical, and sufficient, to assess causality. These are: (1) the strength of the association, (2) the consistency of the observed association, (6) biological plausibility, and (4) the temporal relationship of the association (Reekum et al., 2001).

Obviously, if evidence exists for the remaining five criteria, conclusions about causality will be further strengthened. Notably, the specificity criterion (3) is not considered necessary in neuropsychiatry given that many neuropsychiatric disorders have multiple causal factors. Indeed, any neurological disease in which genes, toxins, or the interaction of the two has been postulated will similarly be included in such a consideration. Specifically, most of the neurological diseases considered in this book do not have to satisfy Hill criterion 3.

As important as satisfying the Hill criteria tends to be, especially in epidemiological studies, they are not actually themselves sufficiently powerful or unbiased to assign definitive causality to *any* outcome. The reasons for this have been thoroughly discussed by Ward (2009) and other authors. Ward stresses that the Hill criteria "are neither inductive nor deductive in character," but rather are more appropriately used as keys to "inference to the best explanation," citing the use of this term from other studies. The latter can serve as a basis for further hypothesis generation and more rigorous experimental and statistical evaluations.

With these criteria and their caveats firmly in mind, it is now worthwhile to consider in brief the evidence for the various proposed etiologies in age-dependent neurological diseases. To do so, I will begin with putative genetic factors in the current chapter, and then consider environmental toxins in the next.

5.3 Actions of Mutant Genes in Neurological Disease

It would likely be fair to say that the search for genetic determinants of neurological diseases is the major theme in the field at present. The successful mapping of the genomes of various species, notably that of human beings, has created a strong trend for both research funding and mentality (and the two are completely interlinked), supporting the view that to find a gene or genes involved in provoking any of the age-related neurological diseases is to find the key to that disease. This applies across the neurological disease domain and includes Parkinson's disease, ALS, and Alzheimer's disease, amongst various others. It has even spread into developmental neurological disorders such as autism spectrum disorder (ASD).

In general, the methods used to search for a genetic basis to neurological diseases involve the following general steps: First, identify some family (ideally *families*) in which the disease is unusually prevalent compared to the general population. Next, perform genetic screens of various types on those in the families affected versus those who are not and/or members of unaffected families to identify chromosomal regions, genes, single-nucleotide polymorphism (SNPs), and so on that may be different. Finally, with the putative genetic variant identified, delineate the biochemical pathways that seem altered in those with the disease. These are all part of the observational aspects of the research.

The reasoning for the next stages is also stepwise: once a study has identified an abnormal genetic variant in a particular disease state and understood, at least in part, what proteins that gene codes for and what these proteins do for a neuronal cell, the pathway(s) leading to neuronal degeneration should be understood. Then, when the pathway has been clearly identified, therapeutics, drugs, or other interventions designed to interfere with this pathway can be designed and employed. All of this now becomes the experimental portion of the research and provides a very logically progressive position. That is, if one accepts the initial assumption that the alleged mutant gene alone determines neuronal dysfunction and/or death.

The problems that arise from this position, however, are several-fold. First, most cases of the age-related neurological diseases under consideration are sporadic, without any identified genetic causes (so far). Of course, the ratios of genetic to sporadic neurological disease cases might change with the discovery of other genes or parts of the DNA not yet identified, and indeed such is the assumption/hope of many of those working in the field.

Another assertion is that even though the overall numbers associated with mutant genes may not be large in relation to the number of cases that are sporadic, the cell-death pathways activated will be consistent across etiologies. Thus, a gene that triggers neuronal cell death by one pathway may mirror a toxin that has the same action by activating the same pathway.

The numbers of purely genetic etiologies vary between ALS and the other neurological diseases, but in no case could it currently be said that a purely genetic etiology plays a causal role in more than about 10% of any of the key diseases in question. Further, within any individual neurological disease, the fraction of so-called familial cases is further subdivided into a variety of different genetic mutations. ALS, for example, lists a large number of such mutations of various sorts ("loss"- or "gain"-of-function mutations). These include mutant *SOD1, TARDBP, FUS, C9orf72, UBQLN2*, and a host of others. Parkinson's disease has α-synuclein and *LRRK2*, amongst others. Alzheimer's disease has *APP* and presenilins 1 and 2 (*PSEN1, PSEN2*). Details of some of the major genes linked to these diseases will be provided in the next sections.

A good place to start in considering genetic determinants of neurological disease is Huntington's disease, in which the genetic mutation was clearly identified years ago. From this, I will show that the success, or lack thereof, in treating Huntington's disease will have implications for the other age-related neurological diseases, if indeed they have clear genetic causalities that can account for more than a fraction of the sporadic forms on their own.

5.3.1 Huntington's Disease

The clearest example of a neurological disease linked to a genetic defect is Huntington's disease which was initially described by its eponymous discoverer, George Huntington, in 1872 (Huntington, 1872). It is worthwhile to briefly consider some of the features of a primarily inheritable neurological disease like Huntington's, especially in the context of neurological diseases such as Parkinson's disease, ALS, and Alzheimer's disease which are considered for the most part to be non-inheritable, sporadic presentations.

Huntington's disease is also known as Huntington's "chorea" – the Latin-derived word "chorea" used to describe the rapid, jerky, uncoordinated movements that are symptomatic of Huntington patients. Huntington's disease occurs at an incidence slightly higher than that of ALS (approximately 2–4/100 000), affecting approximately 3–6/100 000 persons. (Note that as cited in Chapter 2, the incidence numbers vary for ALS across various studies, but this range is adequate for the purpose of this chapter and elsewhere in the book.)

Huntington's disease occurs in those of European heritage and usually begins in middle age. An earlier-onset form can occur before age 20, but this makes up only a small fraction of all cases.

In addition to disturbed motor features, Huntington's disease patients can show psychiatric disturbances, along with deterioration of memory and intellectual abilities.

Clinical signs and symptoms such as these have been described in the medical literature as far back as the early 1500s (as cited by Eftychiadis and Chen, 2001): observations that are in keeping with the notion that the primary causal factors are genetic rather than, for example, environmental (e.g., due to a recent introduction of toxins of human origin).

Early-stage pathological features of Huntington's include damage to the striatum, an area of the forebrain, which is also affected in Parkinson's disease, albeit in a different manner. Other regions of the nervous system can also be impacted as the disease progresses, including the frontal cortex (Selemon et al., 2004).

Huntington's disease appears to arise from an autosomal-dominant mode of inheritance, in that if one parent carries the mutation there is a 50% chance that it will be passed on to the offspring. The probability is greater if the father bears the mutation. However, the sex differences in the cellular processes triggered by the mutation are not well understood.

The gene mutation in Huntington's disease occurs on chromosome 4 in a region that normally makes a protein called HTT or "huntingtin," a molecule which is ubiquitously expressed at low levels throughout the body with the highest levels being found in the brain and testes. The mutation consists of an increase in the number of copies of a "triplet" of DNA nucleotides. In the case of Huntington's, the abnormal sequence of nucleotides is cytosine, adenine, guanine, abbreviated as CAG.

Normal huntingtin protein has a number of cellular functions, including during embryonic development. Huntingtin also acts as an antiapoptotic molecule, controls aspects of the activity of brain-derived neurotrophic factor (BDNF; crucial for striatal neuron survival), and is involved in vesicle transport along microtubules and vesicle release across the synapse. The failure of any single function, or any combination of functions, is able to trigger the death of striatal neurons (Schulte and Littleton, 2011).

5.4 Genetic Mutations Linked to Parkinson's Disease

A number of genetic mutations have been described in the familial forms of Parkinson's disease, many of which have been widely studied in recent years. The key ones are listed in Table 5.1 and some are presented in this section. Two of the most important are those for α-synuclein, a signaling molecule in the central nervous system (CNS), and *LRRK2*.

Table 5.1 Causal genes linked to Parkinson's disease.

Gene	Location	Inheritance	Diagnosis	Clinical features	References
SNCA	4q21-22	AD	Early-onset PD, aggressive course	LBs, atypical in some cases	Polymeropoulos et al. (1997)
LRRK2	12q12	AD	Typical, late onset PD	Pleomorphic, typical LB in most	Zimprich et al. (2004)
GBA	1q21	AD (risk gene)	Typical, late-onset PD	Typical LBs	Sidransky et al. (2009)
VPS35	16q12	AD	Typical, late-onset PD	Unknown	Vilariño-Güell et al. (2011), Zimprich et al. (2011)
EIF1	3q26-q28	AD	Late-onset PD, mild course	LBs	Chartier-Harlin et al. (2011)
CHCHD2		AD	Late-onset PD	Unknown	Funayama et al. (2015)
Parkin	6q25.2-q27	AR	Early-onset PD, slow course	No LBs in most cases	Kitada et al. (1998)
PINK1	1p36	AR	Early-onset PD, slow course	LBs	Valente et al. (2004)
DJ-1	1p36	AR	Early-onset PD, slow course	Unknown	Bonifati et al. (2003)
ATP13AP2	1p36	AR	Juvenile-onset, atypical PD	Ceroid lipofuscinosis	Ramirez et al. (2006)
PLA2G6	22q13.1	AR	Juvenile-onset, atypical PD	Typical LBs, brain iron accumulation	Paisan-Ruiz et al. (2009)
FBXO7	22q12.3	AR	Juvenile-onset, atypical PD	Unknown	Di Fonzo et al. (2009)
DNAJC6	1p31.3	AR	Juvenile-onset, atypical PD	Unknown	Edvardson et al. (2012)
SYNJ1	21q22.2	AR	Juvenile-onset, atypical PD	Unknown	Krebs et al. (2013)

AD, autosomal dominant; AR, autosomal recessive; PD, Parkinson's disease; LB, Lewy body.

5.4.1 α-synuclein

As with mutant superoxide dismutase 1 (m*SOD1*) in ALS, studies of α-synuclein have largely dominated Parkinson's disease research for much of the last 20 years (for a review, see Stefanis, 2012), at least until the discovery of the leucine-rich repeat kinase 2 (*G2019S-LRRK2*) gene mutation. Duplications of the α-synuclein gene are thought to be responsible for a late-onset typical Parkinson's disease. Triplications result in an early-onset and rapidly progressive dementia with the presence of Lewy bodies. As with m*SOD1*, mutant α-synuclein forms inclusions of misfolded protein that are thought to be at least part of the pathological mechanism underlying the loss of neurons in the SN, as cited in Chapter 2.

In vivo animal models have been developed and widely studied in an effort to uncover the pathological mechanisms of action of the mutation. As in Parkinson's disease, the animals expressing mutant human α-synuclein do show some behavioral dysfunctions reminiscent of the disease, and also demonstrate collections of misfolded α-synuclein in Lewy body-like structures in the brain and in other organ systems. Such models sometimes show the loss of SN neurons (Masliah et al., 2000; Giasson et al., 2002; Martin et al., 2006), but not always (Matsuoka et al., 2001). Since such loss is part of the hallmark of Parkinson's disease and most of the parkinsonisms, the variation may be problematic for the view that mutant α-synuclein is always a key causal factor.

5.4.2 *LRRK2*

Mutations in *LRRK2* have been identified in a fraction of families with autosomal-dominant parkinsonism (3–41%) (Zimprich et al., 2004; Di Fonzo et al., 2005). Penetrance appears to vary. The *LRRK2* gene encodes a large protein, dardarin 3 (2527 amino acids), of still unknown function, which belongs to a group within the Ras/GTPase superfamily, termed ROCO. This group is characterized by the presence of two conserved domains named "Roc" (Ras in complex proteins) and "COR" (C-terminal of Roc), together with other domains including a leucine-rich repeat region, a WD40 domain, and a tyrosine kinase catalytic domain.

The *LRRK2* mutation phenotype is broad, with both early- and late-onset features. Lewy body inclusions may or may not be present. Dopaminergic neurons of the SN degenerate in all patients in association with gliosis, but there is considerable variability, even in the same family, in the presence of other pathological markers. In some cases, α-synuclein-positive Lewy bodies may be present in the brainstem and extend into the cerebral cortex, as in diffuse Lewy-body disease. Other cases show tau protein inclusions, the latter normally a feature of Alzheimer's disease or PSP, as cited previously. Some cases of Parkinson's disease show neither tau nor α-synuclein deposits and are thus independent of these abnormal proteins, yet they do show a loss of SN neurons, as demonstrated in a murine model (Kett et al., 2015). These authors have suggested that the key pathology lies in an endolysosomal dysfunction leading to SN neuron loss, rather than one arising from mutations of α-synuclein.

A schematic summary of the key genes linked to Parkinson's disease is provided in Figure 5.1 in order to put these mutations into the overall context of the disease.

Such observations, to be expanded on in later chapters, clearly show the spectrum nature of Parkinson's disease, as cited previously. In this manner, the genetic forms of Parkinson's disease (as well as the sporadic forms) mirror the spectrums that describe ALS and Alzheimer's disease as well.

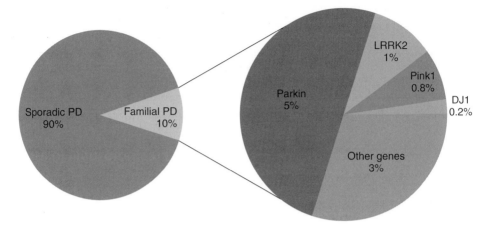

Figure 5.1 Number of identified causality genes in early-onset familial Parkinson's disease. (See color plate section for the color representation of this figure.)

Some authors have attempted to link *LRRK2* and α-synuclein mutations to some types of synergistic pathological outcome in Parkinson's disease (Hyun et al., 2013). One perspective, proposed by Hyun et al. (2013) in their review of the field, suggests that defects in protein degradation by proteasomal malfunction are the primary cause of the disease (see also McNaught et al., 2003), a theme echoed by the ubiquilin 2 studies in ALS (cited in Section 5.5). Other possible mechanisms leading to neurodegeneration include proinflammatory responses amongst microglia, disruption of α-synuclein signaling, abnormalities in vesicle transport, and autophagy.

5.4.3 Lesser Genes Associated with Autosomal-Recessive Forms of Parkinson's Disease

Parkin (Parkinson protein 2, E3 ubiquitin protein ligase), Parkin2 (Parkinson disease, autosomal recessive, juvenile 2), *DJ-1*, and *PINK1* (PTEN-induced putative kinase 1) are thought to be responsible for some autosomal-recessive forms of Parkinson's disease, usually those with an early onset that are not associated with Lewy bodies (Brice, 2005).

5.4.4 Summary

A lot of effort, time, and money has produced relatively little in the way of effective therapeutics based on the genetic models. I will return to this subject in Chapters 13 and 14.

5.5 Genetic Mutations Linked to ALS

Table 5.2 lists some of the causality genes linked to familial forms of ALS. This section presents only the most common of these. Other mutations, such as those impacting motor neuron axonal transport (Holzbaur et al., 2006; Chevalier-Larsen and Holzbaur, 2006), seem to have faded from view and will not be considered here in spite of the fact that the damage such dysfunctions can do is as valid a potential reason for motor neuron death as any other.

Table 5.2 Causal genes linked to ALS.

Gene	Location	Inheritance	Diagnosis	Onset	References
SOD1 (ALS1)	21q22.11	AD, AR, *de novo*	ALS, PMA	Adult	Rosen et al. (1993)
ALS2 (ALS2)	2q33-2q35	AR	ALS, PLS, HSP	Juvenile	Hadano et al. (2001)
SETX (ALS4)	9q34	AD	ALS, AOA2	Juvenile	Chen et al. (2004)
SPG11 (ALS5)	15q21.1	AR	ALS, HSP	Juvenile	Orlacchio et al. (2010)
FUS (ALS6)	16q11.2	AD, AR, *de novo*	ALS, ALS-FTD	Adult	Kwiatkowski et al. (2009), Vance et al. (2009)
Unknown (*ALS7*)	20p13	AD	ALS	Adult	Sapp et al. (2003)
VAPB (ALS8)	20q13.3	AD	ALS, SMA	Adult	Nishimura et al. (2004)
TARDBP (ALS10)	1p36.2	AD, AR	ALS, ALS-FTD	Adult	Gitcho et al. (2008), Kabashi et al. (2008), Sreedharan et al. (2008)
OPTN (ALS12)	10p15-p14	AD, AR	ALS, POAG	Adult	Maruyama et al. (2010), van Es et al. (2009)
VCP (ALS14)	9p13.3	AD	ALS, ALS-FTD, FTD, IBMPFD	Adult	Johnson et al. (2010)
UBQLN2 (ALS15)	Xp11.21	X-linked	ALS, ALS-FTD	Juvenile, adult	Deng et al. (2011)
SIGMAR1 (ALS16)	9p13.3	AR	ALS, FTD	Juvenile	Al-Saif et al. (2011)
DAO	12q24.11	AD	ALS	Adult	Mitchell et al. (2010)
PFN1	17p13.2	AD	ALS	Adult	Wu et al. (2012)
hnRNPA2B1/A1	7p13.2/ 12q13.3	AD	ALS, IBMPFD	Adult	Kim et al. (2013)
TUBA4A	2q35	AD	ALS, ASL-FTD	Adult	Smith et al. (2014)
Unknown (*ALS-FTD1*)	9q21-q22	AD	ALS, ALS-FTD, FTD	Adult	Hosler et al. (2000)
C9ORF72 (ALS-FTD2)	9p21.2	AD, sporadic	ALS, ALS-FTD, FTD	Adult	DeJesus-Hernandez et al. (2011), Gijselinck et al. (2012)
TBK1	12q14.1	AD, sporadic	ALS, ALS-FTD, FTD	Adult	Freischmidt et al. (2015)

AD, autosomal dominant; AR, autosomal recessive; ALS, amyotrophic lateral sclerosis; PMA, progressive muscular atrophy; PLS, primary lateral sclerosis; HSP, hereditary spastic paraplegia; AOA2, ataxia with oculomotor apraxia type 2; ALS-FTD, amyotrophic lateral sclerosis–frontotemporal dementia; SMA, spinal muscular atrophy; POAG, primary open-angle glaucoma; FTD, frontotemporal dementia; IBMPFD, Paget's disease of bone and frontotemporal dementia.

It should be emphasized at the outset that the overall percentage of ALS cases contributed by inherited gene mutations is small – approximately 5%, and certainly not more than 10% – comprising some 20 gene loci (Harms and Baloh, 2013; Marangi and Traynor, 2015). Table 5.2 shows these, and gives a sense of their number within the spectrum of fALS and sALS. They include, in a rough order of percentages: *C9orf72* (fALS: 30–50%; sALS: maybe 10%); the copper/zinc (Cu/Zn) *SOD1* enzyme (fALS: 10–20%; sALS: approx. 3%), TAR DNA-binding protein (*TARDBP*) (fALS: 0–62%; sALS: approx. 2%), and Fused in Sarcoma (*FUS*) RNA-binding protein (fALS: 1–13%; sALS: approx. 2%). These will be described, not in order of their overall contribution to ALS, which is still controversial, but more from a general chronology in the literature.

5.5.1 *SOD1*

I will begin with what are currently the most widely studied and perhaps best known of these mutations in fALS, namely those involving Cu/Zn superoxide dismutase, especially the gene *SOD1*, which codes for the soluble homodimeric metalloenzyme located in the cytosol and in the mitochondrial intermembrane space.

Superoxide dismutase is one of the main antioxidant molecules in mammalian species (the other key ones being catalase and glutathione). In animals, the role of SOD1 as an antioxidant is to catalyze free radicals into hydrogen peroxide and molecular oxygen (Bruijn et al., 2004). The enzyme is activated by post-translational modification, including the binding of copper and zinc ions, dimerization of two identical SOD1 monomers, and stabilization by disulfide bond formation (Vehviläinen et al., 2014).

Mutations in the gene come in about 180 varieties in any of the five exons of the gene encoding SOD1 and result in the substitution of amino acids in the resulting protein (ALS Online Genetic Database: www.alscience.it). Some of these substitutions result in clinically different ages of onset and disease duration (Andersen et al., 1997). In total, these mutations cumulatively affect less than 20% of fALS patients (Byrne et al., 2011).

The mutations in human *SOD1* applied to transgenic animals are described as being a "toxic gain of function," since the loss of *SOD1* in general in *SOD1* knockout experiments does not result in motor neuron loss (Gurney et al., 1994), but a loss of various functions may occur (Saccon et al., 2013). The precise nature of the toxic gain of function is not known, but it may involve a variety of abnormal biochemical pathways, including some involved in increased pro-oxidant activity (Tu et al., 1997). It is clear, however, that oxidative stress is not the sole determinant of overall toxicity to motor neurons or to supporting glial cells.

It would be safe to say that since the first description of mSOD1, this collection of mutations has dominated the ALS field experimentally with numberous investigators using various animal models of mSOD1 to better understand the mechanisms leading to motor neuron death and seeking effective therapeutics to prevent the same.

One claim is that mSOD1-induced fALS is clinically and neuropathologically indistinguishable from sporadic forms of the disease (Kabashi et al., 2007), although a clear case could be made that this convergence refers to an end-state status, not the earlier, and thus largely undetectable, pre-clinical stages.

Concerning the specifics of the *in vivo* models of mSOD1, various transgenic mouse and rat models have been developed to harbor mutations found in mSOD1 patients. Each mirrors the generally progressive nature of the disease, aspects of motor neuron death, and many of the histopathological hallmarks associated with clinical ALS (Kato, 2008; Joyce et al., 2011). A recent study using the G37R mouse model demonstrated that the fALS phenotype and related histopathology are enhanced by an environmental agent that is sufficient for producing a neurodegenerative phenotype alone (Lee and Shaw, 2012).

Several transgenic mouse models of fALS have been generated that include animals harboring the G93A (Gurney et al., 1994), G37R (Wong et al., 1995), G85R (Bruijn et al., 1997), and D90A mutations (Jonsson et al., 2006). While all of these mouse models are characterized by motor neuron loss and similar histopathological findings in general, the G93A and G37R mutations have been – and, as of this writing, remain – the most widely used variants. It should be noted that other vertebrate and invertebrate models using m*SOD1* have also been created.

A key feature of each of the m*SOD1 in vivo* models is that the mutant gene copy number is crucial for reproducing the features of motor dysfunction and motor neuron loss (Zwiegers et al., 2014). This is not the case in human ALS in which one copy of the mutant gene at one locus is found in the various m*SOD1*-related fALS cases. This point will be further discussed in Chapter 8 as it is critical to an overview of neurological disease model systems in general.

In this regard, it is worth noting here that, to date, the various m*SOD1* models have not successfully led to translational advances in treating human ALS. This statement applies whether one is speaking of fALS or sALS (Wilkins et al., 2011). One group evaluating the literature of ALS therapeutics in the context of m*SOD1* murine models was considerably harsher in their conclusion, stating that:

> The presence of these uncontrolled confounding variables in the screening system, and the failure of these several drugs to demonstrate efficacy in adequately designed and powered repeat studies, leads us to conclude that the majority of published effects are most likely *measurements of noise* [my emphasis] in the distribution of survival means as opposed to actual drug effect. (Scott et al., 2008, p. 4.)

One interesting feature of mSOD1 lies in its propensity to change its native conformational shape to a misfolded form following oxidant stress (Rakhit et al., 2002). A result of this misfolding is the creation of protein inclusions similar in some ways to those seen in human ALS.

In ALS research, one view holds that the misfolding of SOD1 in m*SOD1* animal models may propagate to induce further misfolding of normal SOD1 and that such a "prion"-like process underlies the spreading pathology from one part of the motor system to another in human ALS (Grad and Cashman, 2014; Grad et al., 2015).

The similarity of protein malfunctions across neurological disease states has led some investigators to define the mSOD1 mutant protein product and the others in the different diseases as "proteinopathies" (Bayer, 2015), including, for example, α-synuclein in Parkinson's disease and Aβ in Alzheimer's disease, as cited previously.

Various therapeutic strategies have been devised to either reduce the impact of the toxic gain of function itself or remove the misfolded SOD1 (Liu et al., 2012). To date, at least in human patients, none has been successful in slowing or reversing the progression of the disease. The reasons for this lack of translation to patients will be dealt with at length in Chapters 13–15, but at least part of the problem appears to lie the characteristics of the *in vivo* models themselves.

The lack of translation is one reason why m*SOD1* models have begun to lose their dominance in the ALS field in recent years – a dominance that was expressed both in the numbers of experiments done and, crucially, in the share of research funding received. That dominance, both theoretical and financial, now appears to be shifting to more recently discovered mutations in fALS. Whether these newer gene mutations will be any more successful at finding common mechanisms of motor neuron death or in stopping the progression of the disease in a timely way remain uncertain.

5.5.2   *TARDBP*

TARDBP, the gene encoding the TDP-43 (TAR DNA-binding protein 43 or transactive response DNA-binding protein 43) mutation, is linked to an autosomal-dominant form of fALS. The proportions for fALS and sALS are cited at the start of this section.

As an RNA-binding protein, TDP-43 regulates gene transcription, mRNA stability, pre-mRNA splicing, and microRNA biogenesis. In consequence, the *TARDBP* mutation causes mRNA splicing abnormalities, resulting in the absence of certain proteins and the production of aberrant ones (Robberecht and Philips, 2013). In addition, it favors TDP-43 accumulation in stress granules which play a role in forming the ubiquinated cytoplasmic inclusions that are typically seen in upper and lower motor neurons in ALS (Dewey et al., 2012) and in FTD (Neumann et al., 2006). Patients with *TARDBP* mutations exhibit a classical ALS phenotype with a co-occurrence of dementia. There is a trend for earlier disease onset with more common upper-limb onset and a longer duration of disease.

There are various, relatively recent animal models of TDP-43. The murine models expressing the human wild-type gene or the ALS-linked mutant *TARDBP* under the control of the murine prion protein promoter display motor neuron degeneration (Gendron and Petrucelli, 2011; Tsao et al., 2012). TDP-43 mutation models have also been developed other organisms, including zebra fish (Kabashi et al., 2010), as well as simpler models such as *C. elegans* (Ash et al., 2010) and *Drosophila* (Li et al., 2010).

5.5.3   *FUS*

FUS mutations cause autosomal-dominant fALS and account for about 4–6% of cases of fALS (the range given at the start of this section is actually quite large) (linked to 0.7–1.8% of cases of sALS) (Kwiatkowski et al., 2009; Vance et al., 2009). Humans with *FUS* mutations exhibit a conventional ALS phenotype, without cognitive impairment. The clinical time course is diverse, even amongst carriers of the same mutations. The motor neurons of *FUS* mutation patients are characterized by the presence of basophilic inclusions (Bäumer et al., 2010).

FUS is similar in structure and function to TDP-43. In normal physiological conditions, FUS is mainly found in the nuclear compartment where it is involved in various cellular processes, including cell proliferation, DNA repair, transcription regulation, and RNA and microRNA processing. The mutations at the C-terminus disrupt the transport of FUS into the nucleus and result in mislocalization of FUS protein into the cytoplasm, where it is recruited into stress granules which may form inclusions (Kwiatkowski et al., 2009; Vance et al., 2009).

The overexpression of mutant FUS in a transgenic rat model leads to progressive paralysis due to motor neuron axonal degeneration followed by motor neuron loss in the motor cortex. Neurons in the hippocampus can also be affected (Huang et al., 2011). In a transgenic *Drosophila* model, age-dependent progressive motor neuron damage is observed when mutant FUS is overexpressed (Chen et al., 2011). Additionally, wild-type FUS overexpression and mutant FUS overexpression in *C. elegans* and the knockdown of endogenous FUS in zebra fish have been used to study FUS-mediated motor neuron degeneration (reviewed in Lanson and Pandey, 2012).

5.5.4 *UBQLN2*

A relatively new genetic player in the search for mutant ALS-related genes was announced with considerable fanfare in 2011: an autosomal-dominant mutation in *UBQLN2*. This gene codes for ubiquilin 2 (UBQLN2), an ubiquitin-like protein. In the recent study, the mutation was found in 40 individuals from five affected families (Deng et al., 2011).

UBQLN2 is involved in proteasomal activity and any disturbance in the same – according to Deng et al. (2011) – leads not only to motor neuron loss, but also to FTD-like cognitive impairment. The Deng study was hailed as a key to understanding various forms of fALS (including those generated by mutant TDP-43 and C9orf72 (for the latter, see Section 5.5.5)) and perhaps sALS, based on presumably common aspects of proteasomal malfunction. This aspect, similar to one proposed some years ago for Parkinson's disease (as cited earlier), makes this gene and its protein a potential target for translational therapies. In spite of this, a transgenic *UBQLN2* mouse strain did not cause motor neuron degeneration, although hippocampal neurons were negatively impacted (Gorrie et al., 2014).

5.5.5 *C9orf72*

A mutation of chromosome 9 open reading frame 72 (*C9orf72*) is reputedly the most common ALS-causing gene mutation, found in 34.2% of fALS and linked to 5.9% of sALS cases (van Blitterswijk et al., 2012). The causal defect has been identified as a massive hexanucleotide repeat expansion, consisting of $(GGGGCC)_n$ in the intron between non-coding exons 1a and 1b of the gene. Bulbar onset and frontotemporal involvement are frequent, and the penetrance is about 50% at around 60 years of age and nearly 100% above the age of 80 (Majounie et al., 2012).

The mechanism of toxicity of this mutation is currently unclear, and the normal function of *C9orf72* remains unknown.

Initial reports suggested haploinsufficiency due to low levels of *C9orf72* transcripts (DeJesus-Hernandez et al., 2011; Renton et al., 2011). However, in parallel, RNA foci containing the hexanucleotide repeat were identified in patients, suggesting the possibility of a toxic gain-of-function mutation (DeJesus-Hernandez et al., 2011). Some studies have suggested that the consequent pathology may be the result of abnormal levels of a form of toxic RNA acting to disrupt normal transcription by sequestering normal RNA and the proteins involved in transcriptional regulation (Renton et al., 2011). Abnormal protein inclusions have also been found, however any pathogenic role of these aggregates is still unclear (Ash et al., 2013).

Several recent studies have investigated the consequences of the loss or reduction of C9orf72 using mice (Lagier-Tourenne et al., 2013), zebra fish (Ciura et al., 2013), and *C. elegans* (Therrien et al., 2013) models. These studies produced conflicting results that failed to either definitively establish, or rule out, reduced C9orf72 expression as a pathogenic mechanism of motor neuron degeneration in ALS. However, the overexpression of C9orf72 in zebra fish (Lee et al., 2013) and *Drosophila* (Mizielinska et al., 2014) showed repeat length-dependent formation of RNA foci which correlated with cellular toxicity leading to motor neuron degeneration.

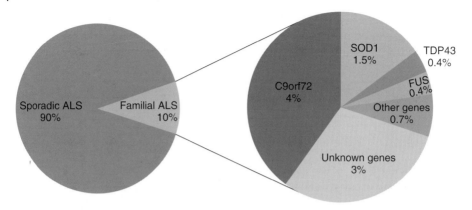

Figure 5.2 Number of identified causality genes in early-onset fALS. (See color plate section for the color representation of this figure.)

5.5.6 Summary

A recent article reports the use of exome sequencing to identify yet another associated gene/protein linked to ALS: TANK-binding kinase (TBK1), which phosphorylates proteins involved in immunity and autophagy (Cirulli et al., 2015). This study illustrates yet again the ongoing hunt for causal genes in ALS (and other neurological diseases), which may now join the nearly endless ranks of things that can induce neuronal death. A schematic summarizing the contribution of mutant genes in ALS is shown in Figure 5.2 for comparison to the total number of ALS cases.

In fALS, further recent studies have implicated *TUBA4A* (Smith et al., 2014) and the gene coding for the protein profilin 1 (Smith et al., 2015); for ALS/FTD, there is the above mentioned *TBK1* (Freischmidt et al., 2015). There will doubtless be more such studies published between the time of writing and when this book goes to print.

Although some in the field would be inclined to disagree, it is difficult from a more neutral perspective to reconcile the relatively large investments in time and money in the genetics of ALS with any significant improvement in the onset, time course, or ultimate survival outcomes of those with the disease. In brief, nothing the field has learned about disease mechanisms in the various genetic models, or indeed in the human disease, has yet translated into effective long-term therapeutics.

I will explore in later chapters why this seems to be true – not least the notion that the genetic models do not in most cases have any clear overlap with the sporadic forms of the disease, in spite of the frequent statements to the contrary. Of course, this could change in the future, and it is clearly the ardent hope of many that such will prove to be the case.

5.6 Genetic Mutations Linked to Alzheimer's Disease

There are considerably fewer genes causally linked to Alzheimer's disease than to Parkinson's disease or ALS (Table 5.3, Figure 5.3).

5.6.1 *APP*

The gene for amyloid precursor protein (*APP*) is located on chromosome 21q21 and encodes a ubiquitously expressed single-pass transmembrane polypeptide of 770

Table 5.3 Causal genes linked to Alzheimer's disease.

Gene	Location	Inheritance	Onset	References
APP	21q21.2	AD	Early (40–60 years)	Goate et al. (1991)
PSEN1	14q24.3	AD	Early (30–60 years)	Schellenberg et al. (1992)
PSEN2	1q31-42	AD	Early (40–75 years)	Levy-Lahad et al. (1995), Rogaev et al. (1995)

AD, autosomal dominant.

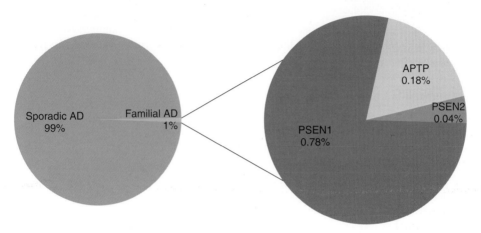

Figure 5.3 Number of identified causality genes in early-onset familial Alzheimer's disease. (See color plate section for the color representation of this figure.)

amino acids. Aβ, the major component of amyloid plaques in Alzheimer's disease brains, is generated from APP by two endoproteolytic cleavage pathways catalyzed by β-secretase and γ-secretase. The former, β-secretase, is now part of a therapeutic strategy to reduce Aβ burden and thus, it is hoped, alleviate Alzheimer's disease progression (Singer et al., 2005).

The most abundant form of Aβ is Aβ40, which is 40 amino acids long; the less abundant form, Aβ42, is longer, and it is this that is associated with Alzheimer's disease (Tandon et al., 2000).

More than 30 different *APP* mutations have been identified to date, of which 25 appear to be pathological and are implicated in autosomal-dominant early-onset (familial) Alzheimer's disease (Cruts et al., 2012). These mutations account for approximately 5% of inherited disease cases (Alonso Vilatela et al., 2012). This general outcome is somewhat analogous to the proliferation of *SOD1* mutations in ALS, with their overall contribution to this disease. Most of the mutations are located at the β- and γ-secretase cleavage sites (exons 16 and 17 of APP), influencing APP proteolytic processing and aggregation.

In addition to the autosomal-dominant mutations, two recessive mutations in *APP* – A673V *and* E693Δ – are known to cause early-onset Alzheimer's disease (Di Fede et al., 2009; Giaccone et al., 2010). A copy number variant mutation has also been found (Hooli et al., 2012).

5.6.2 Presenilin 1 (*PSEN1*)

PSEN1 is located on chromosome 14q24.3 and encodes an integral membrane protein containing nine transmembrane domains with a hydrophilic intracellular loop region (Schellenberg et al., 1992). The protein forms a catalytic core of the γ-secretase complex and localizes to the endoplasmic reticulum and Golgi apparatus where it takes part in protein processing (Kovacs et al., 1996; De Strooper et al., 1998).

More than 180 mutations in *PSEN1* have been reported, accounting for about 50–75% of familial Alzheimer's disease cases (Cruts et al., 2012; Alonso Vilatela et al., 2012). Most of the mutations are missense mutations distributed throughout the *PSEN1* region, and they seem to cause a relative increase in the ratio of Aβ42 to Aβ40.

Although there is phenotypic variability amongst patients with *PSEN1* mutations, the *PSEN1* mutations generally cause the most severe forms of early Alzheimer's disease with complete penetrance and earlier age of onset (age 30–58 years) (Alonso Vilatela et al., 2012).

5.6.3 Presenilin 2 (*PSEN2*)

PSEN2 is located on chromosome 1q31-q42 and has a sequence homology and a similar protein structure to PSEN1 (Levy-Lahad et al., 1995; Rogaev et al., 1995). PSEN2 is also a component of γ-reductase and the *PSEN2* mutations have likewise been reported to increase the ratio of Aβ42 to Aβ40 (Kimberly et al., 2003). To date, 13 dominant, pathogenic mutations have been reported in *PSEN2*, accounting for approximately 1% of inherited forms of Alzheimer's disease (Alonso Vilatela et al., 2012).

The clinical features of *PSEN2*-affected families seem to be different from those found with *PSEN1* mutations. For example, the age of onset is higher (45–88 years) and tends to be highly variable even within the same family (Sherrington et al., 1996; Campion et al., 1999). *PSEN2* mutations also appear to have lower penetrance than *PSEN1* mutations (Bekris et al., 2010). Finally, *PSEN2*-affected patients may also have atypical clinical features (Binetti et al., 2003).

5.7 Genes and Neurological Disease: Some General Considerations

The overall similarities in genomic approaches, general outcomes, gene variants, and overall percentages between the three diseases considered here should be obvious. When combined with considerations of environmentally derived etiologies for neurological disease, the overall variability across individuals makes each a unique presentation.

It is now well known that less than 2% of the human genome is composed of exons that can encode proteins. Given this, the potential is that the vast bulk of DNA in the remainder could, in principle, contribute to the etiology of some forms of neurological disease. The remaining non-protein-coding sequences have commonly been referred to as "junk DNA," originally referring to gene regions that undergo mutations with no subsequent loss of the ability to encode functional proteins (Ohno, 1972). The term has now been extended to include many types of non-coding DNA; that is, any DNA sequence without an apparent functional role in development or physiology (Palazzo and Gregory, 2014).

An emerging view, however, is that rather than being simply "junk," such segments of DNA have a relationship to the coding DNA that may be analogous to the lighting in a house: if the exons are the light bulbs, the introns and other non-coding regions comprise the wiring. The former would not function without the latter, so the notion that mutations or polymorphisms in these portions could contribute to disease outcomes cannot be easily dismissed – nor have they been ignored in analyses of SNPs (Li et al., 2008; International Parkinson Disease Genomics Consortium et al., 2011; Ramanan and Saykin, 2013; Tosto and Reitz, 2013; Renton et al., 2014).

More recent studies have further refined our views of junk DNA. For example, the recently completed Encyclopedia of DNA Elements (ENCODE) project has shown that DNA contains transcripts that play important roles in various cellular processes (The ENCODE Project Consortium, 2012) and that up to 76% of the human genome's non-coding DNA sequences are in fact transcribed. A newer estimate is that over 80% of the genome contains elements linked to actual biochemical functions.

Some of the non-coding DNA includes transposable elements (TEs) which make up approximately 50% of primate genomes. TEs appear able to play a role in changing gene expression by providing cis-regulatory elements such as promoters, enhancers, and transcription factor binding sites (Warnefors et al., 2010; Levin and Moran, 2011). TEs also contribute to transcript diversity and may play a role as a source of small RNAs that control host–gene transcription (Cowley and Oakey, 2013).

Introns, as already noted, increase the diversity of protein products by regulating alternative splicing. The RNAs transcribed from intron sequences are now known to contain codes for modulating alternative splicing (Ladd and Cooper, 2002; Hui et al., 2005). Introns also encode other functional short non-protein-coding RNAs, such as micro RNA (miRNA) (see Chapter 6) and small nucleolar RNA (snoRNA), which are essential for regulating gene expression and the processing of ribosomal RNAs (Mendes Soares and Valcárcel, 2006; Hoeppner et al., 2009; Monteys et al., 2010). A recent study of chromatin-associated RNAs that modify chromatin structure and affect gene expression showed that nearly two-thirds are derived from introns (Mondal et al., 2010).

Additionally, there are a number of pseudogenes in the human genome (around 12 600–19 700) (Pei et al., 2012). Some pseudogenes are transcribed into non-coding RNAs that regulate protein-coding genes. Pseudogenes can decrease the level of gene expression through RNA interference (Meister and Tuschl, 2004; Tam et al., 2008; Watanabe et al., 2008) and increase expression through target mimicry of RNA-degrading enzymes.

An overall consideration in the hunt for causal genetics as a dominant factor in disease is that it is not unique to neurological diseases. Indeed, this same path, both theoretical and practical, has been taken by researchers in a variety of other disciplines, notably oncology. Here, as in neurological disease research, the bulk of funding has gone into trying to identify causal oncology genes, although some of the major efforts in this regard seem to be winding down (Ledford, 2015). Notably, the number of successes in identifying autosomal-dominant genes that cause cancer has been relatively minor, and an emerging view in some quarters is that more random epigenetic mutations, largely unpredictable, are primarily responsible for many expressions of the various cancers. Needless to say, large numbers of these epigenetic mutations may be caused by a variety of environmental toxins acting alone or in synergy with other toxins or with susceptibility genes. The similarities to the dominant gene-based perspective in neurological disease research over the last few decades cannot be overstressed. This point will be addressed in more detail in Chapter 16.

The addition of junk DNA as a potential source of genetic alterations leading to the expression of neurological diseases may seem to increase the likelihood that a dominantly genetics perspective for such diseases is feasible. However, adding the non-coding portions of DNA might just as well bolster the notion that such alterations are part of a disease spectrum composed of unique genetic "snowflakes."

One variant perspective that seems to be gaining support is that rather than DNA linearly providing for RNA and then proteins in a one-way path, gene function is more recursive (as noted in Chapter 1). That is, modifications can occur in both directions. Much of this perspective is new, emerging from the work of Pellionisz et al. (2013).

A final note on genetic causality in age-related neurological diseases is this: in spite of almost heroic efforts, this field seem no closer to finding a dominantly genetic basis for Parkinson's disease, ALS, or Alzheimer's disease, nor for the variant neurological diseases such as ALS–PDC. Emerging Parkinson's disease genetics now acknowledges that, at the very least, a polygenetic etiology is likely (Escott-Price et al., 2015).

In regard to the potential genetic basis for ALS-PDC, Steele et al. (2014) noted that some of the same genes identified for the other neurodegenerative disease are present in this disorder. These authors expressed the hope that additional exome sequencing might still identify genetic risk factors. This view builds on older observations that Parkinson's disease, ALS, and Alzheimer's disease show some shared genetic susceptibilities and tend to overlap in families (Majoor-Krakauer et al., 1994).

The hope expressed by Steele et al. (2014) should be viewed in contrast to an earlier report by Morris et al. (2004), which concluded in relation to the PDC part of the ALS-PDC spectrum that, "This study has not identified a single gene locus for PDC, confirming the impression of a geographic disease isolate with a complex genetic, a genetic/environmental etiology, or a purely environmental etiology" (p. 1889).

The themes raised in this section will be addressed in more detail in later chapters, particularly Chapter 7, where the history and features of ALS-PDC will be considered in more detail.

6

Environmental Determinants of Neurological Disease and Gene–Toxin Interactions

> *"It is indeed easier to unravel a single thread – an incident, a name, a motive – than to trace the history of any picture defined by many threads. For with the picture in the tapestry a new element has come in: the picture is greater than, and not explained by, the sum of the component threads"*
>
> R.R. Tolkien, "On Fairy Stories"[1]

From the Preface

2) The complexity of the nervous system arises due to the interplay between genetic programs and environmental influences. This complexity includes the interactions that lead to neurodegeneration. Gene defects in the germ cell line and in the early developing CNS are likely to be fatal or result in profoundly disturbed neuronal functions. Environmental impacts on the CNS depend crucially on the stage of development: prenatal ones are likely to be of greater impact than those occurring in postnatal life, while early postnatal ones will be more impactful than those later in life. The concept of the "fetal basis of adult disease" used in other fields of study likely applies to neurological disease just as strongly (or even more so) to those disorders with which it is more conventionally associated. Environmental impacts also crucially depend on the number of CNS levels impacted (e.g., from genome to the whole CNS).

3) It is almost certain that gene defects/mutations alone will not explain most types of age-related neurological disease. Nor, for that matter, will obvious environmental stressors/toxins be found to be solely responsible in most cases. Hence, gene–toxin interactions are the likely source of most such diseases, acted upon by a number of other variables across the lifespan.

4) Neuronal compensation for genetic or environmental insults to the CNS will be limited by the type of insult and the stage(s) at which they occurs. Early gene defects, if not rapidly fatal, may be compensated for by redundancy of function of other genes. Environmental impacts, if they do not cross too many levels of organization, may allow for neuronal compensation by unaffected cells or regions. "Neuronal plasticity" is not a simple process, nor one strictly limited to the stage of neuronal development.

Neural Dynamics of Neurological Disease, First Edition. Christopher A. Shaw.
© 2017 John Wiley & Sons, Inc. Published 2017 by John Wiley & Sons, Inc.

6.1   Introduction

The study of putative toxins, demonstrated and presumed, in neurological diseases such as Parkinson's disease, ALS, and Alzheimer's disease comprises a huge literature, not all of which can be encompassed in the following brief presentation.

6.2   Toxins and Neurological Diseases

Several aspects of the literature on neurotoxins are worth dealing with at the outset. First, as noted in the previous chapter, it is well recognized that most cases of the diseases under consideration here are sporadic, that is, they arise from unknown causes that are not genetic, or at least from mutations/polymorphisms/translational errors not yet identified.

Some would argue that as more familial forms of each disease are investigated, additional mutations will be found that will expand the percentages that have a genetic basis and/or identify mechanisms that are common to both familial and sporadic forms of the disease. The first assertion is undoubtedly true, but after several decades of active searching with the bulk of the research funds available, it is hard not to suggest that this approach is reaching some final fixed percentage that is not going to be much higher than that currently demonstrated. The second assertion, that mechanisms of neuronal death in sporadic and genetic forms of the disease are the same, is broadly likely and specifically unlikely, at least so far as is now known.

In broad strokes, it is certainly true that the major means by which neurons can be compromised remain common: oxidant stress, excitotoxicity, mitochondrial damage, the failure of other cellular organelles, and so on. The latter, however, is the neurological disease equivalent of a "motherhood" statement. That the specific pathways that trigger neuron loss are the same across both forms is widely believed, but remains to be clearly demonstrated. Much of the basis for the genetic approach in terms of translational medicine hinges on this belief and on the ultimate demonstration of the same. As discussed in the Chapter 5, this demonstration may come, but to date it has not been convincingly presented except in the most general terms.

The unavoidable conclusion from all of this is the following: based on what is now known from epidemiology and an analysis of risk factors, something that is not purely a genetic mutation triggers most forms of Parkinson's disease, ALS, and Alzheimer's disease. Epigenetic factors, be they toxin-triggered gene-expression changes or toxin-triggered miRNA alterations, will be addressed further later in the chapter.

Only two truly plausible possibilities remain: (i) neurotoxins as key causal factors and (ii) the intersection of neurotoxins with the various known and unknown genetic susceptibility factors.

Chapter 7, on the Guamanian neurological disease, ALS-PDC, will deal specifically with some putative toxins that have been proposed as the source of that disease spectrum. In the current chapter, however, I merely want to make some general notes on the potential of various molecules to induce different forms of neural cell death and thus neurological disease.

The first point to consider in this regard is that there are thousands of toxic molecules, natural and of human origin, in the biosphere, and more are added each year. Many of these, if not most, can, under the right conditions of dose and duration, be damaging to the nervous system, either directly or indirectly. In the latter category, I include molecules that may cause toxic by-products to arise from metabolic or degradative pathways in other organs such as the liver. Whether such molecules actually are the triggers for the onset or progression of sporadic neurological diseases remains uncertain.

Some of the toxins known to damage the nervous system in humans and animals are discussed in this section, but this list is by no means exhaustive. Although most of these molecules are not likely to be the sole cause of the various neurological diseases, the potential exists that in very high concentrations they may be sufficient etiological factors (Shaw and Höglinger, 2008). Similar examples exist for the immune system in regard to the induction of autoimmunity by repeated antigen presentation (Tsumiyama et al., 2009).

6.2.1 Pesticides, etc.

Toxic chemicals used in agriculture of various types, including the following, have been implicated as risk factors in neurological diseases (Franco et al., 2010; Goldman, 2013): rotenone (insecticide and pesticide); maneb (foliate fungicide); paraquat (herbicide), various organophosphates, such as parathion and malathion (insecticides, herbicides, and nerve agents); and organochlorines (dichlorodiphenyltrichloroethane (DDT), dieldren). Organophosphates are also notable in being listed as nerve agents. Organochlorine compounds were banned in North America and elsewhere in the 1970s.

Some of these molecules, alone or in combination, have been linked repeatedly to Parkinson's disease, ALS, and Alzheimer's disease, in part due to their ability to disrupt mitochondrial activity (Guillette et al., 1998; Public Health Agency of Canada, 2015). There is evidence for this in animal models, especially for some of the parkinsonisms (Thiruchelvam et al., 2000; Betarbet et al., 2002).

The widespread addition of glyphosate in commercial agriculture has recently been associated by some investigators with developmental disorders such as ASD (Nevison, 2014; Seneff et al., 2015).

6.2.2 Toxic Metals

Various metals, especially the transition-ion metals, which can induce Fenton-reaction oxidative stress, are linked to neurological diseases. These include iron, manganese, zinc, and lead, amongst others. In regard to manganese, there is a well-documented older literature on what was termed "manganese madness," a form of parkinsonism observed in manganese mine workers (Cotzias et al., 1971, 1974). Zinc has been implicated in some studies of the Guamanian form of ALS-PDC, as will be documented in the next chapter.

Data on the toxic impacts of lead on the central nervous system (CNS) in development and its link to Alzheimer's disease in later life are also known. Much like aluminum (see Section 6.3), lead can alter many biochemical processes and induce, amongst other things, oxidant stress, mitochondrial damage, disruption of calcium homeostasis, and excitotoxicity (Finkelstein et al., 1998; Lidsky and Schneider, 2003; Nicolescu et al., 2010). These effects are not necessarily direct actions, but may follow as consequences of other events (e.g., mitochondrial damage may be a downstream consequence of excitotoxicity and *vice versa*, as previously discussed).

6.2.3 Amino Acids, Natural and Human-Made

Some plant-derived amino acids that interact with ionotropic glutamate receptors as agonists have been associated with one or more of the age-related neurological diseases, as discussed in Chapter 7. These include domoic acid (kainate receptors), BOAA (AMPA receptors), and β-methyl amino alanine (BMAA) (N-methyl-D-aspartate (NMDA) and AMPA receptors).

Amino acids of human origin have also been implicated, including methionine sulfoximine (an inhibitor of glutathione synthesis) (Shaw et al., 1999), monosodium glutamate (a glutamate receptor agonist) (Olney, 1969), and cysteine (also a glutamate receptor agonist) (Olney et al., 1990).

6.2.4 Steryl Glucosides

Molecules such as the various steryl (or, more commonly, but chemically correct, "sterol") glucosides and similar have been implicated in neurological disorders such as ALS-PDC and Guadaloupe PDC in humans (Khabazian et al., 2002; Shaw and Höglinger, 2008), an ALS-PDC phenotype in mice (Wilson et al., 2002), and a parkinsonism phenotype in rats (Shen et al., 2010; Van Kampen et al., 2014b, 2015). It should be stressed that these molecules are not conventionally viewed as neurotoxic, although evidence for such toxicity is emerging, as in the cited references. That some of the steryl glucosides, notably β-sitosterol-β-D glucoside (BSSG), can be toxic must be put into the broader context of the fact that other steryl glucosides appear to be neuroprotective. Concerning the latter, some isolated ginsenosides appear to prevent neuronal degeneration (Van Kampen et al., 2014b). Remarkably, considering they have been known to science for over 100 years, quite little seems to actually be known about the steryl glucosides in general in either health or illness (Vanmierlo et al., 2015).

Binding sites for the various steryl glucosides in the CNS are not definitively known, but some speculation has centered on a subtype of the Liver X receptor (Kim et al., 2008).

6.2.5 Bisphenols

Recently, the potential CNS developmental impacts of the various bisphenol-like compounds and other endocrine disrupters have been studied, including some of the newer versions designed to replace bisphenol-A. A recent report described developmental disorders in zebra fish embryos caused by bisphenol-A and compared the data to a purportedly safer alternative, bisphenol-S (Kinch et al., 2015). Both compounds appeared to have negative impacts on neuronal development.

6.2.6 Summary

There are, of course, many other potential toxin candidates – far too many to list here. Needless to say, not only is the potential list of neurotoxins to which humans are exposed vast, but toxin–toxin additive effects and/or synergies would form a still larger pool. Such toxin–toxin interactions are rarely addressed experimentally, for a variety of reasons.

As I will detail in Chapter 7, one reason to focus on ALS-PDC is that as a so-called "geographic isolate" it limits the range of toxins to test, at least in principle. This relatively simple situation contrasts with the almost limitless number of toxins and their combinations in areas exposed to industrial chemicals for longer periods.

6.3   Aluminum and Neurological Disease

One toxic element to which humans are currently heavily exposed is aluminum, whose ubiquity in the human biosphere has been steadily increasing for well over 100 years. Not only does aluminum toxicity have clear impacts on the CNS of animals and humans, it also negatively impacts other organ systems in both. It can also be toxic to plants (for reviews, see Tomljenovic, 2011; Shaw et al., 2014b).

The scientific literature is replete with examples of such toxicity, some of them going back almost to the earliest exposures to bioavailable aluminum derived from human activity. As noted by William Gies (1911) over a century ago:

> These studies have convinced me that the use in food of aluminum or any other aluminum compound is a dangerous practice. That the aluminum ion is very toxic is well known. That aluminized food yields soluble aluminum compounds to gastric juice (and stomach contents) has been demonstrated. That such soluble aluminum is in part absorbed and carried to all parts of the body by the blood can no longer be doubted. That the organism can "tolerate" such treatment without suffering harmful consequences has not been shown. It is believed that the facts in this paper will give emphasis to my conviction that aluminum should be excluded from food. (p. 816)

Gies was referring to even earlier studies, some from the early 19th century, starting with observations on the parenteral administration of aluminum salts (Orfila, 1814) and with animal studies (Siem, as cited in Döllken, 1897). Döllken (1897) showed instances of degeneration in rabbit CNS following aluminum exposure.

What makes the current state of affairs in regard to the rather clearly demonstrated neurotoxicity of aluminum unique is that the negative effects of this element are widely perceived in the medical and lay communities to have been "debunked," to use a lay/journalistic term (see, for example, Lidsky, 2014). Such views make this as good a place as any in the book to consider two aspects of studies sometimes considered to be invalid, especially by those in industries that might be impacted and/or by some in mainstream media. In the Preface, I noted that any scientific narrative must necessarily choose the material it will use. Usually, this is done to bolster a particular viewpoint, and, as such, some "cherry picking" is inevitable, appearing in the work of many – if not most – scientists from time to time. The second aspect will be considered in more detail in Chapter 8, but briefly it refers to the work of Dr. John Ioannidis and others, who have observed that much of the literature is simply wrong (Ioannidis, 2005).

The operating principles available to deal with these two situations are simple: minimize selective reporting of the literature, or at least acknowledge that it has been done; and bring a critical evaluation to any research, whether it mirrors conventional views – or one's personal views – or not. In addition, special skepticism needs to be applied when the potential for conflicts of interest is present, as, for example, when research is sponsored by industries that stand to profit from the conclusions.

The Lidsky review typifies the latter problem, in that the author is listed as a consultant for the aluminum industry and the paper achieves its conclusions in large measure by ignoring much of the countervailing scientific literature (Lidsky, 2014). The author also descends into *ad hominem* commentary on those who have raised concerns about aluminum and its potential connections to human health. These comments are, at least in my opinion, not appropriate in an unbiased scientific review.

Apart from careless scholarship, there are other reasons leading to the view that aluminum is not involved in neurological diseases. These are often more accurate than those presented by Lidsky, but frequently are based on certain assumptions that are quite demonstrably incorrect. In part, some of the objections have arisen from what was perceived to be a lack of evidence for earlier claims that aluminum from various environmental sources posed a health risk, as promoted by McLachlan et al. (1991). Critics of McLachlan's work contended that human exposure to ionic aluminum exposure was, and remains, fairly minimal under most circumstances, and thus could not play a significant role in neurological diseases.

The McLachlan review, may, however, have been prescient, in that while metallic aluminum is relatively inert, as are the various aluminum–silicate complexes, aluminum ions (Al^{3+}) can be released in acidic environments and are anything but benign.

The release of ionic aluminum can occur in acidic conditions, such as in acidic soil or in food preparation, where acidic solutions are in contact with metallic aluminum. The former includes soils of volcanic origin and, more commonly at present, soils exposed to acid rain. In this context, it is worth observing that acidified soils are an increasing feature of the human biosphere, with the consequence that aluminum has become even more bioavailable than in previous decades (Exley, pers. comm.).

Concerning aluminum in foods, the acidity of some foods cooked in aluminum pans may serve to release ionic aluminum. Additionally, as most "tin" cans are actually now made of aluminum, and have been for a number of years, any acidic solution that breaches the protective epoxy coating, a bisphenol-A epoxy resin, will release potentially large amounts of ionic aluminum (not to mention bisphenol-A). This concern applies to cans containing fruit juices and various "soft" drinks. The structural integrity of the epoxy coating on aluminum cans can also be compromised by mechanical stress and/or heat (Goodson et al., 2004).

Far beyond the possible release of aluminum ions from older cookware and current aluminum cans, aluminum finds its way into a variety of products for human use, as presented in the following subsection. In each case, the relative absence of obvious acute effects has led to a view similar to that which greeted the McLachlan study, namely that human exposure to aluminum from most sources is unlikely to have a significant impact on human health. That this perception is largely incorrect is abundantly demonstrated every 2 years at the Keele University conference on aluminum (Keele University, 2015).

6.3.1 Some Background to Aluminum Chemistry and the Intersection of Aluminum with the Biosphere

Aluminum is the third most common element after oxygen and silicon, and the most abundant metal in the earth's crust. The abundance of aluminum on earth and the recent historical and current ubiquity in the biosphere have fostered attitudes such as that already mentioned: that if it is so common, it cannot be harmful. However, as shown by Exley and colleagues (Exley et al., 1996; Exley, 2003, 2004) and others (Tomljenovic, 2011), this element was not widely bioavailable until recent historical times. In regard to this point, it may be notable that due in part to its historical lack of bioavailability, aluminum seems to have been "selected out" of involvement in terrestrial biochemistry (Exley, 2003). This situation changed with the industrial extraction of aluminum, primarily from bauxite, from the 1820s on, and its myriad current materials applications have brought human beings into ever-increasing contact with various forms of the element.

Chemically, aluminum avidly binds to oxygen, carbon, phosphorous, and sulfur, all key elements in biological systems, and thus provides the potential to significantly impact such systems. In spite of claims often made in the context of aluminum's various industrial and medical applications, the element is therefore certainly not inert – nor, as will be shown later, is it harmless. It is also manifestly not an "essential" element, as claimed by some medical websites (e.g., The Children's Hospital of Philadelphia, 2013).

As already noted, aluminum has been linked to various disorders in plants, animals, and humans (Exley, 2009; Poot-Poot and Hernandez-Sotomayor, 2011; Tomljenovic, 2011; Tomljenovic and Shaw, 2011b; Seneff et al., 2012), not least of which are those involving the CNS in animals and humans.

Aluminum in the biosphere, particularly that which may affect humans, arises from various sources (Saiyed and Yokel, 2005). It has a significant presence in processed foods, both through deliberate addition for its chemical properties and due to contamination during the manufacturing process. Salts of aluminum show up in a great variety of medicinal products, including antacids, various coatings for pills, and some vaccines. In regard to the latter, aluminum salts serve as adjuvants to improve the immunogenicity of antigens (Tomljenovic and Shaw, 2011a). Aluminum salts are also used as mordants in cosmetics and in antiperspirants.

Table 6.1 highlights some of the key sources of bioavailable aluminum to which humans are exposed (excerpted from Tomljenovic, 2011. See original article for relevant references).

Food remains the most common source of human exposure to aluminum (Yokel and McNamara, 2001). The second most common appears to be aluminum vaccine adjuvants (Tomljenovic and Shaw, 2011a). In both cases, aluminum can readily enter the body by way of soluble salts. In the case of food, aluminum is absorbed through the gastrointestinal (GI) system with an average daily human range of 3–10 mg (Yokel and McNamara, 2001). Intestinal absorption is influenced by compounds that increase absorption (e.g., citrate and fluoride) or is decreased by substances such as milk (Strunecká et al., 2002).

Given normal patent kidney function, most dietary/waterborne aluminum ions will be excreted through the kidneys relatively rapidly. An additional major route of aluminum excretion is through sweat (Minshall et al., 2014). Notably, the same is not true for aluminum bound up in fluoride complexes or for aluminum that has a different route of administration, such as by injection into muscle or skin.

Aluminum can appear in drinking water following the use of aluminum sulfate as a flocculant, but its overall impact seems to be low (0.3%) (Yokel and McNamara, 2001), except in unusual circumstances such as the large aluminum sulfate spill into the water supply in Camelford, UK in 1988. High concentrations can also arise naturally in well water near volcanic or acidified soils.

The addition of fluoride to drinking water as part of a campaign against dental caries raises concern from two neurological perspectives, notwithstanding the presumed – and, apparently, incorrect – value of fluoride for the prevention of tooth decay (see Chapter 16 for details). First, fluoride promotes GI disorders (Varner et al., 1998). Second, the joint presence of aluminum and fluoride can form aluminofluoride complexes, which can be extremely toxic to humans as they can act as phosphate analogues (Strunecká et al., 2002).

Aluminum can also enter the body by inhalation, with an estimated daily uptake of 4.4 μg in industrialized areas (Nurchi et al., 2012). Aluminum metal workers may show higher levels in blood, urine, and bone (Ljunggren et al., 1991; Elinder et al., 1991;

Table 6.1 Sources of bioavailable aluminum in humans.

Major sources of Al exposure in humans	Daily Al intake (mg/day)	Weekly Al intake (mg/day)	÷ PTWI[a] (1 mg/kg/bw; for an average 70 kg human, PTWI = 70 mg)	Amount delivered daily into systemic circulation (at 0.25% absorption rate)
Natural food	1–10	7–70	0.1–1.0	2.5–25.0 µg
Food with Al additives	1–20 (individual intake can exceed 100)	7–140 (700)	0.1–2.0 (10)	2.5–50.0 µg (250 µg)
Water	0.08–0.224	0.56–1.56	0.008–0.02	0.2–0.56 µg
Pharmaceuticals (antacids, buffered analgesics, antiulceratives, antidiarrheal drugs)	126–5000	882–35 000	12.6–500.0	315–12 500 µg
Vaccines (HepB, Hib, Td, DTP)	0.51–4.56	NA	NA	510–4560 µg[b]
Cosmetics, skin-care products, antiperspirants[c]	70	490	NA	8.4 µg (at 0.012% absorption rate)
Cooking utensils and food packaging	0–2	0–14	0–0.2	0–5 µg

a) PTWI (Provisional Tolerable Weekly Intake) is based on orally ingested Al. Generally, only 0.1–0.4% of Al is absorbed from the gastrointestinal (GI) tract, but Al may form complexes with citrate, fluoride, carbohydrates, phosphates, and dietary acids (malic, oxalic, tartaric, succinic, aspartic, and glutamic), which can increase its GI absorption (0.5–5.0%). Co-exposure with acidic beverages (lemon juice, tomato juice, coffee) also increases Al absorption, as well as conditions of Ca2+, Mg2+, Cu2+, and Zn2+ deficiency.

b) A single dose of vaccine delivers the equivalent of 204–1284 mg orally ingested Al (0.51–4.56 mg), all of which is absorbed into systemic circulation. Al hydroxide, a common vaccine adjuvant, has been linked to a host of neurodegenerative diseases; it also induces hyperphosporylation of microtubule-associated protein (MAP) tau *in vivo*.

c) The risk from antiperspirants comes both from dermal exposure and from inhalation of aerosols. Inhaled Al is absorbed from the nasal epithelia into the olfactory nerves and distributed directly into the brain. (excerpted from Tomljenovic, 2011. See original article for relevant reference).

Gitelman et al., 1995). Health outcomes of inhaled aluminum can include respiratory tract infections with asthma-like symptoms (Krewski et al., 2007) and cognitive disorders (Riihimäki and Aitio, 2012), the latter implicating uptake into the CNS.

In regard to CNS levels, the amount of aluminum in the normal adult human brain is less than 2 μg/g (Andrási et al., 2005), with the distribution reflecting higher concentrations in gray compared to white matter (Bush et al., 1995). Along with bone, the brain has the highest potential to accumulate aluminum (Exley, 2009). Post-mortem brain samples of individuals exposed during the Camelford incident showed an aluminum concentration of from 0.75 μg/g in frontal white matter to 49 μg/g in the choroid plexus (Exley and Esiri, 2006). The association of aluminum with the hallmark abnormal protein entities in Alzheimer's disease, Aβ plaques and NFTs, has been well documented (Bolognin et al., 2011) (Figure 6.1).

There is disagreement about how much aluminum entering the brain is later removed (Yokel, 2002 versus Khan et al., 2013), although the differences in outcome may reflect the routes of administration. However, retained aluminum seems to be stored in five main compartments: the blood–brain barrier, the brain interstitial fluid, neurons, glia, and such pathological inclusions as Lewy bodies, NFTs, and Aβ plaques (Reusche et al., 1996; Lévesque et al., 2000; Aremu and Meshitsuka, 2005).

Another main source of aluminum, particularly in the very young, is its widespread use as a vaccine adjuvant. There are a variety of aluminum adjuvant preparations, but the two most common are aluminum hydroxide and aluminum phosphate (Brunner et al., 2010). Although a single vaccine may contain only a relatively small amount (usually less than 0.5 mg), aluminum adjuvants may cumulatively constitute an important source of the overall aluminum body burden. For example, the administration of 20 or more vaccines containing 0.5 mg aluminum as adjuvants would add up to an extra 10 mg aluminum in the body burden: equivalent to a normal dietary intake of aluminum of over 4000 mg/day (Nurchi et al., 2012).

Two considerations apply here. First, circumstances in which aluminum from vaccines may be given in such amounts include the typical pediatric vaccine schedule of many Western countries and war-time conditions. In the latter case, it is notable that Gulf War Syndrome was associated, at least in part, with multiple vaccines given to

Figure 6.1 Aluminum and Aβ in neurological disease. Transmission electron microscope (TEM) micrographs of Aβ and Aβ–metal complexes. *Source*: Bolognin et al. (2011), with permission from Elsevier.

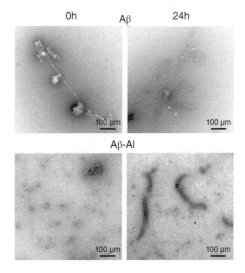

potentially deploying soldiers. Many of these were aluminum-adjuvanted (Hotopf et al., 2000). The second consideration is that aluminum adjuvants are not subject to the same pharmacokinetics as that of dietary/water aluminum exposure and do not seem to be efficiently excreted.

In regard to aluminum excretion, there are two key caveats to consider. The first is that the form in which aluminum is found is a major factor in its potential toxicity. Thus, not all aluminum adjuvants are likely to be identical in their potential impact. Nor have detailed studies compared the various forms (Shaw et al., 2014b). Second, companies making such adjuvants usually employ proprietary forms of these molecules, which may have quite different properties to those that are more commercially available. The neurological pathologies associated with aluminum-adjuvanted vaccines administered to commercial sheep, as described later, do not support the notion that such proprietary forms necessarily have lesser neurological impacts than commercial forms of the same molecules (Luján et al., 2013).

In addition to the early evidence for aluminum toxic actions on the CNS, more recent studies have clearly implicated this element in human neurological disorders. A now-famous example termed "dialysis-associated encephalopathy" (DAE) occurred when kidney dialysis patients were accidentally given dialysis fluids containing high levels of aluminum (Reusche et al., 1996). The outcomes were typically of relatively rapid onset and severity. The resulting neurological signs included cognitive dysfunctions resembling Alzheimer's disease and epileptic seizures. Post-mortem histology showed some of the hallmark pathological features of Alzheimer's disease, including NFTs and Aβ plaques. It is likely that the mechanism by which aluminum ions were transported into the brain involved one or more of the various carrier proteins, including ferritin and transferrin (Sakamoto et al., 2004; Yokel, 2006).

Aluminum has been further linked to other neurological disorders across the lifespan, from Alzheimer's disease (see review by Tomljenovic, 2011) in old age to ASD in children (Tomljenovic and Shaw, 2011a; Shaw et al., 2014b).

A variety of other CNS disorders of an autoimmune nature have also been associated with aluminum. These include macrophagic myofasciitis (MMF) (Gherardi et al., 2001; Gherardi and Authier, 2012), a deteriorating neuromuscular disorder that follows intramuscular injections of aluminum hydroxide. A sequela to MMF is often a form of mild cognitive impairment (MCI) (Rigolet et al., 2014), sometimes viewed in other circumstances as a precursor to Alzheimer's disease. MMF also features a variety of disturbances in interhemispheric functions. Variations on the "autoimmune syndrome/inflammatory syndrome induced by adjuvants" (ASIA) disorders (Israeli et al., 2009; Shoenfeld and Agmon-Levin, 2011), including MMF, may also occur; these are discussed in more detail in Chapter 11.

Animal models of neurological disease using aluminum are available for ALS (Petrik et al., 2007b; Shaw and Petrik, 2009), Alzheimer's disease (Walton, 2006, 2007, 2009a,b; Walton and Wang, 2009; Tomljenovic, 2011), and ASD (Tomljenovic and Shaw, 2011; Shaw and Tomljenovic, 2013; Shaw et al., 2013, 2014b). In the first instance, subcutaneous injections of aluminum hydroxide in young male mice induce apoptotic neuronal death in motor neurons in the spinal cord and motor cortex, accompanied by degraded motor function (Figure 6.2).

Similarly negative CNS outcomes in more extensive experiments have been reported (Crépeaux et al., 2015). In addition, subcutaneous aluminum hydroxide injections in newborn mice induce significant weight increases and a range of behavioral changes

Figure 6.2 Motor neuron degeneration induced by aluminum. NeuN and activated caspase-3 fluorescent labeling in ventral horn of lumbar spinal cord. Green: NeuN; red: activated caspase-3; yellow: co-localization of NeuN and activated caspase-3; blue: nuclear DAPI. (a,b) NeuN labeling in control and aluminum hydroxide-injected mouse lumbar spinal cord sections, respectively. (c,d) Control and aluminum hydroxide mouse lumbar spinal cord sections labeled with caspase-3. (e,f) Merge of NeuN and caspase. Magnification ×40. (g,h) Enlargements of neurons indicated by white arrows in (e,f). Magnification ×100. (i,j) Enlargement of another activated caspase-3-positive motor neuron. (j) Merged image of activated caspase-3 and NeuN. Magnification ×100. *Source*: Petrik et al. (2007), with permission from Springer Science and Business Media. (See color plate section for the color representation of this figure.)

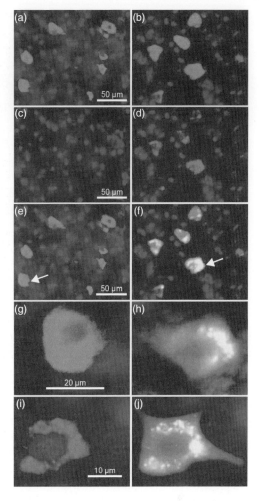

associated with increased anxiety (Shaw et al., 2013). Aluminum-treated mice also showed deficits in social interactions (Sheth et al., 2015) and pronounced changes in gene expression for a range of genes associated with both ASD and Alzheimer's disease (Li et al., 2015, 2016).

Adding yet another species, Luján et al. (2013) reported a neurological disorder in commercial sheep after a mass-vaccination campaign against "blue tongue" (Figure 6.3). The adjuvant in the vaccine was aluminum hydroxide. Chronic adverse effects were observed in 50–70% of flocks, and up to 100% of animals within an affected flock, including features such as restlessness, compulsive wool biting, generalized weakness, muscle tremors, loss of response to external stimuli, ataxia, tetraplegia, and stupor. As with human DAE, coma and death could follow. On histological examination, inflammatory lesions in the brain and spinal cord were found associated with the presence of aluminum. These lesions included multifocal meningoencephalitis, demyelination, multifocal neuronal necrosis, and neuron loss in the spinal cord. The disorder was made worse by cold-weather conditions, perhaps suggesting some synergy with other environmental factors. These initial observations were successfully

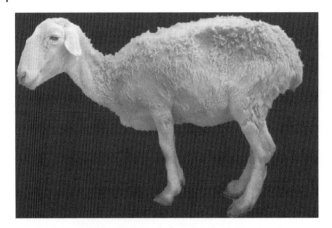

Figure 6.3 Adult sheep affected by the chronic phase of the ASIA syndrome. Note extreme cachexia, poor wool coat, redness of the skin, atrophy of muscular masses, and generalized weakness. The animal also shows abnormal posture. *Source*: Luján et al. (2013), with permission from Springer Science and Business Media.

reproduced under experimental conditions following the experimental administration of aluminum-containing vaccines.

The veterinary studies by Luján et al. (2013) seem largely to confirm the general nature of the negative CNS outcomes in mice following aluminum adjuvant administration. In both mice and sheep, motor and cognitive function changes were noted. Degeneration of neurons in the CNS followed in both cases, particularly amongst motor neurons.

Such studies across species may be of obvious relevance to humans similarly exposed to aluminum from various sources, and the noted CNS pathologies are worth considering in the context of the development of age-related neurological diseases.

A key question is how aluminum might be transported from the site of injection into the CNS. The answer has been provided by the work of a French research group, which showed that aluminum hydroxide administered intramuscularly in mice does not stay localized in the muscle, but rather migrates to different organs. The path by which it does so is now clear from various tracking experiments with fluorescent markers, notably rhodamine- and nano-diamond-labeled aluminum hydroxide. These studies demonstrated that a significant proportion of the nanoparticles escape the injected muscle within immune cells (macrophages), travel to regional draining lymph nodes, then exit the lymphatic system to reach the bloodstream, eventually gaining access to distant organs, including the brain. Such a "Trojan horse" transport mechanism, in which aluminum-containing macrophages enter the brain, predictably results in the gradual accumulation of aluminum, due to lack of recirculation (Khan et al., 2013; Crépeaux et al., 2015). These studies clearly refute previous notions that injected aluminum adjuvant nanoparticles remain localized at the injection site and only act on the immune system through some "depot effect."

The examples in mice and sheep have obvious relevance for human exposure to aluminum adjuvants. In animal models, as demonstrated by Walton (2007, 2009a,b), oral exposure to aluminum through the diet shows neuropathological outcomes resembling those in humans accidentally exposed to high aluminum concentrations in water, such as at Camelford.

This recent *in vivo* work shows that the bioaccumulation of aluminum in the CNS can occur at a very slow rate under many different conditions (e.g., periodic vaccination with aluminum-adjuvanted vaccines) (Table 6.2). Aluminum accumulation may be expected to be equally slow when the source is drinking water or food, and its deleterious eventual outcomes will be the result of cumulative body/brain burden and age. In the latter regard, there is evidence from older literature that aluminum in the brains of the elderly, of Alzheimer's disease patients, and of those with various forms of dementia is often associated with NFTs (Perl and Brody, 1980; Perl, 1985; Perl and Good, 1991; Strong and

Table 6.2 Aluminum's CNS impacts in animals and humans. *Source*: Adapted from Tomljenovic (2011). See original article for relevant references.

Effects on memory, cognition, and psychomotor control	Significantly decreases cognitive and psychomotor performance in humans and animals
	Impairs visuo-motor coordination and long-term memory and increases sensitivity to flicker in humans and rats
	Impairs memory and hippocampal LTP in rats and rabbits *in vivo* (electrophysiological model of synaptic plasticity and learning)
Effects on neurotransmission and synaptic activity	Depresses the levels and activities of key neurotransmitters known to decline in Alzheimer's disease *in vivo*: acetylcholine, serotonin, norepinephrine, dopamine, and glutamate
	Reproduces hallmark cholinergic deficits observed in Alzheimer's disease patients by impairing the activity of cholinergic synthetic and transport enzymes: • impairs acetylcholinesterase activity; • reduces neural choline acetyltransferase; • inhibits choline transport in rat brain and in synaptosomes from cortex and hippocampus; • attenuates acetylcholine levels in rabbit hippocampus and concomitantly induces a learning deficit; • may cause acetylcholine deficit by acting upon muscarinic receptors and potentiating the negative feedback controlling acetylcholine release into the synaptic cleft.
	Inhibits the neuronal glutamate–NO–cGMP pathway necessary for LTP
	Damages dendrites and synapses
	Impairs the activity of key synaptosomal enzymes dependent on Na-K, Mg2+, and Ca2+
	Inhibits glutamate, GABA, and serotonin uptake into synaptosomes
	Impairs neurotransmission by disrupting post-receptor signal transduction mediated by the two principal G-protein-regulated pathways: PLC and AC

(Continued)

Table 6.2 (Continued)

	Inhibits dihydropteridine reductase, essential for the maintenance of BH4, a cofactor important in the synthesis and regulation of neurotransmitters
	Impairs ATP-mediated regulation of ionotropic and metabotropic receptors: cholinergic, glutamatergic, and GABAergic
	Interferes with receptor desensitization by increasing the stability of the metal–ATP receptor complex and causes prolonged receptor activity (by replacing Mg2+ from the metal site)
Effects on G-proteins and Ca²⁺ homeostasis	Alters IP and cAMP signaling cascades by interfering with G-proteins (as AlF), second messengers, and second messenger/Ca2+ targets:

- potentiates agonist-stimulated cAMP production following chronic oral exposure in rats, by inhibiting the GTPase activity of Gs, leading to prolonged activation of Gs after receptor stimulation and increased cAMP production by AC;
- increases cAMP levels by 30–70% in the brains of adult and weanling rats;
- inhibits muscarinic, adrenergic, and metabotropic receptor-stimulated IP3 accumulation by inhibiting Gq-dependent hydrolysis of PIP2 by PLC;
- decreases IP3 in the hippocampus of rats following chronic oral administration;
- inhibits PKC;
- blocks the fast phase of voltage-dependent Ca2+ influx into synaptosomes;
- binds to CaM and interferes with numerous CaM-dependent phosphorylation/dephosphorylation reactions;
- impairs Ca2+/CaM-dependent LTP.

May cause a prolonged elevation in intracellular Ca2+ levels by:

- interfering with desensitization of the NMDA receptor channel;
- delaying the closure of voltage-dependent Ca2+ channels;
- blocking the CaM-dependent Ca2+/Mg2+-ATPase responsible for extrusion of excess intracellular Ca2+.

Elicits a Ca2+-dependent excitotoxic cascade by frequent stimulation of the NMDA receptor, which may result in:

- persistent further activation of the NMDA receptor by endogenous glutamate and exacerbation of glutamate excitotoxicity;
- mitochondrial and ER Ca2+ store overload;
- compromised neuronal energy levels;
- erosion of synaptic plasticity;
- increased susceptibility to apoptosis and accelerated neuronal loss.

Table 6.2 (Continued)

	Perturbs neuronal Ca2+ homeostasis and inhibits mitochondrial respiration in a complex with amyloidogenic A peptide in a triple transgenic mouse model of Alzheimer's disease
Metabolic and inflammatory effects	Inhibits utilization of glucose in the brain
	Inhibits hexokinase and G6PD
	Reduces glucose uptake by cortical synaptosomes
	Alters Fe2+/Fe3+ homeostasis and potentiates oxidative damage via Fenton chemistry
	Alters membrane properties by: • decreasing the content of acidic phospholipid classes PS, PI, and PA in rat brain myelin by 70%; • inducing the clustering of negatively charged phospholipids, thereby promoting phase separation and membrane rigidification and facilitating brain-specific LPO.
	Increases the permeability of the blood–brain barrier by: • increasing the rate of transmembrane diffusion; • selectively changing saturable transport systems.
	Facilitates glutamate transport across the blood–brain barrier and potentiates glutamate excitotoxicity
	Decreases antioxidant activity of SOD and catalase in the brain
	Increases cerebellar levels of NOS
	Augments specific neuroinflammatory and proapoptotic cascades by inducing transcription from a subset of HIF-1 and NF-B-dependent promoters (APP, IL-1 precursor, cPLA2, COX-2, and DAXX)
	Activates microglia, exacerbates inflammation, and promotes degeneration of motor neurons
Nuclear effects	Binds to phosphonucleotides and increases the stability of DNA
	Binds to linker histones, increases chromatin compaction, and depresses transcription
	Inhibits RNA polymerase activity
	Reduces the expression of the key cytoskeletal proteins, tubulin and actin
	Downregulates the expression of the light chain of the neuron-specific NFL gene in 86% of surviving neurons in the superior temporal gyrus of Alzheimer's disease patients
	Upregulates well-known Alzheimer's-related genes: APLP-1 and -2, tau, and APP in human neuroblastoma cells when complexed with A, to a larger extent than other A-metal complexes (A-Zn, A-Cu, and A-Fe)
	Upregulates HIF-1 and NF-B-dependent gene expression

(Continued)

Table 6.2 (Continued)

Effects on MTs, cytoskeleton, and NFT formation	Induces neurofibrillary degeneration in basal forebrain cholinergic, cortical, and hippocampal neurons and accumulates in NFT-bearing neurons
	Causes neurite damage and synapse loss in hippocampal and cortical pyramidal neurons by disabling their capacity for MT assembly
	Directly alters MT assembly by interfering with magnesium and GTP-dependent MT-polymerization mechanisms and actively displaces magnesium from magnesium-binding sites on tubulin and promotes tubulin polymerization
	Decreases the sensitivity of MTs to calcium-induced depolymerisation and effectively disables the regulatory circuits that are set to maintain the sensitive dynamics between the polymerization and depolymerisation cycles of tubulin, and ultimately impairs MT assembly
	Inhibits axonal and dendritic transport mechanisms by depleting MTs
	Induces cAMP-dependent protein kinase phosphorylation of MAPs and NFs in rats following chronic oral exposure and enhances the formation of insoluble NF aggregates. Al-induced hyperphosphorylated NFs are resistant to dephosphorylation and degradation by calcium-dependent proteases (calpain)
	Promotes highly specific non-enzymatic phosphorylation of tau *in vitro* by catalyzing a covalent transfer of the entire triphosphate group from ATP to tau via O-linkage (cAMP-dependent protein kinase phosphorylation sites) at concentrations similar to those reported in Alzheimer's disease brains
	Induces tau phosphorylation and motor neuron degeneration *in vivo* (as a vaccine adjuvant)
	Facilitates cross-linking of hyperphosphorylated tau in PHFs, stabilizes PHFs, and increases the resistance of PHFs to proteolysis
	Inhibits dephosphorylation of tau in synaptosomal cytosol fractions
	Decreases levels of specific MAP isoforms
Effects on amyloidosis	Elevates APP expression and induces senile plaque deposition in 30% of patients subjected to chronic dialysis treatment
	Elevates APP expression and promotes A deposition and amyloidosis in hippocampal and cortical pyramidal neurons in rats and mice following chronic oral exposure
	Binds the amyloidogenic A peptide and perturbs its structure from a soluble helical form to the insoluble random turn–sheet conformation at physiologically relevant concentrations; the neurotoxic A-sheet conformation may be reversed by the addition of a natural Al binder: silicic acid, a promising therapeutic agent for Alzheimer's disease

Table 6.2 (Continued)

Promotes the formation of amyloid fibrils in complex with ATP and induces their aggregation

Induces conformational changes in A and enhances its aggregation *in vitro* in cultured mouse cortical neurons, following chronic (50 M, >3 weeks) but not acute (10–100 M, 1 week) exposure

Appears to be the most efficient cation in promoting A1-42 aggregation and potentiating A1-42 cellular toxicity in human neuroblastoma cells:

- induces a specific oligomeric state of A1-42 and, by stabilizing this assembly, markedly reduces cell viability and alters membrane structure, an effect not seen with other metal complexes (A1-42-Zn, A1-42-Cu and A1-42-Fe) or A1-42 alone;
- strongly enhances the spontaneous increase of A1-42 surface hydrophobicity (compared to A1-42 alone, A1-42-Zn, A1-42-Cu, and A1-42-Fe), converting the peptide into partially folded conformations.

May promote amyloidosis by interfering with the muscarinic acetylcholine receptor-stimulated IP3/PLC-regulated production of the neuroprotective nonamyloidogenic s-APP:

- as fluoroaluminate, blocks DAG/PKC-dependent budding of secretory vesicles containing APP from the TGN, thus inhibiting redistribution of APP toward the plasma membrane, where it would undergo processing by -secretase to produce s-APP;
- may inhibit IP3/Ca2+-dependent production of s-APP;
- may inhibit PKC-dependent APP cleavage by -secretase .

Inhibits proteolytic degradation of A by cathepsin D

LTP, long-term potentiation; NO, nitric oxide; cGMP, cyclic guanosine monophosphate; GABA, gamma aminobutyric acid; PLC, phospholipase C; AC, adenylyl cyclase; ATP, adenosine triphosphate; IP, inositol phosphate; cAMP, cyclic adenosine monophosphate; Gs, stimulatory G protein; PIP2, phosphatidylinositol biphosphate; IP3, inositol triphosphate; PKC, protein kinase C; CaM, calmodulin; NMDA, N-methyl-D-aspartate; ER, endoplasmic reticulum; G6PD, glucose-6-phosphate dehydrogenase; PS, phosphatidylserine; PI, phosphatidylinositol; PA, phosphatidic acid; LPO, lactoperoxidase; SOD, superoxide dismutase; NOS, nitric oxide synthase; APP, amyloid precursor protein; IL-1, interleukin 1; cPLA2, calcium-dependent phospholipase A2; COX, cyclooxygenase; DAXX, death-domain associated protein; NFL, neurofilament; APLP, amyloid precursor-like protein; HIF, hypoxia-inducible factor; NF-B, nuclear factor beta; MT, microtubule; NFT, neurofibrillary tangle; MAP, microtubule-associated protein; PHF, paired helical filament; DAG, diacylglycerol; TGN, *trans*-Golgi network.

Garruto, 1991; Wakayama et al., 1996; He and Strong, 2000). The source of the CNS aluminum in these cases is not known and could be any of those mentioned in this section.

These cumulative data may provide a biological basis for a previous suggestion partially linking aluminum adjuvants in pediatric vaccines to increased rates of ASD in various Western countries (Tomljenovic and Shaw, 2011) (discussed further in Chapter 11).

What will be obvious from a consideration of these data is that while aluminum has the potential to be both acutely toxic, as in DAE, and chronically toxic, as perhaps in Alzheimer's disease, the range of impacts on the CNS can be extremely varied, both in

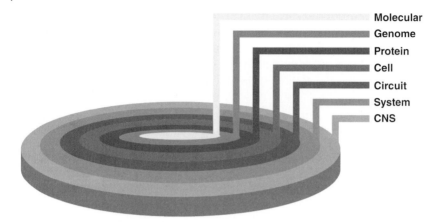

Figure 6.4 Aluminum impacts at various levels of organization in the CNS. *Source*: Redrawn from Shaw et al. (2014a) under the Creative Commons Attribution License. (See color plate section for the color representation of this figure.)

CNS area affected and the time course of any resulting pathology. In this regard, aluminum neurotoxicity is disseminated both spatially and temporally in a manner that may more closely resemble the typical phenotype of multiple sclerosis. What is equally clear is that aluminum has the capacity to impact the CNS at multiple levels of organization, from DNA all the way though to higher systems interactions (Shaw et al., 2014b) (Figure 6.4).

From the preceding, one way to view aluminum neurotoxicity may be to consider it as a generally neurotoxic element with spatial variations in CNS subsystem impacts that are extremely diverse. In this view, the precise outcome may depend on a variety of intrinsic and extrinsic factors. Concerning the former, age, sex, and individual genetic polymorphisms and biochemistries (including the microbiome; see Chapter 16 and Scheperjans et al., 2014) are likely to be key players. Extrinsic factors include the type of aluminum compound, the amount of exposure, and the route of exposure (e.g., by food, water, intramuscular versus other types of injection, inhalation, etc.).

For all of these reasons, the toxicity of aluminum in the CNS appears to depend on a number of variables, which include both direct and indirect cellular mechanisms. In either case, factors include the form of aluminum complex, the size of the particles, the route of administration, and the dose. Dose itself may not be the major consideration (Crépeaux et al., submitted). In animal models, species and even strain may influence aluminum outcomes (Crépeaux et al., 2015). Finally, it should now be apparent that interactions with the immune system, as detailed in Chapter 11, will determine, at least in part, the influence of the other factors.

6.4   Single- vs. Multiple-Hit Models of Neurological Disease: Gene–Toxin Interactions

Most neurological diseases have traditionally been thought to arise from fairly linear, "one-hit" types of process (see discussion of Clarke et al., 2001 in Chapter 9). For example, the initial observations that the hallmark features of Alzheimer's disease are Aβ plaques and NFTs led to decades of research to understand the origin and pathology of these abnormal protein entities. The idea that dominated the field for a long time was that to understand these proteinopathies was to understand the disease. Tied to this, a presumed genetic basis for such proteinopathies made this notion even more attractive to many in the field. Similarly, in Parkinson's disease, the identification of misfolded α-synuclein led in the same direction. In much the same way, the mSOD1 in some cases of fALS drove a huge effort to understand mSOD biochemistry and the "toxic gain of function" impacts on motor neurons and glial cells. Single-hit views of neurological disease origins, whether gene- or toxin-based, as cited in this and the previous chapter, have thus held a dominant position for many years.

In spite of these more conventional perspectives, it has become increasingly obvious that a series of deleterious events, or multiple hits, is involved in driving the neurological disease process toward its ultimate end state. While it has been abundantly clear for years that at the very least genetic and toxic events are almost certainly involved in interactive ways, research into such interactions has tended to be viewed as "unfocused" (and thus often not fundable) by the various granting agencies.

There is now, however, a growing recognition that not only are toxins often playing out their pathological role in the context of various susceptibility genes, but that gene–gene interactions and toxin synergies are likely involved in disease etiology for all of the sporadic diseases considered so far in this book. A schematic of what a single versus a multiple factor/"hit" for neuronal degeneration might look like is shown in Figure 6.5.

In addition, it has become apparent that the eventual neural targets of such gene or toxin impacts – that is, the cells whose death is a hallmark of the disease (e.g., motor neurons in ALS) – are not the only cells involved. Rather, the deaths of particular neurons that are used to characterize the disease end state may be fairly far downstream in the cascade of pathological events which likely involves numerous other cell types at earlier stages.

As cited in Chapter 2, it now seems likely that the early events in any such disease may involve cells in regions not conventionally considered to be involved at all. For example,

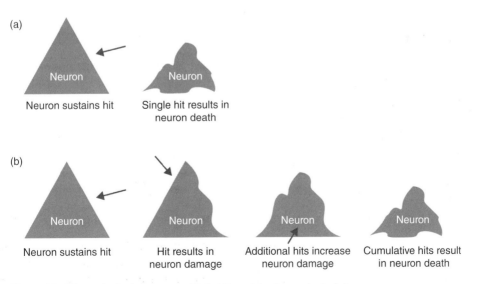

Figure 6.5 Schematic single- versus multiple-hit models of neurological disease.

the loss of some olfactory neurons and function seems to be an early precursor to the loss of dopaminergic neurons in the nigro-striatal system in Parkinson's disease.

In spite of the gaps in current funding, at least some official entities have recognized that the likely future success in identifying risk factors, and therefore potentially successful therapeutics, for neurological diseases may lie in identifying the intersection between genes and environmental factors. In the United States, a subdivision of the National Institutes of Health (NIH), the National Institute of Environmental Health Sciences (NIEHS), created the National Center for Toxicogenomics in 2000. For reasons not totally clear, the Center was closed in 2006 and its responsibilities shifted to other sections in NIEHS. The restructuring put the general subject of toxicogenomics into the Division of Intramural Research – in other words, basically into the general mix of study areas and review panels.

Toxicogenomics also found a new home in the Division of the National Toxicology Program (NTP), particularly in "Toxicology Testing in the 21st Century" or "Tox21" program.

The NTP in general has performed preliminary toxicogenomic studies which suggest that gene expression is often predictive for phenotypic alterations:

> NTP is researching if gene expression pattern analysis can provide indicators of toxicity (1) at earlier time points and (2) at lower doses than is possible for traditional toxicology parameters. Evaluating patterns of gene expression may provide more than just a link between genetics and morphology. It is also expected to provide insights into the pathogenesis of the disease and how different rodent models respond to toxicants.

Tox21, as described on the NIEHS website, seems more concerned with a high-throughput screening of toxic molecules.

The closure of the National Center for Toxicogenomics seems unfortunate. It may represent a truly lost opportunity, at least for the present, to make a focused effort to probe gene–toxin interactions in neurological disease, let alone any disease in which such interactions are likely at play a significant role.

In spite of the demise of the Center, various studies suggest that this may be a fruitful avenue of future investigation. As one example, Lee and Shaw (2012) examined the impact of adding toxic steryl glucoside molecules described in Section 6.2.4 (and in more detail in Chapter 7) to transgenic mice carrying two of the main m$SOD1$ mutations. The mutations alone caused the loss of motor neurons, as expected. The addition of the steryl glucoside toxin changed the rapidity of the morphological changes of astrocytes and microglia without necessarily changing the time course of neuronal degeneration and survival. This outcome was in keeping with the idea that if either genes or toxins induce overwhelming impacts, then the most that the other can do is likely be additive (Figure 6.6. Only the results from astrocyte labeling are shown here).

In contrast, true synergistic interactions would more likely arise in animal models, or in human neurological disease victims, when the genes involved were more of the susceptibility gene type and the toxin concentrations were relatively low.

The latter notion has not yet been widely tested experimentally. Evidence that it might be the case comes from studies looking at the same toxic steryl glucosides in concert with apolipoprotein E (APOE) polymorphisms, in which the level of behavioral and pathological outcomes was dependent on the subtype of gene carried (Wilson et al., 2005)

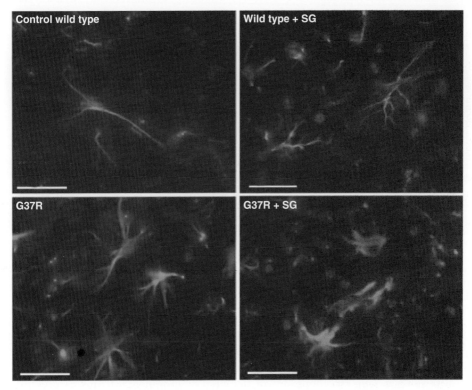

Figure 6.6 Gene–toxin interactions in the m*SOD1* model of ALS. Micrographs of green fluorescent glial fibrillary acidic protein (GFAP) immunostaining for astrocytes in lumbar spinal sections of control-fed wild-type, steryl glucosides (SG)-fed wild-type, control-fed G37R, and SG-fed G37R mice. *Source*: Modified from Lee and Shaw (2012), under Creative Commons Attribution License. (See color plate section for the color representation of this figure.)

(Figure 6.7). These outcomes clearly mirror the risk factors involved in some human neurological diseases. Similar results have been noted by other groups in relation to Liver X knockout mice exposed to various steryls and steryl glucosides (Andersson et al., 2005; Kim et al., 2008).

Given the daunting number of possible gene–toxin combinations, one way to narrow the search for viable interactions might be to take a "reverse engineering" approach, in which candidate toxins are considered in connection to those genes/gene products that might modify their chemical nature, degradation, transport into the CNS, and so on. This has not so far been widely done, but it may be a fruitful means of preselecting genes for study. My laboratory has followed this approach in seeking changes in gene expression following aluminum exposure in a murine model of ASD (Li et al., 2016 accepted for publication, in press), as will be discussed later in this chapter.

6.5 Genetic Susceptibility Factors

Tables 6.3–6.5 list some susceptibility genes linked to age-related neurological diseases. The list should be viewed as preliminary at best, and it is almost certain to grow in the future. Potentially, it could prove to be enormous given the size of the human genome

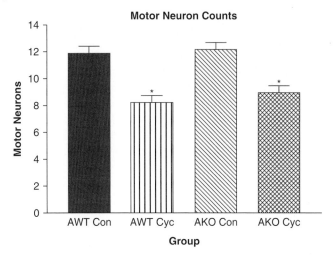

Figure 6.7 APOE–toxin interactions. Ventral horn motor neuron counts in cycad-treated mice with and without APOE expression. Both cycad-fed groups showed significantly decreased motor neuron numbers compared with controls. *$p < 0.05$. AWT Con, APOE wild-type control; AWT Cyc, APOE wild-type cycad-fed; AKO Con, APOE knockout control; AKO Cyc, APOE knockout cycad-fed. *Source*: Wilson et al. (2005), with permission from Canadian Science Publishing.

(approximately 23 000 genes). How many of these genes could contribute to neuron loss if interactions with other genes were to occur, or if they singly or jointly interacted in negative ways with the thousands of potential environmental toxins, is presently unknown.

The eventual outcome of such a line of research is almost certain to be that multiple interactions leading to neurological disease will be found. The likely corollary to this is that the overall numbers of such interactions will not be small. In other words, there are likely to be a very large number of combinations leading to the same general neurological disease end state. This could be a daunting problem from the perspective of translational medicine/therapeutics, and is a topic to be addressed in more detail in later chapters.

6.5.1 Toxin-Triggering Genetic Alterations and Gene Expression Levels

An emerging area of study is that of "epigenetics," or the changes in gene expression regardless of the mutational state of the gene. Epigenetic modifications can occur in several ways. The first is when a stable but reversible alteration of gene function is mediated by histone modification, cytosine methylation, the binding of nuclear proteins to chromatin, or interactions amongst any of these elements. Such modification does not require, or generally involve, any changes in the DNA sequence itself.

A second way epigenetic modification can occur is through "epimutation," or a heritable change in gene expression that does not affect the DNA sequence. Instead, epimutation involves the silencing of a gene that is not normally silenced, or, conversely, the activation of a gene that is not normally active. It is useful in this regard to consider the probability demonstrated in the literature that some factor, perhaps a toxin, can be the trigger of such epigenetic changes, whose net consequence is to cause some gene to under- or overexpress downstream protein production.

A recent example ties back to the discussion of aluminum toxicity and is based on older observations that aluminum can bind to and alter DNA (Karlik et al., 1980).

Table 6.3 Susceptibility genes: Parkinson's disease.

Gene	Location	MAF	OR	References
GBA	1q21	0.01	5.43	Sidransky et al. (2009)
MAPT	17q21.1	0.22	0.80	Pastor et al. (2000), Simon-Sanchez et al. (2009)
RAB7L1	1q32	0.44	0.86	Satake et al. (2009)
BST1	4p15	0.45	0.87	Satake et al. (2009)
HLA-DRB5	6p21.3	0.15	0.80	Hamza et al. (2010a)
GAK	4p16	0.28	1.14	Pankratz et al. (2009), Nalls et al. (2011)
ACMSD	2q21.3	0.19	1.07	Nalls et al. (2011)
STK39	2q24.3	0.13	1.12	Fecto et al. (2011)
SYT11	1q21.2	0.02	1.44	Nalls et al. (2011)
FGF20	8p22	0.27	0.88	van der Walt et al. (2004); International Parkinson Disease Genomics Consortium and Wellcome Trust Case Control Consortium 2 (2011)
STX1B	16p11.2	0.41	1.15	International Parkinson Disease Genomics Consortium and Wellcome Trust Case Control Consortium 2 (2011)
GPNMB	7p15	0.40	0.89	International Parkinson Disease Genomics Consortium and Wellcome Trust Case Control Consortium 2 (2011)
SIPA1L2	1q42.2	0.14	1.13	Nalls et al. (2014)
INPP5F	10q26.11		1.10	Nalls et al. (2014)
MIR4697HG	11q25	0.35	1.11	Nalls et al. (2014)
GCH1	14q22.1-q22.2	0.34	0.90	Nalls et al. (2014)
VPS13C	15q22.2		1.11	Nalls et al. (2014)
DDRGK1	20p13		1.11	Nalls et al. (2014)
MCCC1	3q27	0.14	0.87	Nalls et al. (2011)
SCARB2	4q21.1	0.37	0.90	Do et al. (2011)
CCDC62	12q24.31	0.46	1.13	Nalls et al. (2011)
RIT2	18q12.3		1.19	Pankratz et al. (2012)
SREBF1	17p11.2	0.31	0.95	Do et al. (2011)

MAF, minor allele frequency; OR, odds ratio.

Our own work in this area used tissue samples from various CNS subregions of mice exposed to injected aluminum salts early in postnatal life (Shaw et al., 2013). Real-time polymerase chain reaction (RT-PCR) showed that mice so exposed underwent clear changes in gene expression as determined by semiquantitative RT-PCR (Figure 6.8a,b). These changes were both sex-dependent and CNS region-specific. They persisted at least until 16 weeks of age. Male mice showed various gene-expression alterations in comparison to controls: three were upregulated (chemokine (C-C motif) ligand 2 (*Ccl2*), interferon γ (*Ifng*), and tumor necrosis factor (*Tnf*-α)), two downregulated (acetylcholine esterase (*AChE*) and NF-κB inhibitor β (*Nfkbib*)). Ifng and Tnf-α are both multifunctional proinflammatory cytokines and macrophage activators. Ccl2 is

Table 6.4 Susceptibility genes: ALS. *Source*: Modified from Leblond et al. (2014).

Gene	Location	Inheritance	Diagnosis	References
ANG (ALS9)	14q11.1	AD, sporadic	ALS, ALS-FTD, PD	Greenway et al. (2004, 2006), van Es et al. (2011)
FIG4 (ALS11)	6q21	AD, sporadic	ALS, PLS, CMT	Chow et al. (2009)
ATXN2 (ALS13)	12q24.12	Sporadic	ALS, SCA2	Elden et al. (2010)
DCTN1	2p13.1	AD	ALS	Münch et al. (2004)
CHMP2B	3p11.2	Sporadic	ALS, FTD	Parkinson et al. (2006)
DPP6	7q36.2	Sporadic	ALS	Cronin et al. (2008), van Es et al. (2008)
VEGF	6p21.1	Sporadic	ALS	Lambrechts et al. (2003)
UNC13A	19p13.12	Sporadic	ALS	van Es et al. (2009), Shatunov et al. (2010)
NEFH	22q12.1-q13.1	Sporadic	ALS	Figlewicz et al. (1994), Al-Chalabi et al. (1999)
PRPH	12q13.12	AD, sporadic	ALS	Gros-Louis et al. (2004)
SQSTM1	5q35.3	AD, sporadic	ALS	Fecto et al. (2011)
TAF15	17q12	AD	ALS	Ticozzi et al. (2011)
ELP3	8p21.1	Sporadic	ALS	Simpson et al. (2009)
SMN1	5q13.2	AD, sporadic	ALS	Corcia et al. (2002)
PON1,2,3	7q21.3	Sporadic	ALS	Saeed et al. (2006)
HFE	6p22.1	Sporadic	ALS	Yen et al. (2004)
KIFAP3	1q24.2	Sporadic	ALS	Landers et al. (2009)
APEX1	14q11.2	Sporadic	ALS	Greenway et al. (2004)
PGRN	17q21.31	Sporadic	ALS, FTLD	Schymick et al. (2007)
ITPR2	12p12.1-11.23	Sporadic	ALS	van Es et al. (2007)
PLCD1	3p22.2	Sporadic	ALS	Staats et al. (2013)
ARHGEF28	5q13.2	AD	ALS	Droppelmann et al. (2013)
PFN1	17p13.2	AD, sporadic	ALS	Smith et al. (2015)

AD, autosomal-dominant; ALS, amyotrophic lateral sclerosis; PLS, primary lateral sclerosis; FTD, frontotemporal dementia; PD, Parkinson's disease; CMT, Charcot–Marie–Tooth disease; SCA2, spinocerebellar ataxia type 2; FTLD, frontal temporal lobe dementias.

a macrophage-secreted chemokine. AChE is the degradative enzyme that stops the action of the neurotransmitter acetylcholine. Nfkbib is an inducible transcription factor modifier. Gene-expression alterations were verified at the protein level using Western blots (Figure 6.8c,d). In female mice, an upregulation of *Tnf*-α and downregulation of NF-κB inhibitor ε (*Nfkbie*) were identified. Changes in expression alterations were also confirmed by Western blots.

Table 6.5 Susceptibility genes: Alzheimer's disease.

Gene	Location	MAF	OR	References
APOE	19q13.2	0.14	~2–5	Corder et al. (1993)
TREM2	6p21.1	0.049	2.55	Guerreiro et al. (2013), Jonsson et al. (2013)
CLU	8p21-p12	0.379	0.86	Harold et al. (2009)
PICALM	11q14	0.358	0.87	Harold et al. (2009), Lambert et al. (2013)
CR1	1q32	0.197	1.18	Lambert et al. (2013)
BIN1	2p14	0.409	1.22	Seshadri et al. (2010), Lambert et al. (2013)
MS4A6A	11q12.1	0.403	0.90	Hollingworth et al. (2011), Lambert et al. (2013)
MS4A4E	11q12.2	0.41	1.08	Hollingworth et al. (2011)
CD33	19q13.3	0.307	0.94	Hollingworth et al. (2011), Naj et al. (2011)
ABCA7	19p13.3	0.190	1.15	Hollingworth et al. (2011), Naj et al. (2011), Lambert et al. (2013)
CD2AP	6p12	0.266	1.10	Hollingworth et al. (2011), Naj et al. (2011)
EPHA1	7q34	0.338	0.90	Hollingworth et al. (2011), Naj et al. (2011)
HLA-DRB5 and *DRB1*	6p21.3	0.276	1.11	Lambert et al. (2013)
SORL1	11q23.2–q24.2	0.039	0.77	Lambert et al. (2013)
PTK2B	8p21.1	0.366	1.10	Lambert et al. (2013)
SLC24A4	14q32.12	0.217	0.91	Lambert et al. (2013)
ZCWPW1	7q22.1	0.287	0.91	Lambert et al. (2013)
CELF1	11p11	0.316	1.08	Lambert et al. (2013)
FERMT2	14q22.1	0.092	1.14	Lambert et al. (2013)
CASS4	20q13.31	0.083	0.88	Lambert et al. (2013)
INPP5D	2q37.1	0.488	1.08	Lambert et al. (2013)
MEF2C	5q14.3	0.408	0.93	Lambert et al. (2013)
NME8	7p14.1	0.373	0.93	Lambert et al. (2013)
PLD3	19q13.2	0.06	2.75	Cruchaga et al. (2014)
TRIP4B	15q22.31	0.02	1.31	Ruiz et al. (2014)

MAF, minor allele frequency; OR, odds ratio.

The study also looked at regional expression patterns in the aluminum-treated male and female mice. In male mice, the frontal cortex showed *Tnf*-α, *AChE*, and *Ccl2* changes in expression; *Nfkbib* was changed in the thalamus. In female mice, *Tnf*-α and *Nfkbie* were changed in the cerebellum (Li et al., 2017, in press).

The key point here is to illustrate what may serve as a new way of looking at the interaction between genes and toxins. Genes do not have to be modifiable by their DNA structure in order to be modified in their expression. The fact that some toxins, such as

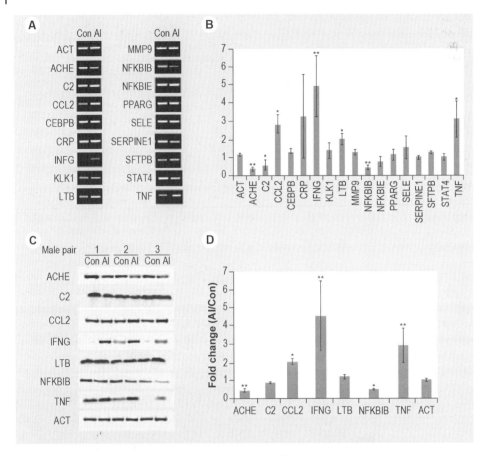

Figure 6.8 Gene-expression alterations in the CNS induced by injected subcutaneously aluminum hydroxide. Aluminum administered to mice in vaccine-relevant dosages altered the expression of genes involved in immunoinflammatory response and neural function. (a) Aluminum-induced gene-expression alterations in the brains of male CD-1 mice. The expression levels of seven neural and innate immunity-related genes were significantly altered in aluminum-injected compared to control male mice, as determined by semiquantitative RT-PCR analyses. β-actin was used as the internal standard. (b) Quantification of the expression change shown in (a). Data are presented as fold difference compared with controls. Histograms report the mean ± standard error of the mean of three independent experiments determined by densitometry. *p < 0.05; **p < 0.01. (c) The protein levels of the seven genes with altered expression levels after aluminum injection were verified by Western blots. (d) Quantification of the protein level change shown in (c). Data are shown as mean signal intensity ± standard error of the mean of three independent experiments. *p < 0.05; **p < 0.01. Al, aluminum-injected male brains; control, saline control males. *Source*: Shaw et al. (2014a), with permission from Future Medicine Ltd.

aluminum, can do so in the CNS may prove to be a factor in the impact of such toxins on neurological disease.

6.5.2 miRNA Alterations in Gene Expression

A less direct means of altering gene expression occurs in the impact that various other genes or molecules may have on the transcriptional machinery of the cell, notably transfer and messenger RNA. RNA transcriptional errors have been implicated in ALS and other neurological diseases (Strong, 2010; Nunomura et al., 2012).

Gene expression is also affected by micro RNA (miRNA), which can act to silence various gene-expression patterns. Again, aluminum may be one of the contributors to this outcome. Changes in miRNA have been implicated in Alzheimer's disease, as one example (Lukiw and Bazan, 2000).

6.6 Biosemiosis (Part 2)

As mentioned previously, in chaos theory the term "butterfly effect" refers to the notion that a very small difference in the initial state of a physical system can make a significant difference to the system at some later time. In lay examples, the term is conceptualized by imagining that a butterfly flapping its wings in the Amazon ultimately causes a hurricane in another part of the world through a series of cascading events.

Nowhere does this concept become more obviously possible than in a consideration of the biosemiotics of the nervous system. As noted previously, "biosemiosis" refers to communication within and between living organisms resulting in biological function. It is literally the study of signs and signals in such systems (Gryder et al., 2013; Oller, 2013).

In a biosemiotic consideration of gene signals, for example, the "sign" is the DNA code, which is mediated and processed as mRNA translated by tRNA/ribosome ("mapping") to form polypeptides: the "object." Needless to say, in a system like the CNS, such biosemiotic considerations may apply at a great variety of levels: DNA to protein, protein to cell function, cell to cell, circuit to circuit, and so on up to communication between individual organisms.

In biosemiosis, the triad is the three subjects just mentioned: sign, mapping, and object (Oller, 2013). Disruption at any step in this sequence has a consequence not only for signaling but also for adverse outcomes. In general, the greatest impacts will be the earliest, as these will progressively impact more downstream events. At the genomic level, signal errors can impact not only mapping, but also epigenetic factors, including DNA self-repair mechanisms.

In a system as highly nested as the nervous system, such errors have the potential to become cascading failures, propagating in both directions back down to the DNA and up to other levels of organization (Shaw and McEachern, 2001). Failures in biosemiosis must therefore eventually, and inevitably result in system entropy and cell death, or at the very least, a form of "pathological plasticity" in which the failed signaling becomes fixed in an incorrect state, as discussed previously.

6.6.1 Aluminum and Failed Biosemiosis

Because the nervous system utterly depends on signaling from the gene (or any part of the DNA that induces protein production) up to neuronal and neural systems outputs, anything that degrades biosemiosis may be highly deleterious. In this regard, aluminum, with its demonstrated potential to impact the various levels of organization, may be one of the more destructive toxins to the CNS from the perspective of biosemiosis.

As cited from our own work, aluminum treatment leads to disruptions in gene expression, thus inevitably impacting protein formation. In turn, altered proteins will impact cellular function. Moving upwards in levels in the CNS, dysfunctional cells cannot help but alter neural circuit function, neural systems function, and, ultimately, behavior. In this manner, aluminum alone may induce a multiple-hit outcome in the CNS on its own, making it perhaps uniquely toxic amongst the various substances known to negatively impact the CNS (Shaw et al., 2014b).

6.7 Gene–Toxin Interactions and Cascading Failures

Regardless of whether mutated genes or chronic or acute toxins are the initiators of neuronal dysfunction, the combination of nested levels of organization with the propagation of biosemiotic errors must inevitably create significant negative feedback loops as the damage makes its way from one level to the next. Damaged neurons will, in turn, affect surrounding cells by releasing various molecules into the microenvironment/niche (e.g., proteases, excitatory amino acids, etc.) and ions (e.g., potassium, calcium). Thus, cell death will disrupt the circuits in which the cell is embedded, and so on through to systems and overall CNS levels above. In such a manner, failure at any level has the capacity to induce cascading failures throughout the CNS. It is thus important to realize that there are reciprocal actions between each level whose cumulative outcomes will impact the system as a whole. In addition, since the CNS does not exist or function in isolation, impacts here will have reciprocal feedback effects on the immune system, as will be discussed in Chapter 11.

It is worth noting, in brief, that due to their nature and general lack of renewal, neurons may be particularly vulnerable to cascading failures. One factor that makes the nervous system uniquely susceptible to disruption is the highly specified differentiation of neuronal activities due to developmental programs. These programs, acting in response to both genetic and environmental instructions, ensure that the loss of functional circuits cannot be easily reversed, since the very milieu in which they might be replaced therapeutically differs in the adult CNS compared to one still within a developmentally critical period. While it is true that critical periods vary between neuronal regions (human association compared to primary cortex, for example), it is also true that younger nervous systems may in some circumstances have a far greater capacity for recovery following injury (Anderson et al., 2011). Part of this capacity for recovery involves the potential for neurogenesis; that is, the birth of new neurons. Although neurogenesis can occur in adult CNS under some circumstances, it is not common, at least not in all areas impacted by the age-related neurological disorders (Winner and Winkler, 2015).

6.8 Genes and Toxins in Neurological Disease: Penultimate Thoughts

The material in this and the previous chapter has highlighted a fraction of the literature on the putative etiologies of the age-related neurological diseases, namely Parkinson's disease, ALS, and Alzheimer's disease. What should be apparent is that these diseases are not likely to arise, for the most part, from simple "one-hit" events, but must in most cases be caused by multiple interacting factors. It is thus likely that the actual origins and mechanisms of neurological diseases will be found within the zone of gene–toxin interactions. It may also be becoming clearer that the multiplicity of such interactions suggests that neurological diseases of the types considered here are all spectrum disorders. This last point will be amplified in the following chapters.

6.9   And, Finally, the Microbiome

No consideration of environmental factors in neurological disease would be complete without factoring in the still-emerging contribution of the microbiome. In humans, a complex microbial community of approximately 100 trillion cells exists, exceeding the number of human cells by a factor of 10. This community comprises something like 800–1000 different bacterial species and more than 7000 different bacterial strains.

Compositional changes in microbiota communities in humans have been associated with certain disease states, such as psoriasis, reflux esophagitis, obesity, childhood-onset asthma, inflammatory bowel disease, colorectal carcinoma, and cardiovascular disease (reviewed in Cho and Blaser, 2012). Whether these disease outcomes are primary or secondary events is not known (Eloe-Fadrosh and Rasko, 2013). However, in general, any such disease state is characterized by dysbiosis of the commensal (beneficial symbionts) microbiota, which can include the loss of such symbionts, decreased microbial diversity, and the emergence of pathobionts, potentially pathological organisms that may, under normal circumstances, be symbionts.

In humans, the infant gut is colonized by microbes of maternal, dietary, and environmental origin, both during birth and shortly afterwards. At weaning, the GI ecosystem is stabilized toward an adult-type phylogenetic architecture (Palmer et al., 2007).

The healthy adult GI microbiota has been considered to be relatively stable throughout adulthood until old age, but recent studies suggest that there may be age-related changes in gut microbiota composition (reviewed in Biagi et al., 2013), primarily for pathological bacteria. A deviation from the healthy intestinal microbiota profile, similarly observed in aging gut microbiota, has been associated with inflammatory disorders such as inflammatory bowel diseases and obesity (Maslowski and Mackay, 2011), but other factors may be involved as well. There are also sex differences in microbiota in humans (Mueller et al., 2006).

A role for the microbiome in neurological disease is a novel and relatively recent area of investigation. However, some preliminary studies have emerged, including one using the m*SOD1* model, which suggests that changes in gut bacteria may have occurred in the transgenic animals (Wu et al., 2015). The overall problems with this model in general, as detailed in various chapters, make these data of uncertain significance.

The studies on toxins, gene interactions, and the microbiome cited in this chapter are useful in setting the stage for a consideration of the major neurological disease spectrum and cluster so far identified. This is the same cluster that may encompass all of the age-related neurological diseases: ALS-PDC.

This often contentious subject, mentioned briefly in preceding chapters, is the one to which I now turn.

Endnote

1 Reprinted in *The Tolkien Reader*, 1966. John Ronald Reuel Tolkien was an English writer, poet, and academic.

7

The Mystery and Lessons of ALS-PDC

"A perfect storm is a rare combination of events or circumstances creating an unusually bad situation. The idiom is derived from the 1997 Sebastian Junger nonfiction book, The Perfect Storm, about a fishing-boat crew encountering a confluence of several storms at sea. The expression fills a gap in the language, as there are few alternatives that convey the same meaning so concisely."[1]

From the Preface

6) At least for Parkinson's disease, ALS, and Alzheimer's disease, there is only one, possibly two, real neurological clusters with a sufficient number of afflicted patients to allow effective epidemiology. The first cluster is ALS–parkinsonism dementia complex (ALS-PDC) of the Western Pacific. This includes the islands of Guam and Rota (where it was first described), Irian Jaya, and perhaps the Kii Peninsula of Japan (whether the CNS disorders in Kii are related to the others is an area of some controversy). The second possible cluster is the form of parkinsonism associated with consumption of the soursop fruit on the French Caribbean island of Guadeloupe.

7.1   Introduction

One solution to the problem of too many potential causal factors is to try to identify a disease cluster. As described in Chapter 3, a cluster is a relatively large number of similar cases of a disease constrained by time and geographical space.

In principle, if enough people get the related signs and symptoms of a disease in a small enough area in a short enough period of time, the search for the disease culprits, either genes, toxins, or their interactions, becomes far more tractable. This is not to say it necessarily becomes easy, as the history of ALS-PDC will indicate.

Typical examples of disease clusters are usually associated with epidemics of infectious diseases to which Koch's postulates can be relatively easily applied. This is rarely the case with neurological diseases, with the exceptions noted in this chapter.

Neural Dynamics of Neurological Disease, First Edition. Christopher A. Shaw.
© 2017 John Wiley & Sons, Inc. Published 2017 by John Wiley & Sons, Inc.

7.2   Neurological Disease Clusters and ALS-PDC

The better-known examples of neurological disease clusters (e.g., prisoner-of-war-camp lathyrism, Minimata methyl mercury contamination, and domoic acid poisoning) were summarized in Chapter 3. However, most age-related neurological diseases have not proven to be so simple.

In fact, with the exception of these clusters, and a few others, when seeking causal factors for most cases of neurological disease – especially in regard to toxins – it seems that the field is dealing with the likelihood that there are chronic exposures to neurotoxins, albeit at relatively low levels. Since the level of the toxin(s) appears to be low, relatively few people go on to show obvious neurological signs or symptoms. Instead, whatever toxins might be contributing to neurological diseases may take years or decades to manifest clinically obvious signs of their cumulative damage. The impact of low-level toxicity thus affects the speed at which both individuals and populations express the disease state.

One consequence of this kind of low to relatively low level of exposure is that real disease clusters do not form. Add to this the additional well-known variables of age, sex, other trauma to the nervous system, variations in genetic susceptibility, individual microbiomes, and so on, and it becomes pretty clear why neurological disease clusters appear to be the exception rather than the rule.

Another complication is that society in the modern industrialized Western world is largely mobile in a way that is vastly different than that of our ancestors only a few generations ago. For example, one may grow up in one part of the country – or even a different country – go to school somewhere else, follow a career or partner/spouse elsewhere again, and finally retire in yet another place.

The lack of geographical consistency and our lack of understanding of when the disease process begins vastly complicate the already complex problems of sifting for answers against a backdrop of low-level toxin exposure. Sporadic Parkinson's disease, ALS, and Alzheimer's disease in North America and Europe may thus fall into a category of nearly unsolvable epidemiological mysteries, at least for now.

This last point was amply reinforced in the previously discussed report that collated the outcomes of some 18 epidemiological studies on neurological diseases (Neurological Health Charities Canada and Public Health Agency of Canada, 2014) (see Chapter 1). What was notable was that for all the effort put into the individual studies and the final report, no clear etiologies emerged for Parkinson's disease, ALS, or Alzheimer's disease or the various disease categories they fell under (e.g., neuromuscular diseases, movement disorders, dementias, etc.). To be fair, most of these studies were more concerned with computing prevalence and incidence for the various disorders and determining how well treatment and care options performed. To some extent, these goals were achieved. It was still surprising, however, that with the level of effort made – where risk factors had to be in the background for most of the research groups – no report, not even the one designed specifically to examine risk factors, was able to derive unambiguous etiological factors. Indeed, apart from those genetic mutations for familial forms of the diseases already clearly established in the literature, nothing of particular consequence for our understanding of the sporadic forms emerged.

The general lack of acknowledged and definable neurological disease clusters equates to a lack of obvious solutions to the problem of causality (unlike for, say, Minimata mercury-induced neurological outcomes). If researchers had at least one real cluster, they would have a place to start the process of sorting through the myriad possible genetic and toxin factors. The success or failure in such as case would have dramatic and far-reaching implications for the disease – or related diseases – outside the cluster.

As it turns out, known clusters for each of the diseases under discussion exist: two for Parkinson's disease, one (maybe two) for ALS, and one for Alzheimer's disease. In one case, it is the same cluster, or spectrum of clusters, although this remains relatively unknown even in scientific circles and is now fading away as a spectrum neurological disorder. The disease in question is none other than ALS-PDC of Guam, as noted briefly in previous chapters.

7.3   History and Features of ALS-PDC

Guam, the southernmost island of the Marianas chain, is roughly 1500 miles northeast of the Philippines and 3500 miles southwest of Hawaii, more or less in a direct line between the two (Figure 7.1). Guam's first known inhabitants were a Malay people who migrated from what are now Malaysia, Indonesia, and the Philippines to settle the Marianas around 1500 BCE.

Their descendants call themselves Chamorros and speak a language described as a Malayo-Polynesian language of the Austronesian family (Safford, 1903). In addition to Guam, the Chamorro people historically inhabited a string of islands further north, including Rota, Tinian, and Saipan.

Two key features of Chamorro history may be relevant to the following considerations of the origins of ALS-PDC. First, during the initial colonization of Guam by the Spanish in the 1600s, the Chamorro population of Guam was significantly reduced by both disease and war, with the result that the population may have been made genetically

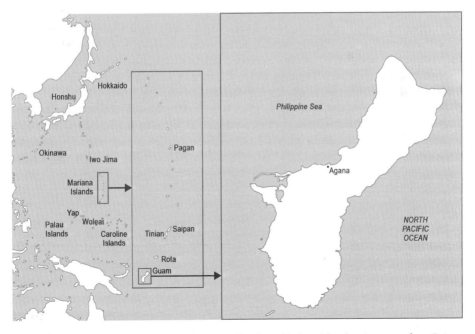

Figure 7.1 Guam, the locus for ALS-PDC. *Source*: Northern Mariana Island regions map from Peter Fitzgerald, Historicair (https://commons.wikimedia.org/wiki/File:Northern_Mariana_Islands_regions_map.png).

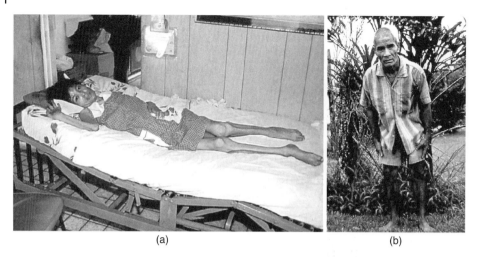

(a)   (b)

Figure 7.2 People with lytico (ALS) and bodig (PDC) on Guam. (a) A woman bedbound with advanced ALS. (b) A man with parkinsonism and dementia. Reference: Used with permission from Dr. John Steele.

more homogeneous. Second, during World War II, many Chamorros were put into labor camps by the Japanese, leading to widespread malnutrition.

It was soon after World War II that American Navy doctors on Guam began to note a large number of cases of a neurological disease manifestation of what appeared, at first, to be one main type. Specifically, it was an almost standard form of ALS (Zimmerman, 1945; Kurland and Mulder, 1954; reviewed in Kurland, 1972, 1988). Known by the Chamorros as "lytico," a variant of the Spanish word "paralytico," or paralyzed, this disease had all of the typical signs of motor neuron disease (Figure 7.2a). These included muscular weakness, beginning often on one side in the legs or less often in the arms, then spreading to the other limbs. The spread from a unilateral to bilateral presentation was much the same as in conventional ALS. The disease showed an ascending pattern, moving upwards in the body to produce prominent neurological signs such as dysphagia and dysarthria. Death, as in ALS in North America, was usually due to respiratory failure, often associated with pneumonia.

Post-mortem analysis of the nervous system showed the loss of motor neurons in the spinal cord. Curiously, lytico also showed non-typical features of ALS, including some features characteristic of Alzheimer's disease, especially the presence of NFTs inside neurons in the hippocampus and frontal cortex. These latter sorts of features in a form of ALS would be rediscovered years later in another neurological disease, FTD, as discussed in Chapter 2.

Lytico on Guam affected men to a far greater degree than women, striking at an average age of 45. The age of onset was particularly notable, since at the time, and to a lesser extent now, this was 10–20 years younger than for ALS in North America and Europe.

A second neurological disorder soon followed the Guamanian form of ALS. This was termed "parkinsonism dementia complex" (PDC), and it resembled a cross between Parkinson's and Alzheimer's diseases. The Chamorros termed it "bodig," from a Chamorro word that means listless or lazy (Figure 7.2b). Like lytico, bodig affected males more than females. A more conventional form of Parkinson's disease alone could also occur, as could a purely Alzheimer's-like disorder termed "Marianas dementia" (Hirano et al., 1961; Kurland, 1972, 1988; Galasko et al., 2002). Where Marianas dementia occurred alone, it was generally found in individuals much older than those afflicted by lytico or bodig, and it strongly favored women by a ratio of over three to one (Galasko et al., 2002).

In general, the brains of bodig victims also showed a loss of neurons in the same regions destroyed in both Parkinson's and Alzheimer's diseases. Neurons containing the neurotransmitter dopamine were lost in the SN, just as in Parkinson's disease. Similarly, neurons were lost in parts of the brain associated with Alzheimer's disease, notably the hippocampus and cortex – those areas associated with learning and memory. Bodig also showed the widespread presence of the same kinds of NFT seen in lytico (Galasko et al., 2002).

Bodig's victims were usually about 10 years older than those of lytico, but much younger than victims of Parkinson's and Alzheimer's diseases elsewhere (Galasko et al., 2002). Curiously, for PDC, there was a nearly complete absence of a feature that is a primary characteristic of Alzheimer's disease, namely plaques composed of the protein Aβ (Galasko et al., 2002).

The initial paper on PDC was by Hirano et al. (1961). It characterized PDC in 47 Chamorros and applied the term "parkinsonism dementia complex of Guam" for the first time. A later review by Steele (2005) described the full characteristic features of PDC, including lack of movement and a mask-like, expressionless face with a "reptilian stare." Patients also showed severe problems in coordination, including skilled actions. Curiously, unlike in typical Parkinson's disease, tremor was not a major characteristic: in over 60% of cases of PDC, tremor was seen only to a mild or moderate degree. PDC patients also showed mental slowness and poor memory (100% of cases). In many cases, this was the primary clinical symptom, with patients appearing disoriented and having memory impairment for recent and past events. Steele noted that:

> Mental changes with memory impairment and disorientation were common, and in a third of cases those changes were accompanied by personality and mood disorders of indifference, depression, and sometimes violent behaviour. Slowness in comprehension, marked difficulty in simple reasoning, increased confusion, and apathy became more obvious as the disease progressed. In 24 of 94 patients (25%) dementia was the only feature of the disease for a variable period, and in 36 cases (38%), it was the dominant feature of illness. Of the 22 patients presenting with parkinsonism, dementia developed in half of cases within 1 year. (Steele, 2005, p. S100).

PDC's aspects of depression thus predated the observation that the same could occur in Parkinson's disease, where it is now a major symptom affecting some 60% of patients, as cited in Chapter 2.

Elizan et al. (1966) examined 94 PDC patients and found many of the same features as the previous Hirano et al. study, adding the observation that none of the patients had a history of prior encephalitis, until then considered a plausible causal factor for the disease, much as it had been for some other forms of parkinsonism. The Elizan study also noted the following features: of those with parkinsonism, half developed dementia within 1 year, and there were more male than female victims.

Steele (2005) went on to note the striking similarity of PDC to another form of parkinsonism, PSP. In both disorders, the signs, behavioral symptoms, and pathological changes within the brain were remarkably similar. However, there were also differences.

PSP is relatively consistent in its clinical expression, while a dominant feature of PDC is the extreme variability in presentation. Also, the abnormal tau protein found in PSP is not the same as the tau in ALS-PDC, the latter being nearly identical to that of Alzheimer's disease. Steele concluded that a PSP syndrome could occur in PDC, and further noted the overlap with some features of corticobasal ganglionic degeneration (CBD) in some Chamorro patients.

All of these observations pointed to the coexistence of PDC, PSP, and CBD in a broad-spectrum neurological disorder whose most common feature was an underlying parkinsonism. It is of interest in this regard that in most aspects a relatively newly described form of parkinsonism, Guadeloupe PDC, resembles both PSP and Guamanian PDC (Caparros-Lefebvre et al., 2002; Shaw and Höglinger, 2008), as previously discussed.

The presence of widespread NFTs in both lytico and bodig was one of the more surprising and intriguing facets of ALS-PDC's pattern of expression. In Alzheimer's disease, where NFTs were first described, the tangles are composed of an abnormal hyperphosphorylated variant of the protein tau, whose normal form helps stabilize microtubules, the cellular structures that regulate the movement of proteins and other compounds inside neurons. In ALS-PDC, NFTs were found not only in those who had the disease, but also in those who appeared to be disease-free (Kurland, 1988).

For those who had ALS-PDC, the distribution of the tangles within the cortex was quite different from that of Alzheimer's disease, involving the upper rather than the lower layers of the cortex. In addition to NFTs, other strange structures were found. One was thought to be unique to ALS-PDC, but was later shown not to be: the odd, rod-shaped structures called "Hirano bodies," after neurologist Asao Hirano, who first described them.

Early in the work on the ALS-PDC spectrum, neuroepidemiologist Dr. Leonard T. Kurland and neurologist Dr. Donald Mulder were amongst the first to document the incredibly high prevalence of ALS on Guam (Kurland and Mulder, 1954). The complementary conclusion of a high prevalence of PDC followed shortly thereafter.

Both Kurland and Mulder seem to have innately recognized the potential global importance of these observations as true clusters of neurological diseases at near epidemic levels. Kurland was later to estimate that Guamanian ALS and PDC were both 50–100 times more prevalent than in North America. In villages such as Umatac in southern Guam, they may have been closer to 400 times greater. Overall, according to Kurland, lytico and bodig were cumulatively responsible for almost 25% of adult deaths during the 1950s and early 1960s (Kurland, pers. comm.).

Kurland, Mulder, and Hirano came to realize that the diseases were not entirely distinct entities, but comprised an extremely wide range of forms with often overlapping symptoms, signs, and pathologies. Some of those initially expressing lytico could go on to acquire bodig as well. The reverse also applied, but was less common.

As documented by later investigators, the numbers were quite telling, as was the changing pattern over time. Guamanian ALS had an incidence of 400 per 100 000 in 1950, dropping to 7 per 100 000 in 1989, then to only 10 patients in total in the years 1997–2000. PDC incidence was 470 per 100 000 in 1960, 22 per 100 000 in 1989, and just 90 patients total in the period 1997–2000 (Galasko et al., 2002) (Figure 7.3).

The large number of victims and the relatively small geographical space were only two of the features that defined ALS-PDC on Guam as a true neurological disease cluster.

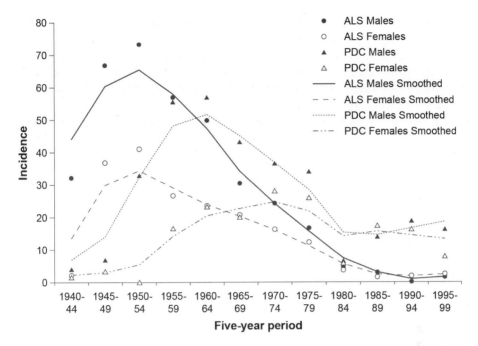

Figure 7.3 Changing rates of ALS-PDC. Average annual incidence of ALS-PDC per 100 000 male and female Guamanian Chamorros per 5-year period from 1940 to 1999. Lines smoothed. *Source*: Plato et al. (2003), with permission from Oxford University Press.

The temporal feature was equally important in the following way: while evidence for something that looked like ALS-PDC went back to the early 1800s, the peak of the disease seemed to occur in the years immediately after World War II.

The diseases of the spectrum tended to cluster in families, with some members having one or the other disease, and some having both (Figure 7.4). Within families in which there were multiple cases of the spectrum, birth order and birth year did not affect the disease phenotype, duration of illness, or age of onset (Steele, 2005).

Adding further to the complexity of the spectrum was the extremely unusual observation that there might be a huge latency between exposure to whatever caused the disease and the expression of clinical signs, which in one case occurred 46 years after the patient left Guam. A study of Chamorros living in California suggested that previous exposure during childhood years to an unknown factor on Guam resulted in a higher rate of ALS-PDC in the Chamorro expatriates than amongst Californians in general (Garruto, 1996).

In regard to age of onset for those remaining on Guam, the youngest documented case of ALS was at age 20, while the youngest of PDC was at age 33. A similar age of onset applied to the other, more recent ethnic populations on Guam, which began to show the disease spectrum at similar ages. For example, some Filipino migrants showed early-onset forms that could arise at 17–26 years of age (Bergeron and Steele, 1990).

The variables of age and disease incidence turned out to be crucially intertwined clues to the origins of ALS-PDC. First, these diseases had a much younger age of onset

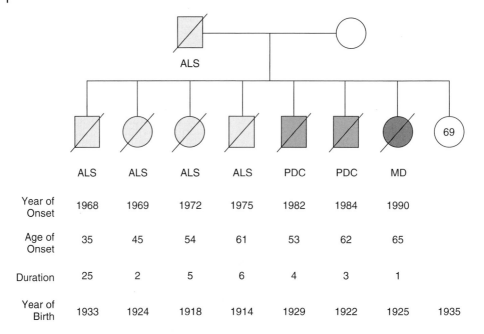

Figure 7.4 Family pedigree of ALS-PDC. Family "T.S.," southern Guam. Years of birth: 1914 through 1933. MD: Marianas dementia. *Source*: Steele (2005), with permission from John Wiley & Sons, Inc.

than equivalent diseases in North America or Europe. As cited in earlier chapters, typical ages for ALS and Parkinson's disease/parkinsonism outside of Guam typically tend to be in the middle to old range. And, as noted earlier, cases of lytico occurred in much younger victims than those who developed bodig. After the 1960s, when disease rates started to decline sharply, lytico declined more rapidly than bodig (Plato et al., 2003).

What made the ALS-PDC cluster most appealing from a neuro-epidemiology perspective was that the historical and ethnic circumstances on Guam vastly limited the number of possible causal factors. Genetic studies in the 1950s and 1960s had been carried out on a relatively homogeneous ethnic population, and environmental studies in those early years had fewer toxic factors to contend with than might be found in the more industrialized countries. All of this changed in the years after the first reports of ALS-PDC. Kurland was later to describe the spectrum of disorders in all of their diversity as an environmental event, unique to Chamorro families.

As with the age-related neurological diseases elsewhere, ALS-PDC showed other organ system involvement (Figure 7.5). One involved skin in the form of collagen disorganization similar to that already cited for ALS (Fullmer et al., 1960). Another involved diaphyseal aclasis or cartilage-capped benign bone tumors (exostoses) (Krooth et al., 1961). Still another involved retinal "tracks" that appeared in the pigment epithelial cell layer of the retina (Cox et al., 1989; Campbell et al., 1993). The latter, however, did not impact visual function. Such types of non-neuronal involvement are suggestive, as discussed previously for the other age-related neurological diseases, of multisystem disorders in which some causal factor(s) target multiple organ systems, but in which the nervous system is the most negatively affected.

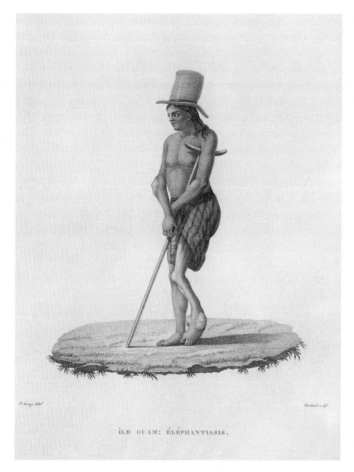

ÎLE GUAM: ÉLÉPHANTIASIS.

Figure 7.5 Guam: a man with elephantiasis? Although the disease listed is elephantiasis, the withered right leg is consistent with a secondary diagnosis of Guamanian ALS. *Source*: "Voyage Autour du Monde sur les Corvettes de L'Uranie 1817–20," engraved by Choubard, published 1825 (engraving), Arago, Jacques Etienne Victor (1790–1855) (after)/Private Collection/Bridgeman Images.

7.4 Cycad and ALS-PDC

Kurland, Mulder, and many others began an intensive search for potential causal factors, and the list, short as it was in comparison to North America, was still large. A genetic basis for the disease was considered and then discarded for lack of evidence, a conclusion that has not changed significantly after an interval of over 60 years (Morris et al., 2004; Steele et al., 2015).

The disease clustered within families, but as before, no clearly inheritable gene could be identified. Families, of course, share far more than genes. Contributory factors could be anything the family members had in common, such as food, water, and living conditions, to name only a few of the most obvious examples. Environmental studies looked at various possibilities. Some examined the effects of radiation from nuclear testing in the Pacific, or of toxic compounds left behind as the debris of the war. Others examined various trace metals in the soil and water and features of the Chamorro diet.

Kurland eventually invited Dr. Margaret Whiting, a nutritionist specializing in indigenous plants of the Pacific islands, to come to Guam to see if she could identify the cause for lytico-bodig. Whiting lived with Chamorro families for a number of months, and her time on Guam shifted the focus in the search for the cause of ALS-PDC. Whiting and other scientists considered numerous foods used by the Chamorros. With the advice of the botanist Dr. F. Raymond Fosberg, she finally began zeroing in on the seeds of an indigenous variety of palm-like trees, the cycad (Whiting, 1963), whose Guamanian subspecies is now classified as *Cycas micronesica* K.D. Hill (Figure 7.6). The link to this variety of cycad has recently been supported by another epidemiological study (Borenstein et al., 2007).

As classified by botanists, cycads are the most ancient order of the seed-bearing gymnosperm class of plants. The order *Cycadales* evolved about 250 million years ago during the Permian and early Mesozoic eras. The order includes three remaining families of 11 genera and 185 species distributed throughout the tropical regions of the world (Stevenson, 1990).

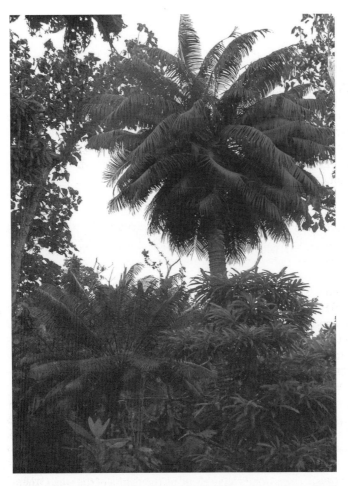

Figure 7.6 Cycad "palm" (*C. micronesica* K.D. Hill) on Guam. *Source*: Dr. Tom Marler. (See color plate section for the color representation of this figure.)

The cycad species native to Guam and other Marianas islands was named after Dr. Kenneth Hill, the botanist who finally identified it as a distinct species. Before this, the Guamanian cycad had been misclassified as *Cycas circinalis*, leading to some confusion amongst both botanists and neurologists.

On Guam and Rota, different parts of cycads in the wild are often consumed by animals and humans. On Guam, the native species of cycad have numerous animal predators. Feral pigs and deer eat the leaves, seeds, and sometimes the stalk. Coconut crabs have been known to consume the seeds. Scarab beetles and fruit bats may feed on the outer spongy later of the seed.

The Chamorros of Guam ate the seeds, and had done so for hundreds of years. They seem also to have chewed the sarcotesta, the soft outer skin, for its liquid content. However, they may not always have used cycad seeds as food, and some reports suggest that cycad consumption did not occur until the Chamorros were taught to wash out suspected toxins by Mexican natives who came to Guam with the Spanish. Much later, as Guam became westernized in diet after World War II, cycad consumption declined, but many older Chamorros continued to use and enjoy "fadang" or "federico," their terms for the flour of the cycad seed. Some Chamorros still do so to the present day, seeing in the use of fadang an affirmation of their cultural identity.

Elsewhere in the Western Pacific, parts of the cycad were historically used as a food or medicine, and neurological disease spectrums resembling that of ALS-PDC of Guam were also apparently found in some of these other locales. On the Kii peninsula of Honshu Island, Japan, seeds of *Cycas revoluta* were used apparently without processing as a miso paste ("sotetsu") and a medicinal balm (Kobayashi, 1972). Japanese and Western researchers spent years considering the possible relationships between cycad use in the two loci and the similarities of the disease spectrums. Current researchers in Japan, however, have tended to deny any linkage between the neurological disease-spectrum disorder in Kii and ALS-PDC of Guam. The reasons for such attempts to delink the two disease spectrums are not clear.

In Irian Jaya of Western New Guinea, the Auyu and Jakai people used *C. circinalis* seed flour ("kurru") without processing as a medicinal poultice. Amongst these populations, neurological disease prevalence was even higher than the average on Guam, coming in at almost 150 times that of North America (Gajdusek and Salazar, 1982). According to these authors, the prevalence of neurological diseases amongst the Auyu and Jakai populations at the time of survey was 97 for ALS and 19 for parkinsonism. As on Guam, the ALS and parkinsonism phenotypes were characterized by quite early ages of onset: 33 and 43, respectively. Based on these population numbers, the overall prevalence of ALS in Irian Jaya would appear to be 116 per 7000, or, in conventional terms, over four times higher than on Guam. PDC was also highly elevated compared to Guam (Spencer et al., 2005a). In Irian Jaya, the incidences of ALS and PDC have both declined to a considerable extent since their peak levels in the 1960s, much like on Guam (Plato et al., 2003; Spencer et al., 2005a).

7.4.1 Human Consumption of Cycad

Human consumption and other use of cycad has often been widespread amongst indigenous cultures in tropical regions around the world, including in Australia (genuses *Cycas*, *Macrozamia*, *Lepidozamia*, and *Bowenia*), India (*C. circinalis*), Southern Africa (genuses *Encephalartos* and *Stangeria*), and the New World (genuses *Zamia* and *Dioon*) (Stevenson, 1990). In Florida, the roots of the indigenous species of cycad, *Zamia floridana*, were ground up for flour by Native Americans long before the arrival of Europeans. Zamia root flour, made from *Z. floridana* and *Z. pumila* (commonly called "Florida arrowroot"), was a major commercial crop in Florida into the 20th century, much of it marketed for infant food in the form of arrowroot biscuits.

Humans have seemingly long been aware that raw cycad seed consumption or medicinal use can have adverse effects, and indeed a number of cycad species seem to contain various compounds that are toxic to humans and animals. Consumption of unprocessed cycad seeds can have acute, even fatal, outcomes, and there are numerous examples documenting cycad toxicity. One of the first such recorded cases occurred during the 1769 visit of Captain James Cook and the crew of the *Endeavour* to Australia. Some of the crew roasted and ate cycad seeds and become seriously ill as a result (The Cycad Pages, 1998–2012).

From such experiences, peoples who employ cycad as a food or medicine have usually developed some process for removing potential toxins. Australian native peoples typically ground up the seeds of *Macrozamia* and other cycad species to make a kind of slurry, which they allowed to sit for days before consumption. In modern Honduras, seeds from species of *Dioon* are harvested, ground, soaked in water containing oak wood ash, dried, and formed into flour to make tortillas. Native Mexicans historically used types of *Zamia* and *Dioon* after simple washing of the seeds, as was later done on Guam by the Chamorros with their own species of cycad.

Once introduced to cycad consumption, the Chamorros adopted it as a cultural icon. Fadang was at some times a dietary staple, at others holiday fare, showing up in either case in tortillas, dumplings, and as a thickener in soups. While many families harvested their own cycad seeds and processed their own flour, a cottage industry in fadang production sprang up that produced flour of different grades of color and consistency. The preparation consisted in cutting open the harvested seeds, extracting the white seed kernel (the gametophyte) from the hard coating, cutting the kernel into "chips," and soaking the chips in a bucket full of water, changed daily for up to 8 days. The washed chips were then sun dried and ground into flour, which was considered ready for consumption (Steele, pers. comm.) (Figure 7.7).

7.4.2 Cycad's Links to ALS-PDC

The notion that the consumption of cycad seeds could cause ALS-PDC seemed both attractive and, at the same time, problematic for Kurland and others studying the disease. One of the main attractions of the so-called "cycad hypothesis" was its simplicity, in that a toxin contained in a food product could cause neuronal degeneration leading to neurological disease if consumed in sufficient quantity.

Much of the then emerging epidemiology of ALS-PDC seemed to fit this hypothesis. For example, something much like lytico and bodig had been reported in local records since at least the early 1800s, and Chamorros had been eating cycad since at least the 1700s. Even given uncertain record-keeping, the temporal sequence seemed reasonable.

However, although cycad was consumed by most Chamorros, those in villages in the southwest such as Agat and Umatac, at the southern tip of the island in Merizo, and in the southeast at Inarajan seemed more likely to develop ALS-PDC than elsewhere on the island. The highest incidence was in Umatac. It was in these same villages, again particularly Umatac, that the disease remained at relatively high levels even as it began to decline on the rest of Guam after the 1960s.

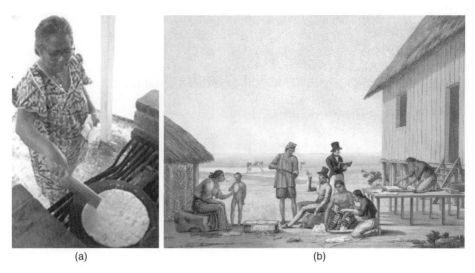

(a)   (b)

Figure 7.7 Chamorro women preparing cycad seed flour. *Source*: (a) Used with permission from Dr. John Steele; (b) From Domestic occupations, Agagna, Guam, Philippines, from "Voyage Autour du Monde (1817–20)" by Louis Claude Desaulses de Freycinet (1779–1842), engraved by Pomel, published 1822–24 (color litho), Arago, Jacques Etienne Victor (1790–1855) (after)/Private Collection/The Stapleton Collection/Bridgeman Images.

The reasons for these patterns of ALS-PDC expression remain uncertain, but they may have had something to do with the relative isolation of these villages, leading to retention of stronger ties to traditional Chamorro culture, including the consumption of fadang. Or there could have been other environmental factors or even subpopulation genetics. Researchers have speculated on different compositions of ions in the soil and water (Garruto et al., 1989) and/or on the presence of other toxic elements, such as aluminum (see Section 7.7).

A major clue to ALS-PDC had to do with what happened to Chamorros on the other islands of the southern Marianas. Guamanians, Rotans, Saipanese, and Tinians are all ethnically Chamorros – essentially one people – yet the first two groups had ALS-PDC and the other two did not, at least not during the 20th century. Disease incidence on the four islands thus fit neatly with the historical fact that cycads grew wild on Guam and Rota and the people there consumed their seeds, while the cycads had been cut down on Saipan and Tinian by the Japanese in the 1920s to make way for sugar cane plantations and the people of these islands no longer had easy access to fadang (Steele, pers. comm.).

Although ALS-PDC was often considered a uniquely Chamorro disease on Guam, Filipino immigrants developed it as well, as did some members of the US military who were resident on Guam. Linking the various ethnic groups was a cultural tie: specifically, participation in traditional Chamorro practices, including the consumption of fadang. Overall, the epidemiology of the ALS-PDC clearly indicated a role for cycad consumption in the disease.

However, there were, and remain, problems with this simple interpretation. Other peoples around the world eat various types of cycad but do not always show a heightened expression of neurological diseases, although cycad use on Japan's Kii Peninsula on the island of Honshu and in Irian Jaya did seem to be linked to neurological diseases very much like ALS-PDC, albeit in the context of different species.

In contrast, Australian native peoples ate the cycad seeds of their own genus of cycad (*Macrozamia* and others) and had no such disorders, while white settlers, including the sailors of the *Endeavour*, often became ill or died. Cattle and sheep grazing on cycad in Australia showed signs of liver and nervous system damage, the latter coupled to a movement disorder in which the back legs became increasingly uncoordinated with ataxia (referred to as the "zamia staggers"). The animals eventually showed complete paralysis of the hind legs (The Cycad Pages, 1998–2012).

7.5 Amino Acid Toxins in Cycad and ALS-PDC

Many questions arose from the early epidemiology of cycad on Guam. For example, if cycad consumption indeed causes lytico and bodig, do the seeds have one toxin that damages all of the neural areas affected in the two diseases, or are multiple toxins, each with a specific neuronal target, to blame? If multiple toxins are present, do they work alone or in synergy? Historically, why were men, on average, usually more affected than women, and why did ALS-PDC strike at younger ages than in related diseases in North America?

The putative link between cycad consumption and ALS-PDC led to a detailed search over a number of years for potential neurotoxins in cycad seeds. The first of the toxins to be identified was cycasin, a glycosylated plant amino compound (Matsumoto and Strong, 1963) (Figure 7.8). The same amino compound with two glucose molecules forms the toxin macrozamin. Cycasin and macrozamin are not particularly toxic by themselves, but removal of the glucose molecules during digestion transforms both into the deglycosylated form, methylazoxymethanol (MAM) (Figure 7.8). MAM is a relatively potent hepatic toxin that, in animals, causes cancer of the liver (Fukunishi, 1973). Various studies have shown that pregnant rats fed MAM give birth to offspring

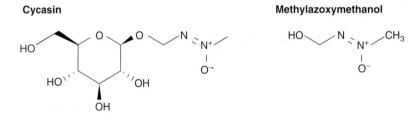

Figure 7.8 Structures of amino acids that have been implicated in ALS-PDC: cycasin, MAM, BOAA, and BMAA.

with birth defects, including retinal abnormalities (albeit not pigment epithelial tracks, as already cited in relation to human ALS-PDC) and damage to the cerebellum, the latter inducing fine motor dysfunctions (for review, see Spencer et al., 2000). Neither retinal nor cerebellar damage, however, is a usual characteristic of ALS-PDC.

In regard to those neural subsystems that are damaged in ALS-PDC, investigators looking at MAM delivered either by food or by injection in adult animals failed to find pathologies similar to the human disorders. In addition, the Chamorro practice of washing the seeds removed virtually all the cycasin/MAM present in them. In regard to this, Kurland was later to write in several review papers statements along the lines that, "The laboratory investigations of *C. circinalis* [actually *C. micronesica* K.D. Hill, as cited earlier] revealed considerable quantities of various glucosides and particularly cycasin, which has striking hepatotoxic and carcinogenic qualities but has repeatedly failed to induce an experimental disorder akin to ALS/PDC" (Kurland, 1988, p. 51).

As cited earlier, after the 1960s, disease incidence for both disorders in the Chamorro population began a sudden decline. The decline fit precisely with social observations that the Chamorros had begun to change their dietary habits to mirror those of the United States. As fast food and a Western diet became the norm in place of the traditional diet, obesity, diabetes, and heart disease became more prevalent and ALS-PDC declined, albeit at a slower rate in the southern villages where it had been more widespread.

During the same general period as the prevalence and incidence of ALS-PDC were changing, neurologists studied lathyrism, as discussed in Chapter 3. *L. sativus* contains the plant amino acid BOAA (Figure 7.8), which is also found in some cycad species, including *C. micronesica* on Guam. Although BOAA does not normally find its way into the diet of humans (again, with the exceptions cited in Chapter 3), at high doses it can be an excitotoxin and can destroy motor neurons. The notion that excitotoxicity through overactivation of glutamate receptors leads to motor neuron death has long been one of the major hypotheses for ALS (Rothstein, 1995). However, the difference between lathyrism and ALS is one of the degree of neuronal dysfunction. In lathyrism, the motor neurons are not typically destroyed; in ALS, motor neuron degeneration is a key end-state feature of the disease. Additionally, BOAA is, like cycasin, washed away by the traditional Chamorro processing of cycad seeds. For these reasons, BOAA was not thought to be the molecule responsible for ALS-PDC.

In 1967, researchers isolated BMAA (Figure 7.8), a free amino acid, from the seeds of the cycad (Bell and O'Donovan, 1966; Vega and Bell, 1967). At the time, it was considered to be unique to cycad. In the years that followed, various groups, including Dr. Peter Spencer and his colleagues, began to revisit the "cycad hypothesis," and in the process took a more detailed look at various cycad-derived excitatory amino acids. Spencer's group initially explored the notion that BOAA could be the cause of ALS-PDC, but quickly realized that the signs, symptoms, and pathologies of the two disorders were quite dissimilar. BMAA seemed a more suitable candidate, in that it activated both AMPA and NMDA subtypes of the excitatory glutamate receptors. NMDA receptor activation had by that time been linked to excitotoxic neuronal death in tissue culture studies (Weiss et al., 1989).

In a series of papers, Spencer's group claimed that feeding BMAA to monkeys reproduced some of the features of ALS-PDC, including muscle wasting and the presence of abnormal, pathological motor neurons (Spencer et al., 1987). There were, however, significant problems with the study's conclusions. First, the dosages needed to produce these effects were extremely high. Some calculations showed that for the Chamorros to have ingested enough BMAA by eating cycad flour, they would have had to have eaten at least 7 kg of unwashed raw cycad seed per day (Duncan, 1991). Second, the actual changes in the nervous system of the BMAA-fed monkeys did not really mimic the signs of ALS-PDC. Specifically, motor neurons did become dysfunctional, but they did not actually degenerate. Additionally, once BMAA feeding ceased, the monkeys showed some recovery.

In tissue-culture studies using isolated neuronal cells, BMAA appears to be a low-potency agonist, which can be toxic, but only at relatively high concentrations.

Studies performed by various investigators showed that BMAA was rapidly removed from cycad seeds by washing, falling to near-trace levels, which were far too low to impact neurons in the nervous system. Other groups tried, and failed, to find ALS-PDC-like outcomes in experimental animals (Perry et al., 1989; Cruz-Aguado et al., 2006).

These latter data and the failure of the Spencer group and others to replicate the initial findings led to a significant weakening of the corollary to the cycad hypothesis, dubbed the "BMAA hypothesis," that BMAA from cycad consumption was the key to the origins of ALS-PDC.

In 2002, the notion that BMAA might indeed be the cause of ALS-PDC experienced a resurgence with studies by Cox and colleagues, who made the additional argument that not only does BMAA from cycad cause ALS-PDC, but BMAA itself from various sources is causal to all the related disorders worldwide (Cox and Sacks, 2002). The various claims, many of them factually incorrect, can be summarized as follows: first, BMAA in cycad is actually not innate to the plant, but rather arises from *Nostoc* (blue-green) bacteria, which can colonize the cycad's roots. This assertion was shown to be erroneous by Marler et al. (2010). Second, *Nostoc*-derived BMAA makes its way through the cycad and into the seeds to be consumed by fruit bats, and is then biomagnified when humans eat the bats (Cox and Sacks, 2002).

Others following in the same vein have gone on to postulate that *Nostoc* bacteria from *any* source, including drinking water in which *Nostoc* blooms have occurred, or even desert dust that once held *Nostoc* blooms, can be the source of toxic exposure to humans and other animals (Caller et al., 2012; Bradley et al., 2013). A crucial part of the overall hypothesis is that BMAA, a free plant amino acid, becomes pathologically incorporated into proteins of the target species, and thereby disrupts various neuronal and other cellular functions. One laboratory has since demonstrated that under certain laboratory conditions, BMAA can indeed be incorporated into proteins (Dunlop et al., 2013). In spite of this, the *in vivo* evidence for ALS-PDC-like outcomes in animal models, at least in vertebrates, has remained marginal at best (as an example, see de Munck et al., 2013).

Newer evidence from the Cox group may have improved the status of the BMAA hypothesis, however (Cox et al., 2016). In their most recent study, the authors have made the claim that vervet monkeys fed BMAA in high doses develop some of the pathological features of ALS-PDC, including NFTs and amyloid plaques. NFTs are a feature of the Chamorro population of Guam, regardless of neurological status, as previously cited. Amyloid plaques, however, are not. Several aspects of this study are notable. First, it may represent the first clear evidence for BMAA-induced pathological features in an *in vivo* model. Second, the number of animals used and the statistics appear to be suitable for a study of this nature. Weighing against this are some features of the study that may suggest it is not demonstrating what it purports to demonstrate.

The first concern is that the dose used is extraordinarily high, in one series of experiments coming in at over 200 mg/kg/day. This would equal almost 12 g/day for an average human, a most unlikely amount that would have to arise from high levels of consumption of either cycad or fruit bats. Second, the pathology shown does not really resemble that of the human disease in terms of the histological aspects of either the plaques or the tangles, and there are considerable levels of artifact in the figures provided. Further, there was no apparent neuronal loss or behavioral abnormality noted. These latter aspects do not support a neurotoxin role for BMAA, unless one wants to postulate, as the authors do, that longer exposure is needed to achieve pathological outcomes. Also, notably, tauopathies can occur following other forms of toxicity, so the results here can hardly be considered specific to BMAA. The authors' continuing insistence on "bound BMAA" as a biomagnified form of the molecule is also a problem for this line of work. In brief, while vastly stronger than those data presented before, these most recent data do not provide increased confidence in the BMAA hypothesis.

The notion that BMAA, or any other molecule for that matter, is causal to ALS-PDC is one that clearly has its adherents. The same applies, as already noted, to the search for universal genetic etiologies in neurological diseases in general. The implications of such viewpoints for the search for the real causal factors in neurological disease are discussed in more detail in Chapter 15.

7.6 Non-Amino Acid Toxins Linked to ALS-PDC

A variety of other molecules have been proposed as causal to ALS-PDC and other neurological diseases. Some of these were discussed in Chapter 6.

Our own work on the subject of cycad toxicity in ALS-PDC led my laboratory to isolate what we believed to be a toxic principal in cycad seeds from Guam (Khabazian et al., 2002). This work resulted in the identification of a series of apparently toxic steryl glucosides – molecules of mostly unknown function, found largely in plants (Figure 7.9).

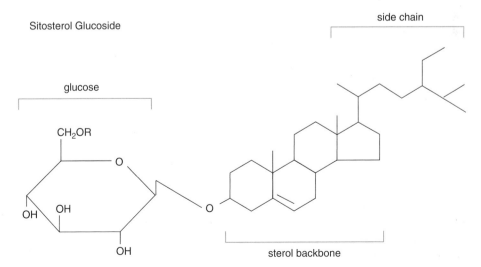

Figure 7.9 Steryl glucosides derived from cycad seeds and other plants.

The molecules are structured around the standard tetracyclic steryl backbone, with an aliphatic chain at one end of the molecule and a glucose moiety attached at the C3 position.

There are now hundreds of plant steryls known to science, many of them glycosylated. For reasons that remain unknown, the glucose molecule may confer neurotoxic properties to some of these. Fairly well-known examples of such toxic steryl glucosides include digitalis and oleandrin (Akihisa et al., 1991).

Removal of the glucose moiety by deglycosylation reactions, as well as the addition of additional glucose molecules beyond a single one, renders the molecules less toxic. Our early studies also demonstrated that a common steryl that has multiple roles in animals – cholesterol – can be made toxic by glycosylation.

A frequent critique of this work is that the three key toxic steryl glucosides that (Khabazian et al. 2002) identified are actually quite common in most plants, although cycad seeds appear to have higher than average levels, which depend rather heavily on the maturity of the seeds. In general, younger seeds have higher concentrations of these molecules than do mature ones (Marler et al., 2006). This last point assumed some potential epidemiological significance with the anecdotal reports that the Chamorros had been forced by circumstance to consume during World War II immature cycad seeds and could thereby have reached a higher toxic body burden of these steryl glucosides, or other toxins, than at other periods in their history.

The toxicity of steryl glucosides is further complicated by emerging evidence that other steryl glucosides are apparently neuroprotective. Some such molecules include several of the ginsenosoids isolated from ginseng (Van Kampen et al., 2014b).

Our additional studies demonstrated neurotoxicity not only *in vitro* but also *in vivo* in both mice and rats. The initial studies by Wilson et al. (2002) on cycad and steryl glucosides given to mice by diet (Tabata et al., 2008) showed motor neuron loss in various regions of the brain and spinal cord (Figure 7.10). Although the behavioral deficits were primarily motor in nature, as was the underlying pathology, the mice would progressively show lesions in the SN, hippocampus, and cortex. These latter pathologies engendered many PDC features, including cognitive deficits (Wilson et al., 2002).

These studies have now largely been replicated in other laboratories (see the work of the Gustafsson group, as cited in articles by Andersson et al., 2005 and Kim et al., 2008, which has linked steryl glucoside's toxic effects to the Liver X receptor, a potential molecular target).

One of the more surprising outcomes is the differences seen with cycad or isolated β-sitosterol-β-D glucoside (BSSG) in mice compared to rats. In mice, as already noted, the dominant feature was a progressive ALS phenotype. In rats, the sole phenotype was that of a Lewy body type of parkinsonism (Shen et al., 2010; Van Kampen et al., 2014b, 2015) (Figures 7.11, 7.12).

What these results seem to suggest is that the same molecule can drive very different neuronal outcomes, which are, in part, species-dependent, in a way that produces the full ALS-PDC spectrum of disorders. Whether this means that the molecule is metabolized differently in mice compared to rats or whether it gains preferential access to particular regions of the nervous system in each species remains unknown. Differences in the ability of the different rodent species to metabolize toxins have been well established in the *in vivo* animal model of Parkinson's disease literature (Jenner and Marsden, 1986).

Another surprising feature of both the mouse and rat studies was that in both cases the animals showed an initially unilateral behavioral response deficit, accompanied by

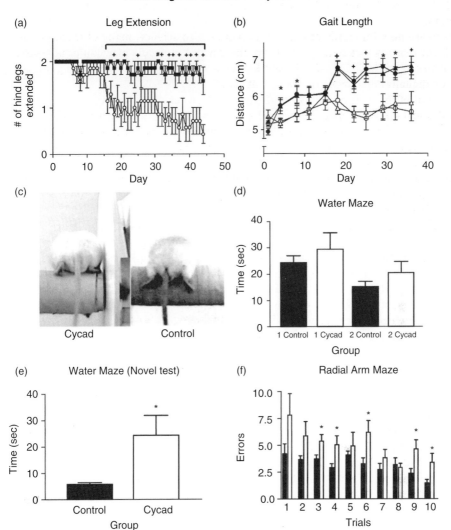

Figure 7.10 *In vivo* data from cycad feeding studies in mice: motor and cognitive effects of cycad feeding. Control animals are indicated by black symbols or bars. Cycad-fed animals are indicated by white symbols or bars. (a) Leg extension as a function of time in days. (b) Gait length as a function of time in days. Circles indicate right stride length and triangles indicate left stride length (both measured as ipsilateral to ipsilateral). (c) Typical body positions of cycad-fed and control mice on the rotarod. (d) Averaged Morris water maze test scores during the entire cycad feeding period. Set 1 includes the first four trials and set 2 the next four trials. (e) Morris water maze following relocation of the platform to a new position. (f) Radial arm maze errors per trial for the same mice at the completion of feeding experiments. Significance: *p < 0.05; +p < 0.0001, ANOVA. *Source*: Wilson et al. (2002), with permission from Springer Science and Business Media.

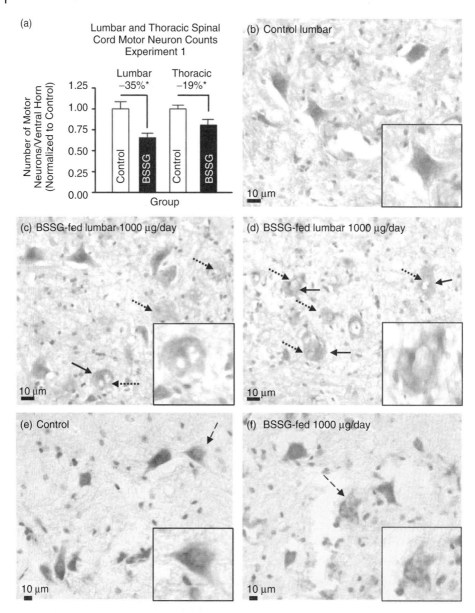

Figure 7.11 *In vivo* data from BSSG feeding studies in mice: motor neuron counts following BSSG treatment. CD-1 mice fed 1000 μg of BSSG/day for 15 weeks. Mice were sacrificed 17 weeks later and lumbar and thoracic spinal cord motor neuron were stained and counted. (a) Lumbar and thoracic spinal cord motor neuron counts; t-test *p < 0.05; (b–d) Normal (control) and abnormal (BSSG-fed) motor neuron morphology visualized with cresyl violet staining in the lumbar spinal cord. (e,f) Cresyl violet staining in the thoracic spinal cord of a control and a BSSG-fed animal. Scale bars, all panels = 10 μm. *Source*: Tabata et al. (2008), with permission from Springer Science and Business Media.

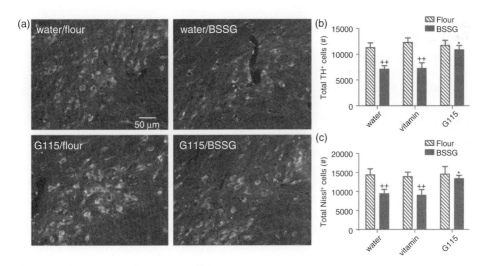

Figure 7.12 *In vivo* data from BSSG feeding studies in rats. (a) Representative fluorescent photomicrographs of tyrosine hydroxulase (TH) (green) and Nissl (red) immunostaining in the SN 35 weeks following initial BSSG exposure. Unbiased stereologic counts of (b) TH + and (c) Nissl + cells in the SN were significantly reduced in those animals treated with BSSG. However, no significant cell loss was observed in those animals treated with G115, a ginseng-derived molecule. In contrast, vitamin supplementation alone failed to alter BSSG-induced nigral cell loss. Each bar represents the mean ($\pm$ SEM, n = 9–12) number of TH or Nissl immunopositive cells counted in the SN. ++sig. diff. from flour control, $p < 0.001$; + $p < 0.05$. **sig. diff. from water control, $p < 0.001$. *Source*: Modified from Van Kampen et al. (2014a), with permission from Elsevier. The caption has been modified from the published article. (See color plate section for the color representation of this figure.)

unilateral spinal cord or brain lesions. Eventually, the effects became generalized to both sides of the spinal cord or brain. This outcome should not, perhaps, have been such a surprise given that this is exactly how Parkinson's disease and ALS present in humans. The issue of initial laterality has already been addressed in Chapter 2 and will be further considered in Chapter 11.

Overall, the notion that various steryl molecules, particularly those that are glycosylated, can be either neurotoxic or neuroprotective is finding additional support from a variety of sources (for a recent review, see Vanmierlo et al., 2015).

As a final note concerning cycad and ALS-PDC, some early (and largely unknown) studies by Dr. Darab Dastur fed cooked and uncooked cycad seed flour to rhesus monkeys. These studies described how he successfully reproduced some aspects of ALS-PDC in terms of both behavioral effects and neuropathology (Dastur, 1964). Many of the data produced, including detailed histological assays, went unpublished for over 25 years (Dastur et al., 1990).

7.7 Aluminum and Ionic Etiologies for ALS-PDC

There has been a considerable amount of work attempting to link purportedly high levels of aluminum in the soil and water of parts of Guam to where ALS-PDC-like disorders appear to be particularly prevalent. Aluminum neurotoxicity was noted in Chapter 6 as a likely factor contributing to some cases of neurological disease, and its neurotoxic potential is now commonly accepted as being established (Tomljenovic, 2011; Exley, 2012).

Garruto et al. (1989) noted high levels of calcium and aluminum in NFTs in the post-mortem hippocampus of ALS-PDC patients. Similar associations between NFTs and aluminum have been noted by other investigators (Perl et al., 1982), including for the disease spectrum in Kii, Japan (Kihira et al., 1993).

The investigators looking at high aluminum on Guam and Irian Jaya postulated that a contributing factor was the low concentrations of calcium and magnesium, which, in their view, led to a secondary parathyroidism causing aluminum accumulation by neurons. This suggestion was reinforced by studies which found low vitamin D levels in males with ALS on Guam, but these studies also noted that differences in calcium were "subtle" (Yanagihara et al., 1984).

In vivo models using monkeys given a high-aluminum/low-calcium diet appear to support the general hypothesis of an aluminum involvement by showing degenerative changes in the motor neurons of the spinal cord and brain stem, as well as neurons in the SN and cerebrum (Garruto et al., 1989). Many of the pathological features of these affected neurons resemble those of ALS-PDC.

It should be noted that the measured ionic concentrations of calcium and aluminum in the soil and water of Guam were not validated by other researchers (Steele and Williams, 1995).

7.8   Still Other Molecules Causal to ALS-PDC

The list of potential toxins involved in ALS-PDC includes a variety of other molecules, both natural and of human origin. These include some toxins associated with fishing using powdered *Barringtonia asiatica*, known as "the fish-kill plant" (Cannon et al., 2004), zinc from galvanized pails used for washing cycad seeds (Duncan et al., 1992), and a host of others.

Part of the search for additional toxins results from the very clear observation that none of those described to date can be said to be the definitive toxin responsible for the disease spectrum on Guam.

Additionally, in spite of the initial hope of Kurland and others that Guam might serve as a model geographic isolate, the search amongst the relatively limited potential causal factors has not proven as easy as they might have wished. In reality, Guam in the years during and after World War II was a very toxic environment due to a number of contaminants that came with the war. This highlights that although Guamanian ALS-PDC may arise from a smaller subset of potential toxins and toxic synergies than is present in North America, the number is still large – likely too large to accommodate a version of the one-hit hypothesis.

7.9   What is the Current View on the Importance of ALS-PDC?

ALS-PDC has historically been a neurological disorder that neurologists, neuroscientists, and epidemiologists either obsessively like or intensely dislike. Those who like it do so because it is mysterious, exotic, and somewhat romantic (due to its location), and it offers the hope of a relatively simple universal toxin or gene etiology that may be applicable to age-dependent neurological diseases elsewhere.

Those who dislike it, however, are far and away the majority, and the reasons for their disdain are relatively simple. There is the obvious observation that ALS-PDC is a "messy" neurological disease: It often combines the features of what are traditionally considered very distinct neurological diseases, in that ALS may occur in an individual who has parkinsonism, but not necessarily at the same time. Further, families can show individuals with one form of the disease spectrum or the other, both, or none.

In some ways, the spectrum of ALS-PDC resembles the overlapping features of ALS and FTD, already cited, and the often overlapping pathologies of Parkinson's and Alzheimer's diseases (Kurosinski et al., 2002). There may also be a temporal lag between exposure to some toxic factor (or the onset of a particular gene product) that makes the correlation to any potential toxin nearly impossible to satisfy using the Hill criteria. In these regards, those seeking a simple etiology for ALS-PDC find that the spectrum does not have one, but rather has a range of likely additive or perhaps synergistic factors.

Next, while there is/was an ethnic factor (i.e., Chamorro heritage/ethnicity), there is no clear genetic mutation or even distinct polymorphism that can be linked to the disorder in any of its multiple manifestations (Morris et al., 2004).

Finally, the various toxin studies carried out have shown disparate, contradictory, and even downright biologically implausible outcomes. In regard to the latter, the current incarnation of the so-called "BMAA hypothesis" is mostly based on observational rather than experimental studies and would likely fail any reasonable evaluation using the Hill criteria.

Perhaps most definitively, a key reason for dismissing ALS-PDC as relevant is that it has been disappearing. No one born after the 1960s has the disease (Galasko et al., 2002), reinforcing the notion that it was, and is, a neurological anomaly, with no particular relevance for understanding any of the other age-related, progressive neurological diseases elsewhere.

All of these reasons are completely valid and understandable. And yet, to a large measure, they miss the key point that ALS-PDC remains the sole widely accepted disease cluster of ALS, parkinsonism, and Alzheimer's disease.

There may, however, be minor and even significant exceptions to this last statement. For example, there may be a subcluster of ALS contained within the broad-spectrum multisystem disorders characterizing Gulf War Syndrome (Haley, 2003). There is also an apparent cluster of a form of parkinsonism associated with consumption of soursop toxins amongst the inhabitants of Guadeloupe in the French West Indies, as cited in Chapter 3. Additionally, ALS-PDC-like disorders have been described for a wider region of the Pacific, including Irian Jaya and the Kii Peninsula of Japan, as also cited previously.

Apart from these examples, there are no other clusters of ALS or Parkinson's disease (or parkinsonism), and none at all for Alzheimer's disease. For these reasons alone, unless the neurological disease field is going to seek answers without first identifying a disease cluster, ALS-PDC remains the most relevant age-related neurological disease spectrum still available.

The study of ALS-PDC had – and maybe still has, in spite of its fading away – some key lessons to teach the world of neurological disease research. Of course, one has to be receptive to these lessons – a perhaps unlikely proposition given the trajectory of the field at present. If one were able to look at the issues objectively, and not solely through a reductionist lens, the following would be the key points to consider:

- None of the main disorders in the ALS-PDC spectrum, neither ALS, parkinsonism (and by extension, Parkinson's disease), nor Alzheimer's disease, is truly independent of the others. First, a reasonably large fraction of those with one have some variation of the others as well. For example, those with ALS and Parkinson's disease often show cognitive dysfunctions as the disease progresses. This is quite obvious for ALS-FTD, but occurs in more classical ALS as well, as cited previously.

- The classical hallmark protein features of Alzheimer's disease, abnormally phosphorylated tau protein and Aβ deposits, however toxic to neurons, are not the key triggering factors. This can be concluded from the fact that abnormal tau deposits can be found in ALS-PDC-free individuals (cited in Kurland, 1988) and that the amyloid deposits so typical in non-Guamanian Alzheimer's are largely absent in ALS-PDC.

- The neuronal diseases in the spectrum can occur in a familial setting, but the expression of one type versus another is apparently dependent on other, still unknown factors. These factors, given a family setting, are not likely to be solely dietary/waterborne (environmental), sex-linked, or genetic mutations of any simple sort. They might, however, be caused by genetic susceptibility factors – polymorphisms within the normal range of expression – which both contribute to the onset of the disorder and further specify which subtype of disease will arise.

- The decline in ALS-PDC incidence suggests that the triggering factor, presumably of environmental origin, has diminished over the same time period. A second and also likely possibility is that since the Guamanian population is now more genetically heterogeneous due to intermarriage with non-Chamorros, genetic susceptibility factors have changed as well.

- These issues point to gene–toxin interactions as key to the etiology of ALS-PDC. This makes it likely that the field could search endlessly (assuming the diseases still exists in a few years) without identifying a clear causal gene mutation, as suggested by Morris et al. (2004). It also means that no environmental trigger, no matter how toxic in model systems, is going to account for the disease spectrum either.

- The impact of the microbiome is likely in the future to be seen as having a profound effect on how toxin and/or genetic mutations affect disease expression. In the context of Guam, it remains important to keep in mind that the homogeneous genetic population prior to World War II and the impact of widespread starvation during the years of Japanese occupation may have contributed in significant ways to disease rates.

- A more productive way to think about gene–toxin/microbiome interactions might be to try to reverse engineer the entire process. Thus, rather than seeking mutations, maybe researchers should be looking at toxin-induced pathways/signaling and asking instead what genes/gene products allow the toxin to have access to the CNS. This topic was addressed, in part, in the studies of aluminum-induced gene expression cited in Chapter 6.

- Finally, unless the field finds another similar neurological disease cluster, or unless it devotes considerable resources to studying ALS-PDC while it is still extant on Guam and Irian Jaya, it is not likely to ever sort through the thousands of potential genetic and environmental factors, let alone the combinations of the same, that may be involved.

The primary difference in perspective between those who like the challenge of ALS-PDC and those who find it merely an annoying anomaly is basically one of reductionism. Put another way, will a reductionist approach that learns more and more about less and less achieve greater success than an approach that takes a more macroscopic view of disease origins and time courses?

In some ways, this is the fundamental question this book seeks to address. The arguments on both sides of this issue will direct a large part of the conclusion that any complex adaptive system, with its propensity to break in a process of cascading failures, needs more the macro than the micro perspective.

7.10   Complexity of Neurological Diseases as Viewed from Guam

As discussed in previous chapters, complexity is a fundamental part of the nervous system in development and in function, both in health and illness. It is clear that the rules governing the organization of the nervous system are many, that there are multiple stages, and that interactions of cellular and systems elements are the norm. Except in the case of utterly traumatic CNS injury, it is also clear that the processes by which the CNS is altered for the worse cannot help but be equally complex.

As I will show in Chapter 16, the ultimate therapeutic approach is almost certain to be prophylaxis. Restoration of a partially, let alone a widely destroyed neural system would be unlikely to succeed, if only because of the vast number of things that would need to be fixed or restored. Halting degenerative cascades, depending on stage, may prove nearly as difficult.

Prophylaxis thus remains the key, as it does in other diseases. This will be the focus of later chapters in which I will review the status of current and prospective neurological disease treatments. In regard to the latter, the relative success, or failure, of such treatments will better make the ultimate case for a prophylactic approach.

Before delving into current treatment paradigms, however, it is important to consider how they are compromised by the limits of the model systems approach. This is the subject of the next chapter. And, beyond this, the additional factors of development, age, and interactions with other biological systems must be considered in any attempt to truly understand the progressive neurological diseases.

Endnote

1 Grammarist: http://grammarist.com/usage/perfect-storm/ (last accessed September 23, 2016).

Part II

Age and Time Lines of Neurological Disease

8

Neurological Disease Models and their Discontents: Validity, Replicability, and the Decline Effect

> *"Insanity: doing the same thing over and over again and expecting different results."*
> Attributed to Albert Einstein

From the Preface

10) Any models of neurological diseases, no matter what kind of model or for which disease, are at best a limited means of understanding the complexity of the particular disease. They are even less effective in developing therapeutic approaches to early or late disease states.
11) Many of the data in the literature in any of the subfields of neurological disease research are likely to be wrong, and thus highly misleading. Each subfield needs a thorough review to cull such incorrect material. This is not likely to happen.

8.1 Introduction

The chapters in Part I have introduced the major age-related neurological diseases and put them into the context of complexity in general and the complexity of the central nervous system (CNS) specifically. The studies thus far discussed on putative gene and toxin etiologies have arisen from the only two sources possible: observational and anatomical/biochemical studies of humans with such diseases and model systems.

Before proceeding to deal with additional contributory factors to neurological diseases, such as those arising from age, sex, and interactions with other organ systems, it is important to understand the limitations in design and interpretation of both human studies and the models used to understand human diseases.

Concerning the latter, any attempt to understand neurological diseases, either in terms of origins and underlying mechanisms or in regard to the testing of potential therapies, ultimately has to rely on model systems of the disease state. Herein lies an inevitable, and perhaps largely fatal, flaw in neurological disease research. Some of the same concerns almost certainly apply to research into diseases of other organ systems.

Neural Dynamics of Neurological Disease, First Edition. Christopher A. Shaw.
© 2017 John Wiley & Sons, Inc. Published 2017 by John Wiley & Sons, Inc.

8.2   Modeling Human Neurological Diseases: Possibilities and Pitfalls

If researchers want to study human neurological diseases, their origins, progression, and, ideally, the means to alleviate them, they can only really do so in one of two ways. The first is by observation, the second by experimentation.

Observation is the basis of empiricism, the forerunner to the scientific method, and is still the basis of much of what scientists know – or think they know – about most things in the natural world. Experimentation, which was formalized by Roger Bacon in the 13th century, building on the work of others, has become a powerful means of discovery, with the scientific method being one of the most effective ways humans have invented of understanding nature. It is not, however, the only way of doing so, nor one that is suited to all forms of inquiry. Nor is it necessarily a methodology that "must inevitably provide answers for all questions," as some might assert. The latter notion will be discussed in more detail in later chapters.

Observation has been the basis for the initial descriptions of the various neurological diseases, and continues to contribute to a large part of the existing literature. As such, it is subject to the caveats cited in Chapter 5 in the context of the Hill criteria.

The eponymous diseases, Alzheimer's, Parkinson's, Huntington's, and others (including, of course, ALS, more properly be called Charcot's disease, rather than Lou Gehrig's disease), followed from the observations of the scientists who first wrote up case reports or case series on patients with the features of each. Observation in all of these cases has been powerful in that it has made lists of signs and symptoms and assigned people to categories based on how many of each that they exhibit. It has also provided information on disease progression post identification and lists of the various comorbidities.

What observation cannot do, however, is provide much information about the mechanism(s) involved in the disease process. This is not to say that observation combined with post-mortem studies cannot tell researchers something about the key hallmarks of any disorder (e.g., the presence of NFTs and Aβ plaques in Alzheimer's disease). It cannot, however, tell researchers much of anything about pre-disease states; that is, when a disease originates or what the susceptibility factors leading to it might be. Nor can it provide much insight into the stages leading to the eventual clinical presentation of the disease or how it progresses to its eventual end state.

One can, of course, assume how such things come about, and further assume that the point of observation accurately reflects the disease, but these assumptions are not likely to be correct. In fact, such assumptions may be wildly invalid, and only serve to mislead the field. One could almost term such incorrect assumptions an example of a neurological version of "Holmberg's mistake."

As described by Charles C. Mann in his book *1491* (Mann, 2005), Allan R. Holmberg was a doctoral student who spent time in the early 1940s amongst the Sirionó people of the Beni province of current Bolivia. The Sirionó appeared to Holmberg to be quite primitive in their cultural and material skills, and he depicted them in this way in his published writings. This depiction led to the assumption that such a condition was consistent with a simple, close-to-nature state of being for such groups. Subsequent anthropological and archaeological studies were to demonstrate, however, that the modern Sirionó were not primitive because they and their ancestors lived close to nature, but rather because they were the small surviving remnant of a vastly larger and more sophisticated culture that had collapsed due to invasion and disease. In other words, by taking a picture out of context in a time frame of events and assuming that it was representative of an initial starting point, Holmberg had created an illusion of the Sirionó and people like them that bore little or no resemblance to their actual history.

What Holmberg did with his observations of the Sirionó would be the equivalent of looking at Jewish concentration camp survivors at the end of World War II and assuming that they were representative of a vibrant pre-war European Jewish culture.

Holmberg's mistake misled generations of anthropologists, and no doubt continues to do so, although Holmberg himself apparently acknowledged the issue in later years (see Mann, 2005).

As discussed in previous places in this book, much of medical science is largely reductionist in its basic nature. It is also highly sectarian. Given the latter, it is perhaps likely that relatively few of those working in the various disciplines, including those in neurological disease research, will be aware of Holmberg's mistake or the potential for something similar to occur in their own domains. Instead, it is more than likely that a conceptually similar snapshot out of time and sequence has occurred in neurological disease research in the past, and could again in the future, leading the field in a wrong direction.

One way out of this possible type of mistake would be to create an accurate time line of events that begins long before the snapshot is taken and extends far beyond it. Indeed, if Holmberg had enjoyed the benefits of knowing in advance the anthropological and archaeological discoveries to come, he might have been able to create such a time line and thus avoid the assumptions that were to prove so dramatically wrong for him and the field of cultural anthropology.

In terms of neurological diseases, one can imagine that if researchers could intensively observe and test, perhaps with biomarkers or imaging, a significant fraction of the population longitudinally – in a neurological equivalent to the epidemiological Framingham cardiovascular study – they could use observation alone to understand many aspects of the progression of neurological diseases. The Framingham study, to be described in more detail in Chapter 9, involved a very large number of participants and was designed to examine the time line of progression of cardiovascular disease and the emerging potential risk factors from onset until the end of the participants' lives.

There are, however, two problems with trying to make neurological diseases approachable by such methods. The first is that barring a major shift in governmental priorities, a project of this scope and cost is simply not going to happen in neurological disease research. The second is that neurological diseases such as Alzheimer's, for all their increasing prevalence (and maybe incidence), simply do not occur often enough in the population to be studied in this way (see Chapter 2). The justification for the Framingham study was that with cardiovascular disease impacting roughly 50% of the population by age 50, studying it at random in presymptomatic individuals would eventually lead to a significant patient population with and without such disease. In contrast, Alzheimer's disease, the most common neurological disorder apart from epilepsy, has an age-dependent prevalence ranging from just 2.8 to 1275.0 per 100 000 (see Chapter 2). Researchers would thus need to study a vast number of subjects who would never show the disease in order to find a future patient population that would. Of course, the number of those afflicted with Alzheimer's increases with increasing age, but it is important to remember that what is really wanted is to see the initial stages of the disease, not just the late or end states.

For neurological diseases with lower prevalence, the problem of numbers becomes even more acute, and thus even less feasible. In ALS, for example, researchers would have to examine 100 000 individuals to get just 2–4 cases at some future time point.

At such a ratio, it would have to study a vast number of people to obtain even reasonable numbers of ALS cases for an exploration of the range and diversity of the disease.

One can make back-of-the-envelope calculations here, but to get Framingham-like numbers for Alzheimer's, the number in the initial presymptomatic study population would be something on the order of hundreds of times higher; for ALS, it would be closer to thousands of times higher. Given the spectrum nature of both diseases, the numbers would probably have to be higher still.

Perhaps if epidemiology had successfully identified more disease clusters like ALS-PDC to bolster the numbers, such a study would be feasible. In their absence, it is not. Further, ALS-PDC is vanishing, so that particular line of attack is closed as well.

All of these issues tie back to the financial aspects of such a study, and the inevitable conclusion that observational studies alone as a means of understanding the origins of neurological diseases are simply not going to be feasible.

This conclusion brings the discussion back to experimentation as a means of evaluating neurological diseases. Leaving aside the ethical concerns, who will be experimented on? Presymptomatic individuals are obviously not suitable. Those already diagnosed with the disease might be, but they alone cannot tell us much, if anything, about disease origins. Nor, judging by the routine failures of therapeutic trials (see Chapters 13 and 14), will they tell researchers much about the myriad disease mechanisms or the cascading failures that have led to the current disease state.

In regard to this last point, it is quite instructive to go to various symposia, or read various articles, which employ genomic, proteomic, or metabolomics techniques. Apart from the technical competence of such studies, one can clearly see the actual dimension of the problem at play in such presentations. For example, what is one to make of the notion that literally hundreds of genes and molecules are different in end-state disease from controls? Leaving aside for now the issue of replicability – a huge problem, to be discussed in Section 8.4.2 – what can be known from the changed molecules in such studies about disease progression? What can be known about which are part of the disease process and which might be bystanders or even part of compensatory events? What therapeutic approaches can be imagined to address the tens, hundreds, or thousands of altered genes, proteins, and metabolites?

The blunt answer to these questions is that even if researchers could address them, there is little to be done therapeutically for the large numbers of genes and molecules that are impacted at the late-stage time point after clinical diagnosis, or even later.

8.3 Considerations Regarding Model Systems

The preceding considerations bring researchers ultimately to the technique that many in neurological disease research have chosen as the means to understand these diseases: model systems. Of these, there are basically three types: computer modeling, *in vitro* methods using some sort of cell-culture preparation, and *in vivo* methods using various non-human animals. Of these, *in vivo* methods are arguably the best, as they allow both for presumed reasonably close comparisons to humans and for invasive means of examining biological processes that cannot ethically be performed on human subjects.

Regardless of the type of model contemplated, it should attempt to satisfy some basic criteria. Three of these are as follows, although there are variants and alternatives described in the literature (Belzung and Lemoine, 2011):

- *Face validity*: Does the model system and its response to the experimental manipulation mirror the thing/disease state that is being modeled? These considerations apply to underlying molecular and cellular mechanisms, as well as to such aspects as the initial unilateral presentation in Parkinson's disease and ALS. The extent to which these issues are satisfied makes any model more or less valid. This criterion has come under recent scrutiny in regard to ALS models, as detailed by Cox (2011) and others (Seok et al., 2013). Genetic and toxin models in which the respective neural subtypes do not actually and routinely degenerate would (or should) fail this criterion.
- *Construct validity*: Does the model accurately measure what it is intended to measure. In a model of Parkinson's disease or ALS, for example, the system should provide predictable, time-dependent neuronal losses in areas known to be affected in the human disease, and, crucially, these should be induced in similar ways. For example, construct validity in models of ALS-PDC would be accompanied by neuronal degeneration in the respective neural subareas and induced by a cycad diet, not by intravenous injections of putative cycad toxins.
- *Predictive validity*: Does the model accurately predict outcomes in other organ systems, especially in human patients which are not yet known? Or, does the model provide an outcome that may have been observed in humans but has not been addressed because it was deemed to be anecdotal? As before, both Parkinson's disease and ALS often present unilaterally in the early stages before becoming bilateral. A predictive animal model would do the same. Another predictive aspect would be to find the involvement of other organ systems, as in the human disease: collagen abnormalities in the skin of ALS patients would be one example.

Another criterion, not often considered, might be that of *epidemiological* validity. For example, if cycad toxins delivered through diet induce ALS-PDC in humans, the model of the disease should preferably use cycad fed to the experimental animal, rather than another source of the toxin or another toxin altogether. This criterion might be viewed as more a corollary of face validity than a stand-alone measure of validity.

Finally, there is the need for reproducibility, or replicability. This is not a trivial concern, as demonstrated in the work of Ioannidis (2005) and discussed in Section 8.4.2.

8.4 Model Systems and their Discontents

Obviously, the value of a model depends on the extent to which it satisfies each of these criteria. Models that do not satisfy them, at least in part, are not likely to be functionally valid for understanding and treating human diseases.

The concept of *ceteris paribus*, Latin for "with all other things the same" (or "all equal"), is relevant for what follows. A *ceteris paribus* assumption in any model is that most or all of the variables that must be controlled for are, in fact, controlled for, at least under "normal" conditions. How often this applies is questionable, as some of the following will make clear.

The accuracy of computer models (also termed "*in silico* models") depends on the accuracy of the biological data on which they are based. These data can only come from human observational studies or various *in vitro* and *in vivo* models. As will be discussed in more detail later, such data are notoriously unreliable for a variety of reasons (see Ioannidis, 2005; Young et al., 2008). As an example, the models on which they are based may not be valid, or the data themselves may not be representative of the overall condition. Less commonly, there may in some cases be actual instances of scientific fraud. Each of these issues can thus become a fundamental problem, rendering the computer model irrelevant. The common phrase, "garbage in, garbage out," can easily be applied to *in silico* methods and is something to be aware of.

In vitro models do not fare much better. While they are attractive from a reductionist perspective in attempting to control most experimental variables, they may not actually do so. In addition, the almost total artificiality of such models in the context of a real neurological system renders many of them nearly useless for actually mirroring the disease state. For example, neuronal cell cultures routinely use late fetal or early postnatal cells in the culture dish. The developing CNS and the adult CNS are completely different places in terms of structures and connections, synaptic development, types and subtypes of receptors and other molecules expressed, regulatory mechanisms, and so on. One example will suffice: The glutamate receptor subtype of the AMPA receptor shows age-dependent changes in structure and hence the ions fluxed by neurotransmitter activation of the neuron (Burnashev et al., 1992; Pagliusi et al., 1994). Attempting to use an *in vitro* model to study the role of AMPA receptors in age-dependent neurological disease would run the risk that the types of event that impact AMPA receptor activation and turn on sodium currents in young neurons would not be the same as those that drive calcium currents in adult neurons. There are numerous other examples.

For reasons such as these, trying to model adult CNS disorders and employ experimental therapeutics in a culture preparation, and expecting to have these data translate into effective treatments *in vivo* in humans, is not realistic. This point comes across quite forcefully in studies in neurological disease, as well as in other diseases.

In addition, the cells in the culture preparation are not in a normal context to other cells normally found in the CNS: in trying to culture a particular type of neuron, one routinely attempts to avoid the presence of the various types of glial cells. This is not completely possible, and thus limits the effective life span of the culture, because not doing so runs the risk of having the undesired glial cells overrun the culture dish.

There is also the deeper problem that a large part of the underlying mechanisms in various neurological diseases likely arise from abnormal neuron–glial interactions; that is, the non-cell-autonomous mechanisms already cited. If this is not modeled in the dish, then the relevance to the human *in vivo* disease is, at best, very questionable. In the worst case, it is likely to be irrelevant.

How do *in vivo* models compare? This is sort of a crucial question, since, as already mentioned, the field does not have much else to fall back upon. The answer is complex, and there are a range of issues to address, many actually never given much scrutiny by numerous investigators.

First, needless to say, the various tests of validity need to be satisfied to a greater rather than lesser degree in *in vivo* models. Then there are some even more fundamental concerns.

The first of these has to do with the species to be employed. Ideally, one would work with humans for the study of human diseases. However, invasive *in vivo* studies of humans are rarely possible, for a variety of reasons – truly invasive ones are not likely to be ethical. The next best option is to use primates, but such experiments come with their own set of problems. One is expense; another is the increasing opposition from animal rights activists. Both problems lead to a justifiable reluctance by researchers to use primates in almost any experimental scenario. Another problem, one rarely addressed, is this: Primates are obtained for research either by capture or by breeding them in captivity. Unlike established rodent colonies, colony-bred monkeys are much closer to a "wild type" in genetic expression – as, incidentally, are humans. What this means for primate studies is that one can expect greater variability with a monkey population, especially in experimental treatments involving any form of drug, than with a colony rodent population. The solution to this problem is to increase numbers, as is done in human drug trials, but this then runs into the previously mentioned problem of cost. Alternatively, the experimenter can try to overcome the wild-type genotype/phenotype by using drug doses beyond those humans might reasonably experience. The latter becomes an obvious problem in its own right.

A recent example will illustrate the nature of the primate problem. Curtis et al. (2015), in an attempt to examine the potential impact of pediatric vaccines as a hypothesized causal factor in ASD, subjected early postnatal-age male macaques (*Macaca malatta*) to a vaccine injection schedule comparable to that given to young human children. The study seemed well done in general, and the numbers (12–16 per group) should have been sufficient to provide a clear statistical analysis. The results seemed to suggest that there were no significant impacts of the vaccines on the neurobehavioral development or any structural features of the injected monkeys.

The problem lay in the nature of the model in comparison to the epidemiology of the human disease. Roughly 1 in 68 children in the United States has one of the disorders within the ASD spectrum (Centers for Disease Control and Prevention, 2016). Thus, to correctly model a wild-type human population with a wild-type monkey population, the researchers should have used vastly more monkeys in each treatment group. No doubt they had done a proper power analysis to calculate the number of animals needed, but the very fact that it was a wild-type population made this otherwise very reasonable effort problematic in terms of the final interpretation.

If such problems attend the use of primates, what about more common experimental species, such as mice and rats? These have the advantage that they are less likely to suffer from wild-type population issues, but this becomes a problem in its own right as they are not likely to be representative of humans in two regards. First, they are far removed in the mammalian family tree from primates and can exhibit quite different biochemical and metabolic processes, not only from humans, but from each other (see, e.g., Sundström and Samuelsson, 1997 on MPTP toxicity in rodents and Seok et al., 2013). Second, while amongst humans individual genetic variations in expression can be quite different (as can variations in living conditions, types of food, conditions of water, etc.), laboratory animal colonies minimize all of these aspects.

Most of this is well known. The problem that arises is that these issues are typically not dealt with in the design of experiments, at least in most mammalian studies.

One solution to issues of variability in neurological disease studies is to increase the levels of the putative causal factor, be it genetic or molecular. In the former case, there is the clear example provided by the (mSOD1) studies used to model ALS, in which the transgenic animals have extremely high copy numbers of the mutant gene. In contrast, in fALS in humans, a single copy of m*SOD1* is sufficient to induce motor neuron degeneration (see Zwiegers et al., 2014 for citations). Similarly, toxin studies often employ much higher concentrations of the suspected substances than most human neurological disease victims would likely be exposed to.

All of this plays out dominantly, albeit not uniquely, in ALS *in vivo* animal studies. It is thus instructive for this discussion to consider again the various genetic models of ALS, which often generate a discernible ALS-like phenotype of altered motor behavior and loss of motor neurons.

Dr. Gregory Cox of Jackson Laboratories gave an illuminating talk at an ALS/motor neuron disease (MND) meeting in Sydney, Australia in 2011 in which he compared the workhorse model in the field, m*SOD1 in vivo*, to a variety of newer genetic models derived from other genes involved in fALS (Cox, 2011). Cox's analysis showed that, to a great extent, most of the extant genetic models failed, at least in part, a significant fraction of the tests of validity. All of this was put into the humorous context of whether ALS itself was a good model of ALS: his conclusion was that it was not, in large part due to the spectrum nature of the disease.

None of this should have been news to those working in the field. And yet the widespread near consensus, at least that voiced publicly, is that while the models may not be "perfect," they are the best that the field has. Indeed, this was Cox's own conclusion as well.

The "best we have" is a pretty thin basis for understanding disease mechanisms, let alone designing effective, targeted therapeutic interventions for human patients. This last point is perhaps crucial for understanding why apparently successful animal studies almost never turn into successful outcomes in human trials. In ALS, to date, they never have, as will be discussed in detail in Chapter 13.

One recent report in the literature illustrates why such a disconnection in so-called "translational" medicine may arise. Seok and colleagues compared the genes activated by various kinds of trauma (scald burn, endotoxemia through lipopolysaccharide (LPS) injection, and haemorrhagic trauma) in humans to those in male C57/B/6J laboratory mice (Figure 8.1). The human subjects showed a broad similarity in response to trauma; mice showed little similarity across the conditions, and only a random similarity to activated human trauma genes overall (Seok et al., 2013). These outcomes have been critiqued, mostly on methodological grounds (Cauwels et al., 2013 and others), but they do raise significant concerns for how widely applicable some model systems are to the human diseases/disorders they are intended to model.

While the Seok study specifically dealt with gene expression following various kinds of trauma, there is no reason to suppose the same general outcomes (i.e., species variations in gene expression) would not be found for diseases of the nervous system, let alone for models of any other human condition.

As already mentioned, while a number of investigators acknowledged the potential problems posed by the Seok study, the response in the neurological disease literature was distinctly muted. Nevertheless, the Seok et al. data seem to be broadly applicable to animal modeling for neurological diseases. For example, Burns et al. (2015) compared genes involved in the age-related neurological diseases to mouse models of the same

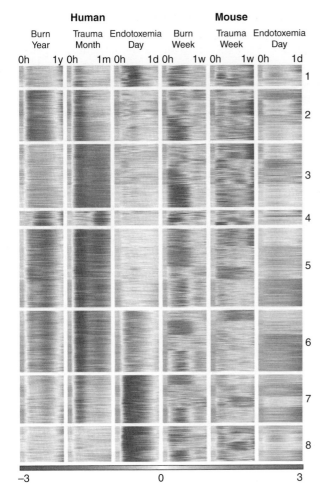

Figure 8.1 Illustration of genomic variation following trauma in mice versus humans, showing comparisons of the time-course gene changes for human burns, trauma, and endotoxin treatment and murine models of the same. K-means clustering of 4918 genes responsive to human systemic inflammation over time. Time interval for the human conditions: burns = up to 1 year; trauma = 1 month; endotoxemia = 1 day. Time intervals for mouse models: trauma and burns = 1 week; endotoxemia = 1 day (endotoxemia). *Source*: Redrawn from Seok et al. (2013). (See color plate section for the color representation of this figure.)

(Parkinson's disease, ALS, Alzheimer's disease, and Huntington's disease) and found that only 3 of 19 such models showed significant correlations.

Perhaps most researchers who did note the Seok and Burns studies did not want to believe them. Or, perhaps, consciously or unconsciously, they believed that these outcomes would lead to a dangerous conclusion, specifically that some, or many, such models do not really model the disease/condition they are attempting to model.

Clearly, such a conclusion would not be particularly welcome for researchers who had devoted years to such models – and who held grants based on them – to contemplate, let alone act upon. And, in the absence of acting on the issue, perhaps by seeking other models, scientific and professional inertia might instead lead to rationalizations and the continued use of models that can be summarized as "not perfect, but the best we have." The latter seems a common refrain, at least in neurological disease research.

8.4.1   Age and Time in *In Vivo* Models as a Function of Species

Before I tackle the more formidable problems of replicability and the decline effect, it is important to address several issues that almost never get seriously considered, or at least adjusted for, in animal models. The first is the animal's sex. Sex, as a potentially contributory variable, is simply often ignored, in spite of the fact that most neurological diseases show a sex-based difference in incidence and/or prevalence, as cited in Chapter 2. However, is not uncommon to find that male and female animals have been merged in *in vivo* studies, or, almost as often, that the sex of the animals in not mentioned at all.

Other studies do acknowledge the potential for problems arising from this omission, but given the realities of cost and the logistics of having large numbers of animals, some investigators sensitive to the potential problems posed by animal sex solve them by studying either males or females alone. Given the differential expression of human neurological diseases in human males and females, the picture that emerges from *in vivo* studies that report only the results of one sex is, at best, incomplete. The studies that merge the two sexes, in contrast, are likely to generate frankly misleading outcomes.

The next issue concerns the impacts of age and time. If an experimenter uses a mouse neuron to model a similar type of human neuron, say a motor neuron in the spinal cord, the time frame of the different phases of synaptic transmission between axon and muscle is going to be broadly very similar. Similarly, the transport of various molecules up and down the motor neuron's axon, the neurotransmitters used, the types of electrical potentials, and so on are going to be mostly qualitatively similar as well. This will be true for adult motor neurons between the two species. Indeed, it will generally be true across most mammalian species, other vertebrates, and in some cases even invertebrates.

However, it is only an assumption, and likely not a very good one, that the same will apply across different ages of mice and humans. Mice are sexually mature at 1 month of age and dead by 2 years; humans are sexually mature in their early to mid-teens and can easily (at least in some countries) live well into their 80s, and beyond. Given this, few researchers would try to model a 1-month-old human spinal motor neuron by looking at a 1-month-old mouse motor neuron.

In spite of this, researchers routinely assume that one can model age-related neurological disease conditions in various model systems regardless of their age in relation to humans presenting the disease. One assumption that seems to prevail is that a young to middle-aged mouse motor neuron/motor system in which researchers have induced some form of neurodegeneration will resemble that of a human with ALS in the typical age range of expression of middle to old age.

This problem is common in the neurological disease literature in general, but seems particularly problematic in the m*SOD1* model of ALS using mice and rats, regardless of the specific mutation line being used. In brief, the field does not know much about ALS progression from pre-clinical stages to clinical stages, but apart from some very rare examples in which onset appears to have a time frame of days to weeks (Huang et al., 2009 – if these cases were indeed ALS), the processes leading to motor neuron death do not necessarily occur rapidly, and certainly not with the time frame seen in mouse m*SOD1* models. For example, the G93A m*SOD1* mouse model shows an extremely rapid progression of the disorder, leading to death by about postnatal day 130; the

G37R model shows death occurring by about 1 year. While the case can be made that the m*SOD1* model is designed to mirror early-onset ALS in humans, what is ignored is that it is not simply enough to attempt to adjust equivalent ages: if humans live approximately 40 times longer than mice, is it reasonable to assume that a 2-year-old mouse is the equivalent to an 80-year-old human in terms of neuronal characteristics? While this might be true proportional to overall lifespan, it is almost certainly not true in terms of the various biochemical processes that necessarily occur over time. In other words, an 80-year-old motor neuron has had an extra 78 years to accumulate various toxic burdens, mitochondrial or gene damage, high levels of reactive oxygen species, aberrant biochemical cascades, and so on. This could well be the reason that mice and other mammals do not routinely show outcomes resembling human neurological diseases in the CNS as they age. The same caveat obviously applies equally to gene and toxin models of the various neurological diseases. In both cases, researchers can certainly induce neural damage that appears in many ways to resemble that found in human diseases at end state, but not the time it takes to arise in humans.

In regard to putative genetic or toxic factors used to induce the desired outcome within the lifespan of a mouse or rat, researchers often have to use copy numbers of mutant genes or toxin doses much higher than those experienced by humans, sometimes introduced by routes that are quite implausible for humans. In regard to the latter, to mimic the potential for the herbicide rotenone to induce parkinsonism features in rats, high doses had to be administered by jugular vein injection (Betarbet et al., 2000). Other Parkinson's models have routinely used MPTP, often directly injected into the striatum, to lesion dopaminergic terminals of the SN. Others have used 6-hydroxy-dopamine in the same manner, a toxin that lesions both dopaminergic and noradrenergic terminals (Blum et al., 2001). While both produce a loss of neurons in the SN and induce some behavioral features resembling Parkinson's disease, these methods cannot be truly said to mimic the likely etiological conditions preceding human Parkinson's disease.

Needless to say, dose and time are not simple trade-offs, certainly not in the context of the myriad other changes that accompany the aging process. These issues in the modeling of human neurological diseases may not always arise, but they often do, and they are thus problematic for a significant fraction of the existing literature.

8.4.2 Replicability and the Problems Created by the Absence of the Same

Another problem that bedevils much of the biomedical research literature, including that concerning human neurological diseases and models of the same, is replicability. One should first note that relatively few experiments are currently actually repeated by other scientists, so the full extent of the problem is not known. The reasons for an absence of experimental replication have been addressed by Ioannidis and others in some detail (Ioannidis, 2005), but they basically arise from a constellation of fairly mundane factors, notwithstanding that replication is supposed to be one of the key pillars of the scientific method.

One of the reasons cited for researchers not attempting to replicate the work of others is that, at present, there is little potential for career advancement in a repeat of someone else's discovery. The reason for this is that a repeat study is not likely to show up in a top-rated journal and thus is not likely to lead to tenure or promotion, let alone future grants.

The problems with the lack of replicability run deeper than a researcher not wanting to reproduce the work of others, however. At one end of the spectrum there is outright fraud, where results are either made up or at least significantly "massaged" to give a desired outcome. Such data obviously cannot be replicated except by blind chance, or by further fraud.

It should be stressed that fraud is not likely to be the largest factor in the failure of replicability. Far more likely, somewhere in the middle of the factors leading to the problem are poor initial study design, misapplied statistical methods, and "cherry-picked best" results, all combined with faulty interpretations. A famous example of the latter occurred in the magnetic resonance imaging (MRI) world when a deliberately misapplied method of analyzing data appeared to show neural activity in a dead salmon (Bennett et al., 2009) (Figure 8.2). In this case, the investigators were attempting to demonstrate that badly applied methodologies could lead to clearly absurd results, an outcome that should suggest caution in a variety of experimental fields, including the neurosciences.

At the far end of the spectrum is chance: the results reported might just be a statistical anomaly that does not routinely occur under the experimental conditions used; that is, *ceteris paribus* is not in play.

It cannot be stressed enough that all of this seems to apply not only generally in biomedical research, but also more specifically in neurological disease research.

The net result of the general lack of replicability leads to the suggestion that a very large fraction of peer-reviewed, published data, perhaps even the majority, is simply not valid. There is no reason to suppose that the situation is any different in the neurological disease literature.

Overall, such nonreproducible results suggest two possibilities. The first is that the initial findings were simply incorrect due to some chance outcome in the experiments, especially in cases where animal numbers are on the smaller side. Such outcomes may well have achieved statistical significance under the particular conditions first employed, but the unique circumstances simply cannot be repeated by others. Sometimes, the initial studies cannot even be repeated by the same investigators, in a phenomenon known as the "decline effect." The other possibility, as already mentioned,

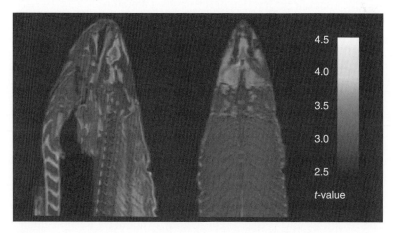

Figure 8.2 The "dead salmon" MRI and faux neural activity. *Source*: Bennett et al. (2009), under Creative Commons Attribution License. (See color plate section for the color representation of this figure.)

is that the initial findings were fraudulent and did not actually exist outside of the creative manipulation of the originators.

8.4.3 The "Decline Effect"

Researchers in a variety of fields have noted what has come to be termed the "decline effect," in which previously apparently robust, statistically significant outcomes decline over time with repeated experimentation, sometimes declining to chance levels (Lehrer, 2010; Schooler, 2011) (Figure 8.3).

The decline effect seems to appear in various scientific disciplines, but for the subject of this book those that occur in relation to experimental models of neurological disease are most relevant. A prime example is a study of rotenone, which initially seemed to create a quite pronounced parkinsonism outcome in rats (Betarbet et al., 2000). The model certainly looked convincing at first as it contained many of the behavioral and pathological features of the human disease. With time, however, fewer and fewer investigators could duplicate the findings. Indeed, the original investigators appear to have had problems doing so themselves.

My laboratory has experienced much the same effect with our steryl glucoside/cycad model of ALS-PDC (cited in Chapters 5 and 7). Initial studies gave robust effects, many of which have been replicated by other investigators (Shen et al., 2010; Van Kampen et al., 2014b). Over time, however, we sometimes began to lose the effect, although it seems still to be robust in the hands of other investigators (Van Kampen et al., 2014b, 2015). Thus, one could consider this a partial decline effect.

The reasons for the decline effect seem to be multifaceted. Some involve the factors cited by Ioannidis in his various studies of replicability in science. Notably, these include, in addition to poor study design, the tendency, often inadvertent, to find exactly the results one is seeking. Small sample sizes exacerbate the problem, even when a formal power analysis suggests that the numbers should be adequate. When the decline effect occurs in the same laboratory that previously had robust outcomes, however, the reasons are much less clear.

Various authors attribute the decline effect in a field, versus that in any one laboratory, to publication bias and selective reporting. In the first case, apparently spectacular outcomes in some experiment may spur other researchers, not to try to reproduce the initial

Figure 8.3 Schematic illustration of the "decline effect."

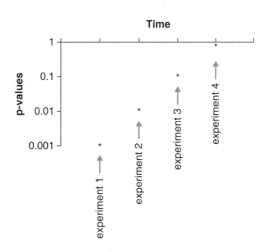

findings, but to elaborate upon them. Once a significant outcome has been published, publication bias sets in, such that only positive results that support a now established or popular outcome get into the scientific journals. In general, negative results are rarely considered publishable, although some granting agencies and journals are increasingly expressing concerns that this imbalance has in many cases misled some disciplines. For example, negative results in *in vivo* models that call into question what have been considered promising therapeutics for neurological disease may not be reported. If only positive outcomes are published, costly human trials may be conducted that would not have been attempted had the negative results been published as well.

Regardless of the reasons for a lack of replicability, the fact that the problem exists raises significant issues for understanding disease states, the mechanisms by which they arise, and, most crucially, the design of potential therapeutic applications.

What does the neurological disease field really have to fall back upon in the attempt to understand the truly daunting complexity of neurological disease? The bad news is that much of what has been relied on for such an understanding in the past is simply wrong and needs to be discarded and/or rethought. The somewhat better news is that once there is a re-evaluation of the literature – *if it ever happens* – including replication of the key aspects of it, what remains may make the now confusing picture of neurological disease origins a great deal clearer. In fact, this may be the only way to move forward.

8.5 Is There an Ideal Model for Studying Neurological Diseases? General Considerations

As discussed earlier, in his talk on the m*SOD1* model of ALS compared to the newer genetic models, Cox commented that ALS is a poor model of ALS. Although he said this tongue-in-cheek, he noted that ALS is really a spectrum disease, such that any one case cannot be considered to mirror any of the others. Much the same applies in Parkinson's disease (Sherer and Mari, 2014), and likely Alzheimer's disease as well. The notion that these neurological disorders represent multiple variations along some continuum of disease features has been considered for some time, but is only now beginning to find more widespread acceptance.

The spectrum nature of each disease raises two key questions: First, how does one model a spectrum disorder with only one mutant gene or one principal toxin? Second, how can effective therapy be applied when the features of different individuals' disorders vary along this spectrum? The latter question will be addressed in Chapter 15.

The answer to the first is itself problematic and, inevitably, leads to problems with the second question and with the appropriate therapeutics to use in each case.

The neurological disease field shows no inclination to give up a model systems approach to the diseases considered in this book. Nor should it, since from the preceding discussion it is clear that no other approach offers any realistic hope of defining etiologies, mechanisms, or potential treatments. It does, however, force researchers to consider just what the best possible model would look like.

The minimal criteria for such a model would include the measures of validity discussed at the beginning of this chapter. The model would also have to address some of the fundamental mysteries that each of the diseases offers. Perhaps the easiest of these criteria, by no means actually easy, would be to define why some cells die while others do not when faced with the same mutant gene or systemic/relatively systemic toxin. In the former case, the assumption is that the mutation is a germ-line mutation, not a somatic one; in the latter, any toxin that could access only one cell type would not be particularly mysterious. I note, however, that mutations leading to particular types of neuron dying have not been identified in the extensive literature on genetic etiologies; further, many putative neurotoxins do not target only selected neuronal populations.

In spite of this, in ALS, α-motor neurons are more negatively impacted by the genetic mutations identified to date than are γ-motor neurons or sensory neurons. The same holds true for toxins preferentially damaging α-motor neurons. Clearly, there must be something different about these neurons, but exactly what that something is remains unknown. Possible answers may lie with neuronal metabolism, the types of membrane receptors, or glial–neuronal interactions, to name only a few of the most obvious possibilities.

In regard to this, metabolic differences are key aspects to be aware of in model systems, as they can be wildly different across species. A now classic example is that of the toxin MPTP, which when injected intravenously in humans induces a form of parkinsonism (Langston et al., 1983). It does the same in rats, but not in mice, as cited earlier. Similarly, cycad toxins seem to be a key epidemiological factor in the Guamanian disorder, ALS-PDC, as cited in Chapter 7, but give very different outcomes in mice, which develop a dominant ALS phenotype, compared to a purely parkinsonism phenotype in rats.

Next, the observed aspect of the initial unilateral presentation of damage, at least in Parkinson's disease and ALS, would have to be addressed. One suggestion for why a unilateral presentation later becomes bilateral is that something moves across the sagittal plane between the two sides, but what that might be is not known.

The question is similar in ALS to asking why the disease appears to move up, or down, the neuraxis from its initial point of presentation. Some reasonable hypotheses have been generated in this regard (e.g., the spread of misfolded mSOD acting as a seed to the further misfolding of normal SOD, as suggested in Chapter 5), but these remain largely unverified.

Next, the long-known "cross-talk" between neurological diseases would have to be accommodated. As cited in Chapter 2, there is considerable overlap between the various neurological diseases considered here, such that Parkinson's disease and ALS have dementia features similar to those of Alzheimer's disease. Why this would be true overall and the staging of the various presentations, as in ALS-PDC, have to be addressed.

In addition, the comorbidities found in most neurological disorders would also have to be addressed. As cited in previous chapters, these can include skin collagen changes in ALS, platelet and other systems changes in Parkinson's disease, insulin-receptor alterations in Alzheimer's disease, and changes in both bone and skin in ALS-PDC. Some of these are not new observations – those in ALS have been known since the time of Charcot (1880). There are, almost without a doubt, additional systems alterations in each neurological disease that are not yet identified.

That these other organ-system changes in the disease state are not addressed is not a matter of their not existing. Rather, since the extraneuronal features are not an obvious part of the nervous system pathology, they tend to get shunted aside in the attempt to deal with the very real crisis caused by neuronal degeneration. However, the skin changes associated with ALS might turn out to be a crucial clue to disease origin and progression. A model system that does not find and seek to address such multisystem features is not going to prove an adequate model for human neurological diseases.

Finally, since neurological diseases are progressive, the model would have to address changes in the CNS over time. Time-line studies are essential, but are rarely done, for reasons that will be discussed in Chapter 9.

As ideal as all of this is, the reality, based on both theoretical and logistic grounds, is that creating such a model is very difficult, and very expensive. Indeed, models of the diseases under consideration in this book, and of the various other neurological conditions, such as epilepsy, multiple sclerosis, schizophrenia, and ASD, have not been able to do more than satisfy some of the basic validity concerns and study a fraction of the items listed in this chapter. This is not due to lack of interest, but rather an issue of costs, resources, and time.

8.6   Specific Considerations for Ideal Model-System Approaches in ALS

It is worthwhile considering ALS model systems in regard to all of the foregoing, primarily for the reason that none of the models, so far, has generated useful therapeutics capable of significantly slowing the progression of the disease, let alone reversing it.

Some of the concerns and items that must be addressed mirror those given in the preceding section:

- ALS is progressive in nature. Regardless of which group of motor neurons is initially affected, the pathological process spreads to other – but not all – groups, ultimately killing some motor neurons throughout the ventral spinal cord and usually in the motor regions of the brain. Laterality of initial presentation is as discussed earlier, but does not appear to reflect dominant-handedness.
- In spite of the limited evidence for genetic causality factors in the vast majority of ALS cases, as cited in Chapter 5, over the last 20 years the field has focused almost entirely on the *SOD1* mutation in humans, or, in terms of a model-systems approach, in transgenic animals expressing the human mutation. The newer mutations identified in fALS have recently become more prominent and are thus receiving more of the research dollars allocated to ALS by the various granting agencies. One rationale for this situation is that the neurodegenerative pathway triggered by the mutant *SOD1* gene (or those of the other mutations) will turn out to be identical to the pathway(s) triggered by unknown environmental toxins. Increasing evidence suggests that this rationale is not necessarily valid, but it would have to be in order for genetic models to be considered valid for sporadic forms of the disease.
- Overall, the field admits to two ALS clusters. The first is ALS-PDC, as described in Chapter 7. The second is a subgroup of patients with Gulf War Syndrome. Epidemiological studies for the latter suggest a roughly twofold increase in ALS levels in military personnel, whether deployed to the Gulf in 1991 or not. The age of onset in this cohort is considerably younger than in classical ALS. This is also a major characteristic of ALS-PDC on Guam and in Irian Jaya, as cited previously. For these reasons, age would have to be a crucial part of any ideal model.
- The m*SOD1* model is usually considered to reflect the underlying pathological processes in human ALS in a "pure" form; that is, with only motor neurons in various parts of the brain and spinal cord affected. There is, however, increasing evidence that this is not the case, either in models (Petrik et al., 2007a) or in humans. The latter is

demonstrated by an older – and apparently largely forgotten – scientific literature, as cited earlier. Models based on genetics or toxins would have to mimic these features.

- As with Parkinson's disease, ALS was for years considered to be a completely distinct entity with no crossover to either Parkinson's or Alzheimer's diseases. The field now knows that this view is, in large measure, incorrect. As in Parkinson's disease, a form of dementia affecting the frontal lobes occurs in at least 20% of all ALS patients. FTD induces profound personality change and shows up neuropathologically as deposits of tau protein in the frontal cortex (Hughes et al., 2003; Rademakers et al., 2004). In addition, as in Alzheimer's disease, classical ALS occasionally shows deposits of abnormal tau protein in various regions of the nervous system (Strong et al., 2005). An appropriate model of ALS would have to include cognitive decline at some stage of the progression of overall neuronal dysfunction.
- In ALS, a genetic susceptibility factor has been identified in the form of genes coding for variant forms of the cholesterol transport protein, apolipoprotein E (APOE), in much the same way as in Alzheimer's disease (Raber et al., 2000). A similar susceptibility gene variant in ALS models would have to provide the same outcomes.
- Finally, in ALS, whatever is causing the disease also appears to have an impact on other organ systems. For example, the patients' skin collagen seems to be altered. These findings have not been widely considered nor funded by granting agencies in North America and Europe. These outcomes too would have to be duplicated in a model.

8.6.1 ALS Considered from the Perspective of Model Systems: Lost in Translation

Little of the preceding has been accomplished. Instead, the general trend since the first descriptions of mutant *SOD1* in some cases of fALS (Gurney et al., 1994) has been to try various drugs in the model in the hopes that one might prevent, or at least delay, motor neuron loss. Within the *in vivo* literature, the outcomes of these studies have been decidedly mixed, in that some drugs do not work at all while others appear to show a limited ability to delay the eventual end state. Many of these efforts, particularly those where the copy number of the mutant gene is not known, are difficult to interpret (see Zwiegers et al., 2014) (Figure 8.4).

Numerous translational approaches based on the positive outcomes in some studies using m*SOD1* models have not been successful in the clinic. The reasons for this state of affairs can be summarized as follows: First, the m*SOD1* model does not truly model the disease in all of its complexity as a spectrum disorder. Second, at a technical level, copy-number variations may have made various studies irrelevant for human trials. Indeed, had this issue been properly addressed, true negative outcomes would have saved vast amounts of money and time by not moving apparently ineffective drugs forward to clinical trials. By the same token, negative outcomes in the animal model may have prematurely discarded drugs that might have been beneficial, at least in principle. Finally, the problem may extend beyond flawed model systems and instead highlight a deeper issue concerning the limits of applying highly reductionist thinking to complex systems like the CNS, which, in the latter case, is undergoing a complex breakdown.

A clear example of such thinking resides in the various experimental approaches that have sought to grow motor neurons *in vitro*, with the goal of putting them into the spinal cord to restore motor function (Toma et al., 2015). Each such experiment neglects what could be termed the "so what" question. For example, assuming one could get motor

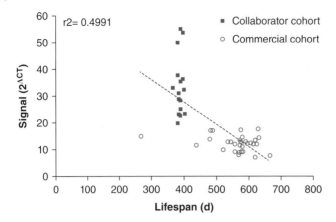

Figure 8.4 m*SOD1* copy-number variations in mice and delayed neuronal degeneration. Transgene dosage effects on lifespan in m*SOD1* mice. Linear regression analysis reveals a negative correlation between relative m*SOD1* copy number and lifespan ($p < 0.0001$). Collaborator n = 16; commercial n = 28. *Source*: Zwiegers et al. (2014), under Creative Commons Attribution License.

neurons grown *in vitro* to survive, and then transport them and correctly reconnect them inside the cord, how would this allow the axons to grow out to the muscles that are now denervated? Since this has not even been accomplished in cases of spinal cord trauma (but see Chapter 15), one has to wonder how the investigators who are engaged in such transplantation studies envision it succeeding.

There are likely two answers to this question, the first trivial and the other philosophical. The trivial answer is that overly reductionist thinking simply does not address this concern at all. The philosophical answer is to take the view – which many have – that eventually science will solve every problem. I will consider the last viewpoint in Part IV.

8.7 Alternative Views of Neurological Disease and Model-Systems Approaches: Multiple-Hit Etiologies

Most neurological diseases, ALS included, have traditionally been thought to arise from fairly linear, "one-hit" sorts of processes. As already noted, the identification of m*SOD1* as a contributor to motor neuron loss in fALS continues to drive a huge effort to understand mSOD1 biochemistry and its "toxic gain of function" actions. In Alzheimer's disease, the identification of Aβ plaques and NFTs led to decades of research on the origin and pathology of these abnormal and/or misfolded proteins. The idea that dominated the Alzheimer's disease field for decades was that to understand these "proteinopathies" was to understand the disease. Similarly, in Parkinson's disease, the identification of misfolded α-synuclein has led in the same direction.

In spite of these efforts in each of these diseases, it has become increasingly apparent that no matter how deleterious a mutant gene product may be, it is not the sole factor driving the loss of neurons in that particular region of the brain or spinal cord. In the same fashion, no single toxic hit, whether it be a natural toxin or one of human origin, is going to do so either. What instead seems to be coming to the fore is that a series of genetic or toxic events – multiple hits – are involved in driving the neurological disease process toward its ultimate end state.

Whether these multiple hits represent gene–gene, gene–toxin, or toxin–toxin interactions is not known, but they are likely to include all of them in some measure. Nevertheless, the fact remains that the whole subject matter of multiple-hit interactions remains at the very early stages of funding, and thus investigation.

There is, however, a growing recognition that not only are toxins often playing out their pathological role in the context of various susceptibility genes, but gene–gene interactions and toxin synergies are likely involved in neurological disease etiologies. In addition, it has become apparent that the eventual neural targets of such toxic impacts – that is, the cells whose death is a hallmark of the disorder (e.g., motor neurons in ALS) – are not the only cells involved and, indeed, may be fairly far downstream in the cascade of pathological events, which may involve numerous other cell types and CNS systems. It now seems far more likely that the early events in any such disease might involve cells in regions not conventionally considered to be involved at all. For example, the loss of olfactory neurons and function appears to be an early precursor to the loss of neurons in the nigro-striatal system in Parkinson's disease. Similarly, at least for animal models of fALS, with all their constraints, muscle end plates may be impacted in some cases *before*, rather than only *after*, motor neuron loss in ALS.

Additionally, as discussed in Chapter 3, not only neurons are involved in the processes underlying neurological diseases. Non-cell-autonomous interactions between neurons and various glial cell types, microglia, astrocytes, and oligodendrocytes are increasingly seen as a crucial part of a dynamic degenerative process in the overall pathological picture of any neurological disease.

Paradoxically, at least for those coming from a purely reductionist frame of reference, it is in the non-cell-autonomous domain that any potential future remediation of neuronal degeneration will arise. If neuron destruction were the sole factor in neurological diseases, then once the neurons primarily affected in the various disorders were dead, few therapeutic options would remain. Basically, the realistic choice would be limited to efforts to try to replace the lost neurons in the most feasible way. The problems with this approach have been discussed in this chapter and will be revisited in Chapter 15. However, if a non-cell-autonomous process is instead the primary cause, then targeting the interaction between neurons and glia might rescue any neurons that are merely dysfunctional, rather than dead.

It is important to recognize in the latter context that the field has no way at present of distinguishing in a living patient (or animal) non-responding dysfunctional versus dead neurons. If the latter were a reasonable fraction of the overall neurons affected, and could be addressed at an early enough time point, then an ability to halt the overall degenerative cascade might exist. There is evidence that this might in part be the case and that neuroprotective agents such as progranulin, amongst others, might serve in this manner. This possibility will be discussed in Chapter 14.

To determine the actual status of neurons at various disease stages, time-line studies in humans or animals become essential. It is thus to this topic that the next chapter turns.

9

The Progression and the Time Line of Neurological Disease

"It appears that these mice can come back from a very severe level of disease progression. This is a very important finding because humans are usually diagnosed when the disease has already progressed relatively far."

Dr. Oded Singer[1]

From the Preface

5) For all of these reasons, neurological diseases that are age-related (e.g., Parkinson's disease, ALS, Alzheimer's disease, and others) are going to be complex as well. The same applies to neuronal disorders at the other end of the age spectrum (e.g., autism spectrum disorder (ASD)).

9.1   Introduction

This statement is here to reinforce the point that the diseases in question are complex and that part of their complexity lies in the progressive nature of each. Given this complexity, trying to understand any of them really requires an understanding of their respective time lines.

The problem is illustrated by the following study: In 2005, Singer and colleagues at the Salk Institute published an article in *Nature Neuroscience* in which they described how in an *in vivo* transgenic model of Alzheimer's disease they had apparently reversed key biochemical events thought to be active at an early stage of the human disease. The basic idea was that if they could target an enzyme (β-secretase) involved with amyloid precursor protein (APP) accumulation in control mice compared to transgenic mice expressing human APP, they could then reduce subsequent neurodegeneration. Using a lentiviral delivery of small interfering RNAs to silence β-secretase, these researchers claimed to have reduced APP cleavage, reduced neurodegeneration, and, in the process, improved spatial learning (Singer et al., 2005).

As of this writing, the techniques used in mice still have not been applied to Alzheimer's disease patients. Possible reasons for this will be presented later in the book when dealing with gene therapies. A more mundane reason, however, may be this: there is still no complete time line of disease progression in humans, nor even in animal models of neurodegenerative diseases.

Neural Dynamics of Neurological Disease, First Edition. Christopher A. Shaw.
© 2017 John Wiley & Sons, Inc. Published 2017 by John Wiley & Sons, Inc.

9.2   Creating Disease Time Lines: The Framingham Study

In the mid part of the 20th century, the National Heart Institute, now the National Heart, Lung, and Blood Institute, noted a dramatic increase in cardiovascular disease in the first half of that century. From about 10% of all deaths in the United States in the early part of the century, rates climbed to 25% in 1940, and, later, to almost 40% by 1960.

In 1948, the Framingham Heart Study was begun in Framingham, Massachusetts in order to provide a population-based prospective examination of the development of cardiovascular disease and its risk factors, with a focus on arteriosclerosis and hypertension.

The study population consisted of 2336 mostly white males and 2873 mostly white females, all in an age range between 30 and 59 years of age. The study examined medical histories, performed physical examinations, and ran laboratory tests to evaluate various potential risk factors including age, sex, blood pressure, cholesterol level, body weight, diabetes, smoking, physical activity, and alcohol consumption (Dawber et al., 1951, 1959; Dawber, 1980). The study continued in 1971 with the offspring and spouses of the original participants and was designed to investigate familial and genetic factors that might be associated with cardiovascular disease. A third-generation cohort (children of the offspring cohort) was recruited in 2002 to continue to look at genetic factors and other precursors to cardiovascular disease (Splansky et al., 2007).

Since 1948, over 1000 papers have been published from mining the Framingham data base. The analyses of these data have led to shifting perceptions about the causes of cardiovascular diseases and the value of prophylactic measures (Kannel, 2011). The early and subsequent articles clearly listed some of the key risk factors, including hypertension, being overweight, cigarette smoking, and high serum cholesterol for arteriosclerosis (reviewed in O'Donnell and Elosua, 2008).

The Framingham Heart Study is still being expanded into other areas, such as the discovery and validation of biomarkers for cardiovascular disease and the development of imaging tools. Of interest to this book, the study has even been used to explore aspects of stroke and dementia (Wolf, 2012).

9.3   Time Lines of Neurological Disease

Could the same rationale that led to the cardiovascular Framingham study be a boon to neurological disease studies as well? If, as in the Framingham study, it were possible to identify a sufficiently large patient base and monitor it for a prolonged period for signs of neurological disease, it might provide the basis for understanding the disease vastly better than the field currently does.

For example, moving from a healthy, neurologically disease-free population and watching the early stages of the disease emerge would provide a solid basis for identifying casual factors, as opposed to our still incomplete understanding of the various somewhat amorphous "risk factors" (see, for example, Public Health Agency of Canada, 2015) (Figure 9.1). From this knowledge would come, at least in principle, policies to seek prevention by prophylaxis by eliminating causal factors to the extent that they are fully or partially environmental or behavioral. In the latter case, the intersection of genetic susceptibility factors and the identified toxins/behaviors would be indicated.

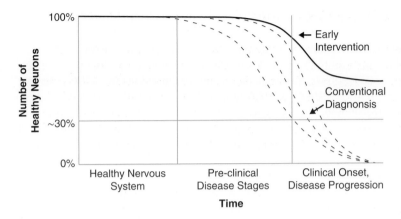

Figure 9.1 A more complex hypothetical time line of neurological disease.

The former would come from the personalized genetic screening that participants in the study would have had.

Where prophylaxis was not possible, researchers would still know the disease stages from onset to end state. With this knowledge, they could target strategically, and selectively, the stage of the disease process in any individual with the hope of halting it before further damage was done.

In some ways, the latter goal is like a discussion of polio compared to ALS (Figure 9.2). In polio, the disease process is largely self-limiting once the initial infection is controlled by the immune system. Obviously, if the same could be done for ALS, the patient might not be like he/she was before the onset of disease, but at least would not progress further toward the inevitable end state. This point will be amplified in Chapters 14 and 15.

Finally, knowing the full course of the disease would allow researchers to know when it had progressed beyond any reasonable hope of treatment. As disappointing – indeed, tragic – as such an outcome might be to patients and caregivers alike, at least it would then serve to focus clinical efforts on quality-of-life care.

At present, none of this can be done. The reasons why this statement is correct are both financial and theoretical. The latter point was briefly considered in Chapter 8.

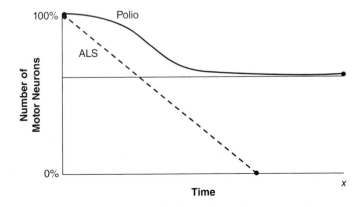

Figure 9.2 Schematic of the differences between ALS and polio.

Concerning the former, governments will likely not do anything much about figuring out the actual time lines of disease in the foreseeable future – a point to be discussed in greater detail in Chapter 16.

The theoretical aspect puts limits to what could be accomplished even if the overall costs were not an issue. Given, however, that costs are an issue, the theoretical concerns are likely moot, but they may be worth considering anyway in order to frame a full consideration of the problem.

The issue basically comes down to a discussion of the scale of the time line of neurological disease progression from inception through to end state. In humans, the starting point cannot be inferred – at least, not so far – from the latter clinical stages of the disease process. The latter focuses on "staging," mostly after clinical diagnosis. In other words, what happens to the diseased parts of the central nervous system (CNS), and in which sequence. Needless to say, the further along this process one precedes, the more complicated is the picture that emerges. This point is amply illustrated in any scientific talk on the genomics, proteomics, or metabolomics of any of the diseases in question, as cited previously.

By way of illustration of what can be done post diagnosis, the pathological staging for Parkinson's and Alzheimer's diseases will be discussed in Section 9.4. A detailed neuroanatomical knowledge is not required in order to understand the basic notion that the disease process spreads within the primarily affected parts of the CNS to include different regions.

9.3.1 Braak Staging for Parkinson's Disease

The Braak staging classification scheme categorizes Parkinson's patients into six stages based on the presence of Lewy bodies and Lewy neurites (Braak et al., 2003).

- *Stage 0*: Pre-clinical (and here is the *precise* problem that this is very much a "black box," about which very little is known).
- *Stage 1 (affected region – medulla oblongata)*: Lesions in the dorsal IX/X motor nucleus and/or intermediate reticular zone.
- *Stage 2 (affected region – medulla oblongata and pontine tegmentum)*: Pathology of Stage 1 plus lesions in caudal raphe nuclei, gigantocellular reticular nucleus, and coeruleus–subcoeruleus complex.
- *Stage 3 (affected region – midbrain)*: Pathology of Stage 2 plus midbrain lesions, particularly in the SNpc.
- *Stage 4 (affected region – basal prosencephalon and mesocortex)*: Pathology of Stage 3 plus prosencephalic lesions. Cortical involvement is confined to the temporal mesocortex (transentorhinal region) and allocortex (hippocampal CA2–plexus). The neocortex is unaffected.
- *Stage 5 (affected region – neocortex)*: Pathology of Stage 4 plus lesions in higher-order sensory association areas of the neocortex and prefrontal neocortex.
- *Stage 6 (affected region – neocortex)*: Pathology of Stage 5 plus lesions in first-order sensory association areas of the neocortex and premotor areas. Occasionally mild changes in primary sensory areas and the primary motor field.

Various researchers believe that some CNS regions that are not part of the nigro-striatal system –those that cause the primarily movement disorders – are also affected. In many cases, these other aspects, pathological and behavioral, may occur prior to those pathological features cited by Braak et al. (2003). They include the loss of olfactory function

(Hawkes, 2003) and behavioral manifestations arising from damage to regions of the hypothalamus (Sandyk et al., 1987).

9.3.2 Braak Staging for Alzheimer's Disease

The pathological staging for Alzheimer's disease is based on the spread of NFT distributions (Braak and Braak, 1991). The same considerations as for Parkinson's disease apply here. (Note that "Pre" in the following stands for one of the subunit layers of the entorhinal cortex (there are four, including a molecular layer and the lamina dissecans) and the external principal statum. "Pri" indicates another layer, the internal principal stratum. The two principal layers of this structure can be subdivided into α, β and γ sublayers.)

- *Stage 1 (transentorhinal stage)*: NFTs and neuropil threads (NTs) are found in Pre-α projection neurons in the transentorhinal region. A few isolated NFTs may occur in the entorhinal layer Pre-α, in hippocampal field CA1, in the magnocellular nuclei of the basal forebrain, and in the anterodorsal nucleus of the thalamus.
- *Stage 2 (transentorhinal stage)*: Pathology of stage 1 plus numerous NFTs and NTs in the transentorhinal Pre-α. The hippocampal CA1 region is affected by modest numbers of NFTs. A few isolated NFTs may be found in isocortical association areas.
- *Stage 3 (limbic stage)*: Severe involvement of layer Pre-α in the transentorhinal and entorhinal regions. Modest involvement of CA1 hippocampus. The isocortex is devoid of changes or is only mildly affected. Mild changes of the magnocellular forebrain nuclei, anterodorsal nucleus of the thalamus, and amygdala are seen.
- *Stage 4 (limbic stage)*: Severely affected Pre-α area in transentorhinal and entorhinal regions. There is considerable involvement of layers Pri-α and Pre-β. There are numerous NFTs in the hippocampal formation. The isocortex is mildly affected.
- *Stage 5 (isocortical stage)*: Severe changes in Pre-α and Pri-β. Pre-β and Pre-γ layers are also distinctly affected. Virtually all components of the hippocampal formation are involved. The isocortex is severely affected, with high packing density of NFTs and NTs in anterobasal portions of the insula and orbitofrontal cortex. Primary sensory areas are still more or less spared. The primary motor field is mildly affected. Thalamus and amygdala are affected.
- *Stage 6 (isocortical stage)*: Loss of nerve cells in Pre-α and Pri-α. Severe changes in the hippocampal formation. Severely affected isocortical association areas are noted. The presence of dense a network of NTs is contrasted by only small numbers of NFTs in layer V of the primary sensory areas. No severe changes are seen in the primary motor field. There is severe involvement of subcortical nuclei and the extrapyramidal system. NFTs are found in the medium-sized nerve cells of the striatum and the melanin-containing neurons of the SNpc.

9.3.3 Problems in Post-Clinical Staging

In animal models, the starting point for an experimentally induced disease state is easy to know since it is likely to be the experimental treatment used to start the degenerative process in the first place. What happens afterwards is more speculative, and thus problematic, since no model has an infinite capacity to allow researchers to look into all possible time scales. This is an important point because, as per the two-hit model described in Section 9.4, neurological diseases are quite unlikely to be the consequence of only one factor whose impacts simply accumulate until enough neurons have died. Rather, the interconnected nature of neural organization means that each element affects all others in its micro- and macro-environment, and this occurs at all scales of organization. Within a neuron (or a glial cell), damage to one organelle (e.g., by reactive oxygen species) will ultimately impact other organelles, and eventually the entire cell. By the same token, the reality of the non-cell-autonomous nature of the CNS means that as one cell is damaged or altered, other cells are negatively impacted in turn. The wave of non-cell-autonomous impacts thus spread outwards, bifurcating at each step, from whatever triggering event, to eventually encompass larger areas of the nervous system.

This latter aspect now becomes the sort of crucial event that I have discussed previously; that is, a cascading failure. No model system, nor any combination of overlapping model systems, is likely to be able to view and coordinate *all* of the time frames to accurately capture *all* of the events of a critical nature that might occur in the disease progression toward some end state. For example, an *in vivo* model, if detailed enough, might show that molecule "X" precedes the creation of molecule "Y." However, to get the precise molecular steps between the two, one would have to go to an *in vitro* model. To do so would bring in the potential problems of coordinating two very different sorts of information between two model systems. Each model would also come with its own caveats for use, as detailed in Chapter 8.

Could such a complementary approach work at all? Such a prospect is, at best, doubtful. The likely cost in money and resources, and the lack of the same, make it even more so. Again, this is a topic that will be addressed in greater detail later in the book.

Lastly, in terms of therapeutic application, even were the precisely right stage of the disease known, identifying it in any individual would require a level of precision that is currently difficult to imagine and would be even more difficult to implement.

9.3.4 Staging of Clinical Features and Pathology

As discussed earlier, Parkinson's and Alzheimer's diseases have their various staging criteria. These are not the same as a time line, however; that is, they are not the neurological equivalent of the Framingham study, since they are largely derived from histology done in the early and progressive stages of the disease, post diagnosis and/or post mortem. While of great value in their own right for understanding some of the expression stages of the diseases, they do not have the capacity to tell researchers much about pre-clinical aspects. For example, those studying the diseases can learn little, if anything, about etiologies and early pathological processes from such staging studies, nor can useful prophylactic therapeutics be effectively designed or applied.

9.4   Back to a Multiple-Hit Disease Consideration

As noted briefly in Chapter 6, Clarke et al. (2001) proposed a one-hit model of inherited forms of neurodegeneration after examining 17 types of neurological disease. Their analysis of these cases suggested exponential kinetics for neuron loss, which they interpreted to suggest that the risk of any neuron's death was constant, random, and independent of the state of other neurons in the same system. This conclusion seemed to lead to the notion that neurodegeneration was the by-product of what they termed to be a single, intracellular biochemical event of a "catastrophic" nature. The contrasting notion, as portrayed by these authors, was a more gradual cumulative kind of damage, such as might occur with increasing levels of free radicals.

In regard to their interpretations of the kinetics data, various lines of evidence suggest that while the initial neuron that dies may be a random event in any population of related types of neuron, the rate is hardly constant, as demonstrated by the cascading-failure features of most progressive neurological diseases. Nor, given the emerging perspective that cell death is often the result of a non-cell-autonomous process, can the death of any neuron be considered to be independent of the death of other neurons, regardless of whether such cell death is mediated by way of other non-neuronal elements.

In terms of multiple hits, a variety of sources support the notion for various neurological diseases. In Parkinson's disease, a variety of events seem to be involved, including dopamine metabolites, mutant/misfolded α-synuclein, and mutant parkin, as well as an inflammatory response (Sulzer, 2007). In Alzheimer's disease, some investigators have linked oxidative stress and abnormal mitogenic changes in cell cycle in the early phases of the disease (Zhu et al., 2004, 2007).

Developmental disorders such as schizophrenia are also thought to arise from a variety of gene–toxin interactions, which provide the multiple hits: one in early development, one or more in adolescence or adulthood (Maynard et al., 2001).

9.5 Haecceity and Quiddity in Context to Biosemiosis and Multiple Hits

The Latin-derived terms "haecceity" and "quiddity" will occur in various places in this book, for the reason that, in my opinion, they describe key features of human beings and their nervous systems in health and disease. "Haecceity" refers to the essence of a person or thing that makes it a particular person/thing. Each human is thus an haecceity in that he/she is totally unique in terms of the combined weight of genomic expression, phenotype based on genome and environmental influences (the latter including more than just toxin exposures), life-time experiences, microbiome, and so on. An analogy to snowflakes all being different while all still being capable of making snowmen would not be misplaced. The same applies, for much the same set of reasons, for each individual's nervous system in health, as well as in disease.

"Quiddity," often used synonymously with "haecceity," is actually somewhat different. It refers to the "whatness" of a person/thing, and may be used to compare the common aspects of individuals of the same general type. For example, humans share with one another broadly similar nervous systems compared to other animals, even though individual human haecceity differs. Further, the similar things that damage these nervous systems may be broadly similar as well (e.g., certain toxic substances), but they may not be specifically so.

The haecceity and quiddity aspects of human neurological diseases tie into the time-line discussion in that it may be nearly impossible to know the exact trajectory by which any one person goes from a state of nervous system health to one of a specific neurological disease. The multiple hits do not even need to be common for all cases. Indeed, it is likely that they are not.

Even the stages described in this chapter for Parkinson's and Alzheimer's diseases post diagnosis are merely general descriptions along some continuum within a population and cannot be applied to any individual – certainly not while that individual is still alive.

In the future, biomarkers may provide some boundaries to the state of any individual post diagnosis, but they will of necessity be vague, in part because of the increasing chaos in the degenerating nervous system. Pre-clinical diagnosis, as per the preceding, will remain difficult or impossible to accomplish, for reasons already discussed.

It is always important to keep in mind that the haecceity of any nervous system relates to the fact that it is a signaling device whose overall complexity depends on species, age, state, and so on. As such, biosemiosis – signaling within and between living organisms – again becomes a key issue.

As already described, signaling within the human CNS is enormously complex and, to a large extent, individual. This includes all stages of signaling, from gene to cell, cell to circuit, circuit to system, and on through to expression in behavior. Generally, the earlier in these steps that the biosemiotic mis-signaling occurs, the worse the general outcome will be (Gryder et al., 2013). For example, biosemiotic mistakes in DNA coding and in transfer RNA tend to be catastrophic, especially if such mistakes also compromise intrinsic DNA repair mechanisms. Once cascading failures begin, they cannot be overcome, at least not by anything medical science now knows how to do.

The problem in some sense becomes one of trying to push back against the emerging entropy of the affected parts of the nervous system. As mistakes propagate and bifurcate, the chaos in the system grows by some power law function.

As will be discussed in Chapter 16, while it is possible to contemplate reversing such catastrophic processes in the CNS, such dreams may be more the substance of science fiction than science reality. This is hard to accept for many in the field, as it seems to go against ingrained philosophical perspectives about the innate power of science.

The actuality may be that the best that can be done in treating neurological disease lies in the dual strategies of prevention in general and, failing this, extremely early detection. Depending on the state of the cascade at some early point, treatments might be able to succeed in halting the degenerative processes. In order to do so, however, one would need to understand the early stages in neurological disease, and this would mean beginning to appreciate the role of early development and its impact throughout the life span. This is the subject of the next chapter.

9.6 Some Final Thoughts on Time Lines of Neurological Disease: Differentiation and Neurogenesis

An observation of still unknown significance in relation to the time lines of neurological disease appearance and neuronal differentiation is the following: the neurological diseases considered here emerge temporally within certain peak age windows. As cited in Chapter 2, ALS tends to arise clinically primarily in the 50–70 age range, with an average age at onset of 55 years (ALS Association: www.alsa.org); Parkinson's disease somewhat later, at an average of 60 years of age (but ranging from 20 to 80) (Parkinson's Disease Foundation: www.pdf.org); and Alzheimer's disease later still, with early-onset forms between 30 to 65 and later forms up until the 90s. Alzheimer's disease is actually more complex in the age of presentation, perhaps highlighting its spectrum nature. For example, one source shows onset for familial Alzheimer's varying with the driving mutation: *APP*, 29–56 years old; *PSEN1*, 30–58; *PSEN2*, 40–85. For sporadic Alzheimer's disease, the age range is 60–100 years of age (Gómez-Isla et al., 1999). In ALS–PDC of

Guam and Irian Jaya, the age of onset historically was shifted downwards in all cases (see Chapter 7).

Why these time windows exist at all is not clear, but the general pattern holds even with a spectrum disorder such as ALS-PDC, in which the ALS phenotype typically appears before the others in individuals who develop PDC as well.

What is curious about this is the fact that the respective groups of neurons affected in each disease begin to differentiate in fetal development and early postnatal life in much the same temporal order as that of disease onset: motor neurons differentiate in spinal cord at about fetal day 28, neurons of the SNpc at about fetal day 50, and neurons of the cortex and hippocampus from fetal day 56, peaking at 28 weeks after birth (Supèr et al., 1998; Clowry et al., 2005; Clancy et al., 2007; Bystron et al., 2008). In other words, as one moves up the neuraxis rostrally, differentiation occurs at progressively later times. It is as if there is a set time point for the degeneration of certain susceptible neuronal populations that is roughly based on the age of differentiation.

The same sort of time line was observed in the mice fed the ALS-PDC-linked cycad seed flour cited in Chapter 7. In these studies, ALS phenotypes preceded parkinsonism phenotypes and cognitive decline. In general, neuronal differentiation in mice follows the same caudal-to-rostral pattern as in humans, so the link between fetal age of neuronal differentiation and later neuronal degeneration in mouse and human manifestations of neurological disease is, at the very least, intriguing.

It thus seems as if developmental features of the CNS are followed by degenerative events in terms of time lines. It is therefore important to consider, in brief, aspects of CNS development, and in this way seek further clues to neurological disease origins.

Endnote

1 From an interview about an article written by Singer et al. (2005): http://www.news-medical.net/news/2005/09/26/13300.aspx (last accessed September 23, 2016).

10

Development, Aging, and Neurological Disease

"Autism is a neurological disorder. It's not caused by bad parenting. It's caused by, you know, abnormal development in the brain. The emotional circuits in the brain are abnormal. And there also are differences in the white matter, which is the brain's computer cables that hook up the different brain departments."

Prof. Temple Grandin[1]

From the Preface

The various items cited previously apply to this chapter.

10.1   Introduction

Postnatal neural development in humans, as with all mammals, is characterized by rapid changes in neuronal and glial numbers and vast modifications in synaptic numbers, types, and distributions (Webb et al., 2001). However, compared to other mammals, humans are born vastly more neurologically, and thus behaviorally, immature. Much of this has to do with the dynamics of birthing and the size of the female pelvic opening in relation to the size of the newborn human's head.

During early postnatal life, neurons and their connections are added continuously, albeit at a low rate, until very late adolescence. Neurogenesis can continue throughout life in some central nervous system (CNS) regions (Winner and Winkler, 2015). At the same time, in early postnatal life, "exuberant" connections and many prenatal neurons are pruned by apoptosis (Paolicelli et al., 2011; Stephan et al., 2012). In the case of ASD, connectivity in some regions, such as the corpus callosum, is not as completely reduced (see Chapter 11), and the "normal" ratio of excitatory to inhibitory synapses in some areas appears to be altered to favor greater excitation (Pettem et al., 2013).

The biochemistry of the early mammalian postnatal CNS is also quite different from that of later life. Various molecules, such as the antioxidant glutathione, rise dramatically (Wang et al., 2005). Neurotransmitter and neuromodulatory receptors change their characteristics, subunit compositions (as well as during later aging), and distributions (see Burnashev et al., 1992 and Pagliusi et al., 1994 for subunit changes during postnatal life and aging, and Shaw et al., 1986 on altered receptor distributions).

Neural Dynamics of Neurological Disease, First Edition. Christopher A. Shaw.
© 2017 John Wiley & Sons, Inc. Published 2017 by John Wiley & Sons, Inc.

Most of these postnatal alterations in structure and biochemistry are qualitatively common to other mammalian species, with some exceptions. Concerning the latter, a key hallmark of humans and other primates (and perhaps some cetaceans) is the expansion of the so-called association areas of the neocortex from which more complex functions arise (e.g., language, abstract thought, and, more generally, higher-order consciousness itself).

There are a host of other, more detailed changes in the CNS, both in normal development and in developmental disorders, whose full descriptions are beyond the scope of this book. As an example of the latter, juvenile schizophrenia is obviously relevant, as the triggers and outcomes seem to be multifaceted. While this disorder is not discussed here in any detail, some discussion of the factors leading to ASD is warranted given the apparent synergy of genetic and environmental influences. These will be addressed in this chapter.

10.2   The Fetal Basis of Adult Disease Hypothesis

An epidemiological study by Barker and Osmond (1986) noted that low birth weight with small head circumference and low ponderal index (mass/height^3) at birth significantly correlated with an increased risk of developing coronary heart disease and hypertension later in life. This became the foundation of the "fetal basis of adult disease" (FeBAD) hypothesis, which postulates that certain events occurring during prenatal life have a profound, but delayed, impact in later adult life. This study was replicated by other investigators and has been broadened to include type 2 diabetes (Hales et al., 1991), breast cancer (Michels et al., 1996), and childhood leukemia (Hjalgrim et al., 2003), amongst other diseases. Possible mechanisms in these cases may include hormonal signals and epigenetic modifications (Lau et al., 2011).

In some ways, the notion is similar to the two-hit/multi-hit hypothesis discussed in Chapter 6, where the initial hit is considered to be some prenatal factor and the second hit is the secondary event later in life, often of the same type, which builds upon the first to create the expression of the disease state.

This concept has not drawn a great deal of attention in regard to neurological diseases, but the data that do exist seem to support the view that similar processes can operate in the nervous system as well. This was proposed in a talk by Prof. Andrew Eisen at an ALS meeting, when he suggested that ALS may arise in part due to fetal neuronal insults of unknown types (Eisen, 2010). Eisen was speaking about sALS, where the notion of toxin-induced motor neuron degeneration is more readily accepted. At this talk, however, his comments were delivered to a heavily pro-m*SOD1* audience, amongst which his speculations seemed to have had little traction. Nevertheless, Eisen's perspective has found some support in the neurological disease literature. Studies by Barlow et al. (2004) employed a murine model of Parkinson's disease in which a pregnant dam was exposed to low doses of common agricultural chemicals (maneb and paraquat) that had been shown previously to induce parkinsonism-like phenotypes following adult exposure (Thiruchelvam et al., 2000). The most striking finding was that pups exposed *in utero* were more likely to develop the parkinsonism phenotype when exposed a second time as adults to doses lower than normally required to produce neuronal degeneration. A second observation was that male mice were more affected than the females.

Very similar outcomes were observed in my laboratory using the toxic steryl glucosides that had been used to create a model of ALS–PDC in mice, as discussed in Chapters 6 and 7. In these studies, low doses of these molecules were administered by diet to the

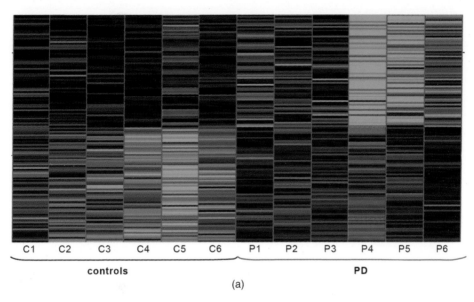

C1 C2 C3 C4 C5 C6 P1 P2 P3 P4 P5 P6

controls   PD

(a)

Figure 1.2 Typical examples of genomic/proteomic differences in neurodegenerative disease victims compared to control patients. (a) Relative expression levels of the 137 genes differentially expressed in Parkinson's disease (PD) samples relative to controls. Only genes that met the criterion of being altered by a factor of 1.5 relative to control and which passed the Wilcoxon test at the significant level of $p < 0.05$ were included. Genes are clustered by their relative expression levels over the 12 samples. Expression levels are color-coded relative to the mean: green for values less than the mean and red for values greater than it. *Source*: Grünblatt et al. (2004), used with permission from Springer Science and Business Media. (b) Genes differentially expressed in the motor cortex of sporadic ALS subjects: 57 of 19 431 quality-filtered genes (0.3%), represented by 61 probes, were differentially expressed (corrected $p < 0.05$), with each row in the matrix representing a single probe and each column a subject. Normalized expression levels are represented by the color of the corresponding cell, relative to the median abundance of each gene for each subject (see scale). Genes are named using their UniGene symbol and arranged in a hierarchical cluster (standard correlation) based on their expression patterns, combined with a dendrogram whose branch lengths reflect the relatedness of expression patterns. For each gene, the fold-change (diseased vs. control) and corrected p values are given. *Source*: Lederer et al. (2007), used under Creative Commons Attribution License.

Neural Dynamics of Neurological Disease, First Edition. Christopher A. Shaw.
© 2017 John Wiley & Sons, Inc. Published 2017 by John Wiley & Sons, Inc.

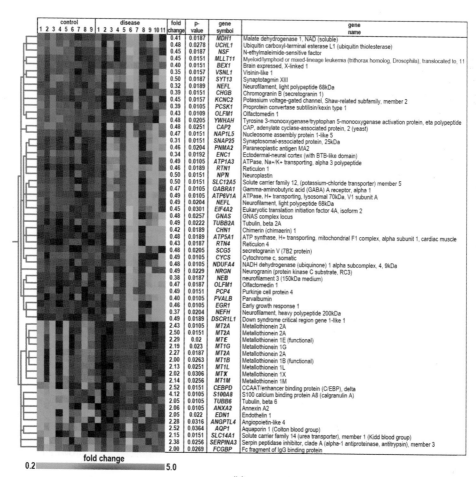

control	disease	fold change	p-value	gene symbol	gene name
		0.41	0.0187	MDH1	Malate dehydrogenase 1, NAD (soluble)
		0.48	0.0278	UCHL1	Ubiquitin carboxyl-terminal esterase L1 (ubiquitin thiolesterase)
		0.45	0.0187	NSF	N-ethylmaleimide-sensitive factor
		0.45	0.0151	MLLT11	Myeloid/lymphoid or mixed-lineage leukemia (trithorax homolog, Drosophila), translocated to, 11
		0.40	0.0151	BEX1	Brain expressed, X-linked 1
		0.35	0.0157	VSNL1	Visinin-like 1
		0.50	0.0187	SYT13	Synaptotagmin XIII
		0.32	0.0189	NEFL	Neurofilament, light polypeptide 68kDa
		0.39	0.0151	CHGB	Chromogranin B (secretogranin 1)
		0.45	0.0157	KCNC2	Potassium voltage-gated channel, Shaw-related subfamily, member 2
		0.39	0.0105	PCSK1	Proprotein convertase subtilisin/kexin type 1
		0.43	0.0109	OLFM1	Olfactomedin 1
		0.48	0.0205	YWHAH	Tyrosine 3-monooxygenase/tryptophan 5-monooxygenase activation protein, eta polypeptide
		0.48	0.0251	CAP2	CAP, adenylate cyclase-associated protein, 2 (yeast)
		0.47	0.0151	NAP1L5	Nucleosome assembly protein 1-like 5
		0.31	0.0151	SNAP25	Synaptosomal-associated protein, 25kDa
		0.46	0.0204	PNMA2	Paraneoplastic antigen MA2
		0.34	0.0192	ENC1	Ectodermal-neural cortex (with BTB-like domain)
		0.49	0.0105	ATP1A3	ATPase, Na+/K+ transporting, alpha 3 polypeptide
		0.46	0.0189	RTN1	Reticulon 1
		0.50	0.0151	NPN	Neuroplastin
		0.50	0.0151	SLC12A5	Solute carrier family 12, (potassium-chloride transporter) member 5
		0.47	0.0105	GABRA1	Gamma-aminobutyric acid (GABA) A receptor, alpha 1
		0.49	0.0105	ATP6V1A	ATPase, H+ transporting, lysosomal 70kDa, V1 subunit A
		0.49	0.0204	NEFL	Neurofilament, light polypeptide 68kDa
		0.45	0.0301	EIF4A2	Eukaryotic translation initiation factor 4A, isoform 2
		0.48	0.0257	GNAS	GNAS complex locus
		0.49	0.0222	TUBB2A	Tubulin, beta 2A
		0.42	0.0189	CHN1	Chimerin (chimaerin) 1
		0.48	0.0189	ATP5A1	ATP synthase, H+ transporting, mitochondrial F1 complex, alpha subunit 1, cardiac muscle
		0.43	0.0187	RTN4	Reticulon 4
		0.48	0.0205	SCG5	secretogranin V (7B2 protein)
		0.49	0.0105	CYCS	Cytochrome c, somatic
		0.48	0.0105	NDUFA4	NADH dehydrogenase (ubiquinone) 1 alpha subcomplex, 4, 9kDa
		0.49	0.0229	NRGN	Neurogranin (protein kinase C substrate, RC3)
		0.38	0.0187	NEB	neurofilament 3 (150kDa medium)
		0.47	0.0187	OLFM1	Olfactomedin 1
		0.49	0.0151	PCP4	Purkinje cell protein 4
		0.40	0.0105	PVALB	Parvalbumin
		0.46	0.0105	EGR1	Early growth response 1
		0.37	0.0204	NEFH	Neurofilament, heavy polypeptide 200kDa
		0.49	0.0189	DSCR1L1	Down syndrome critical region gene 1-like 1
		2.43	0.0105	MT2A	Metallothionein 2A
		2.50	0.0151	MT2A	Metallothionein 2A
		2.29	0.02	MTE	Metallothionein 1E (functional)
		2.19	0.023	MT1G	Metallothionein 1G
		2.27	0.0187	MT2A	Metallothionein 2A
		2.00	0.0263	MT1B	Metallothionein 1B (functional)
		2.13	0.0251	MT1L	Metallothionein 1L
		2.02	0.0306	MTX	Metallothionein 1X
		2.14	0.0256	MT1M	Metallothionein 1M
		2.52	0.0151	CEBPD	CCAAT/enhancer binding protein (C/EBP), delta
		4.12	0.0105	S100A8	S100 calcium binding protein A8 (calgranulin A)
		2.05	0.0105	TUBB6	Tubulin, beta 6
		2.06	0.0105	ANXA2	Annexin A2
		2.05	0.022	EDN1	Endothelin 1
		2.28	0.0316	ANGPTL4	Angiopoietin-like 4
		2.52	0.0364	AQP1	Aquaporin 1 (Colton blood group)
		2.15	0.0151	SLC14A1	Solute carrier family 14 (urea transporter), member 1 (Kidd blood group)
		2.38	0.0256	SERPINA3	Serpin peptidase inhibitor, clade A (alpha-1 antiproteinase, antitrypsin), member 3
		2.00	0.0269	FCGBP	Fc fragment of IgG binding protein

fold change

0.2 ———————— 5.0

(b)

Figure 1.2 (*Continued*)

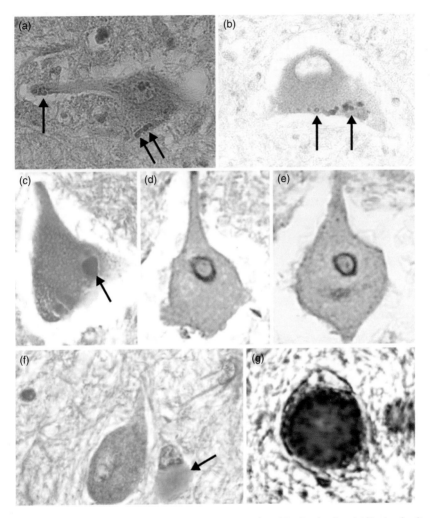

Figure 2.2 Key cellular features of ALS. (a,b) Light micrographs of Bunina bodies. (a) Bunina bodies in an anterior horn cell of an sALS patient. Bunina bodies are small eosinophilic inclusions (approximately 1–3 μm in diameter) that stain bright red with hematoxylin–eosin (H-E). They are observed within the cytoplasm (double arrows), arranged in a chain-like formation, and within dendrites (arrow), appearing as a cluster. (b) Cystatin C immunostaining. Bunina bodies are positive for cystatin C (double arrows). A Bunina body (indicated by the center arrow) appears as a round structure with a central-lucent core, which corresponds to a cytoplasmic island containing neurofilaments and other micro-organelles at the ultrastructural level. (c–e) Light micrographs of neuronal Lewy body-like hyaline inclusions (LBHIs). (c) A round LBHI (arrow) is observed in the cytoplasm of the anterior horn cell, composed of an eosinophilic core with a paler peripheral halo. A small, ill-defined LBHI (arrowhead) is also seen in the cytoplasm of the anterior horn cell, consisting of obscure, slightly eosinophilic materials. H-E staining was used. (d,e) Serial sections of a neuronal LBHI in a spinal anterior horn cell immunostained with antibodies against (d) m*SOD1* and (e) ubiquitin. An intraneuronal LBHI is clearly labeled by the antibodies to *SOD1* and ubiquitin. The immunoreactivity for both *SOD1* and ubiquitin is almost restricted to the halo of the LBHI. (f) Light micrograph of an astrocytic hyaline inclusion (Ast-HI) in the spinal-cord anterior horn. The Ast-HI (arrow) is round and eosinophilic. The astrocyte bearing the Ast-HI is morphologically different from the adjacent neuron. The nucleus of the cell bearing the Ast-HI resembles that of a reactive astrocyte (double arrowheads), and not that of an oligodendrocyte (arrowhead). H-E staining was used. (g) A neurofilamentous conglomerate inclusion, showing intense immunohistochemical positivity for phosphorylated neurofilament protein. Scale bar: (a–e,g) 30 μm; (f) 10 μm. *Source*: Kato (2008), used with permission from Springer Science and Business Media.

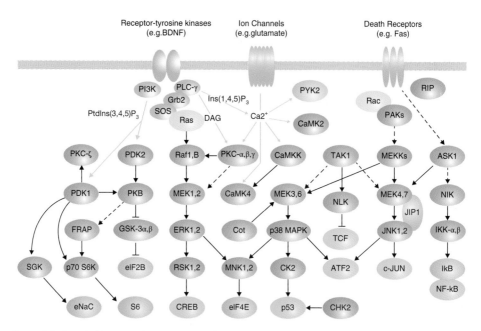

Figure 3.3 Protein kinase pathways activated in ALS and animal models (*mSOD1*) of ALS. In this example, activation of receptor tyrosine kinases can occur via an increased release of growth factors from neurons and non-neuronal cells produced as a regenerative response in ALS (Wagey et al., 1998). Tyrosine-specific protein kinases are shown in pink and serine/threonine-specific protein kinases and mitogen-activated protein kinase (MEK) isoforms are shown in blue (see color plates). Transcription factors are shown in green, monomeric GTPases in yellow, and other in brown. Direct activation is indicated with solid black arrows, whereas indirect activation is indicated by dashed arrows. Actions of second messengers are shown by green arrows. ATF2, activation transcription factor 2; BDNF, brain-derived neurotrophic factor; CHK2, checkpoint kinase 2; CK2, casein kinase 2; Cot, cancer Osaka thyroid; DAG, diacylglycerol; eIF, eukaryotic initiation factor; eNaC, epithelial Na× channel; FKBP, FK506 binding protein; FRAP, FKBP-rapamycin-associated protein; Grb2, growth factor receptor-bound protein 2; GSK-3a, glycogen synthase kinase 3a; IKKa, IKB kinase a; Ins(1,4,5)P3, inositol (1,4,5)-trisphosphate; JIP1, JNK-interacting protein 1; JNK1, c-JUN N-terminal kinase 1; p38 MAPK, p38 mitogen-activated protein kinase; MEKK, MEK kinase; MNK, MAPK-interacting kinase (MAPK signal integrating kinase); NIK, NF-kB-inducing kinase; NLK, Nemo-like kinase; PAK, p21-activated kinase; PDK, 3-phosphoinositide-dependent kinase; PI3K, phosphatidylinositol 3-kinase; PdtIns(3,4,5)P3, s phosphatidylinositol (3,4,5)-trisphosphate; PKB, protein kinase B; PLC-g, phospholipase Cg; PYK2, proline-rich tyrosine kinase 2 (phosphotyrosine kinase 2). *Source*: Krieger et al. (2003), used with permission from Elsevier.

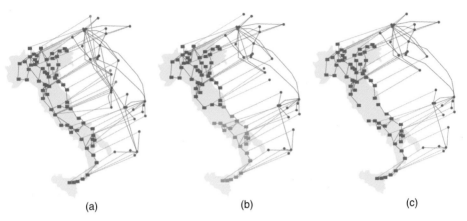

(a)   (b)   (c)

Figure 4.1 Example of a cascading failure: Italian power grid collapse. Illustration of an iterative process of a cascade of failures using real-world data from a power network (located on the map of Italy) and an Internet network (shifted above the map) that were implicated in an electrical blackout in Italy in September 2003. The networks are drawn using the real geographical locations, and every Internet server is connected to the geographically nearest power station. (a) One power station is removed (red node on map; see color plates) from the power network, and as a result the Internet nodes that depend on it are removed from the Internet network (red nodes above the map). The nodes that will be disconnected from the giant cluster (a cluster that spans the entire network) at the next step are marked in green. (b) Additional nodes that were disconnected from the Internet communication network giant component are removed (red nodes above map). As a result, the power stations depending on them are removed from the power network (red nodes on map). Again, the nodes that will be disconnected from the giant cluster at the next step are marked in green. (c) Additional nodes that were disconnected from the giant component of the power network are removed (red nodes on map), as are the nodes in the Internet network that depend on them (red nodes above map). *Source*: Redrawn from Buldyrev et al. (2010), used with permission from Macmillan Publishers Ltd: [*Nature*].

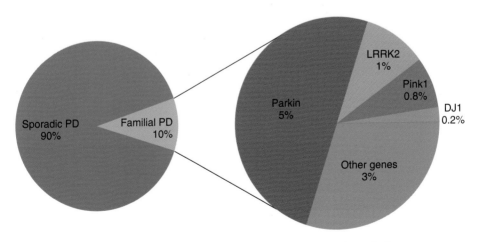

Figure 5.1 Number of identified causality genes in early-onset familial Parkinson's disease.

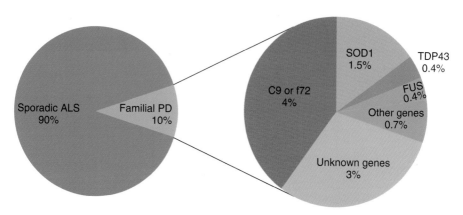

Figure 5.2 Number of identified causality genes in early-onset fALS.

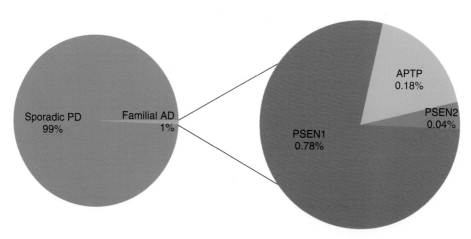

Figure 5.3 Number of identified causality genes in early-onset familial Alzheimer's disease.

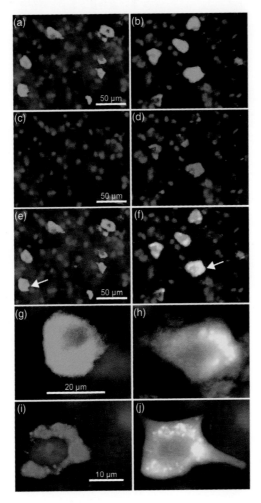

Figure 6.2 Motor neuron degeneration induced by aluminum. NeuN and activated caspase-3 fluorescent labeling in ventral horn of lumbar spinal cord. Green: NeuN; red: activated caspase-3; yellow: co-localization of NeuN and activated caspase-3; blue: nuclear DAPI (see color plates). (a,b) NeuN labeling in control and aluminum hydroxide-injected mouse lumbar spinal cord sections, respectively. (c,d) Control and aluminum hydroxide mouse lumbar spinal cord sections labeled with caspase-3. (e,f) Merge of NeuN and caspase. Magnification ×40. (g,h) Enlargements of neurons indicated by white arrows in (e,f). Magnification ×100. (i,j) Enlargement of another activated caspase-3-positive motor neuron. (j) Merged image of activated caspase-3 and NeuN. Magnification ×100. *Source*: Petrik et al. (2007a), with permission from Springer Science and Business Media.

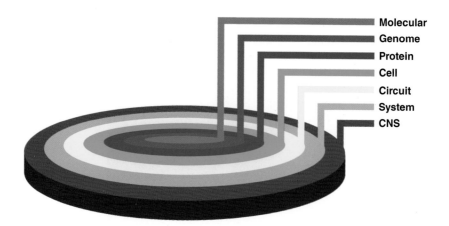

Molecular
Genome
Protein
Cell
Circuit
System
CNS

Figure 6.4 Aluminum impacts at various levels of organization in the CNS. *Source*: Redrawn from Shaw et al. (2014a) under the Creative Commons Attribution License.

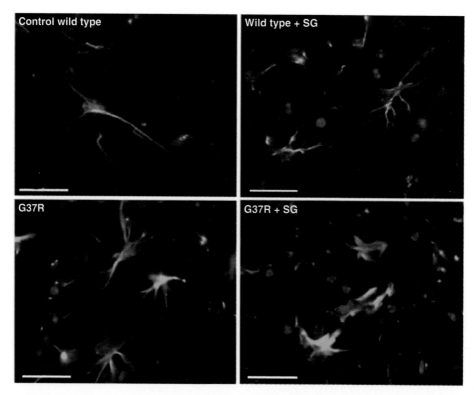

Figure 6.6 Gene–toxin interactions in the m*SOD1* model of ALS. Micrographs of green fluorescent glial fibrillary acidic protein (GFAP) immunostaining in lumbar spinal sections of control-fed wild-type, steryl gluocosides (SG)-fed wild-type, control-fed G37R, and SG-fed G37R mice. *Source*: Modified from Lee and Shaw (2012), under Creative Commons Attribution License.

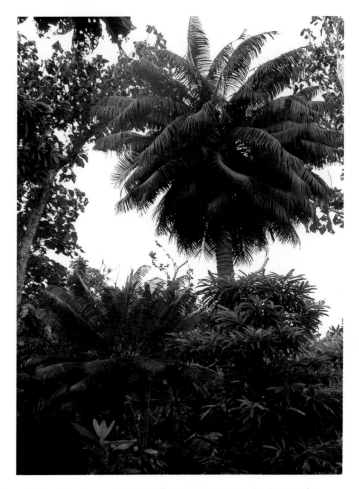

Figure 7.6 Cycad "palm" (*C. micronesica* K.D. Hill) on Guam. *Source*: Dr. Tom Marler.

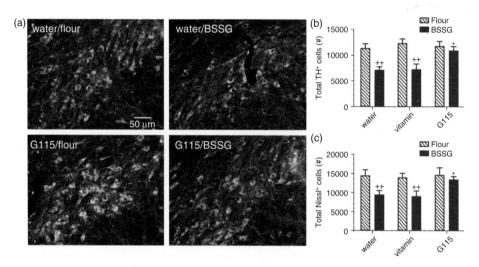

Figure 7.12 *In vivo* data from BSSG feeding studies in rats. (a) Representative fluorescent photomicrographs of tyrosine hydroxulase (TH) (green) and Nissl (red) immunostaining in the SN 35 weeks following initial BSSG exposure (see color plates). Unbiased stereologic counts of (b) TH + and (c) Nissl + cells in the SN were significantly reduced in those animals treated with BSSG. However, no significant cell loss was observed in those animals treated with G115, a ginseng-derived molecule. In contrast, vitamin supplementation alone failed to alter BSSG-induced nigral cell loss. Each bar represents the mean (± SEM, n = 9–12) number of TH or Nissl immunopositive cells counted in the SN. ++sig. diff. from flour control, p < 0.001; + p < 0.05. **sig. diff. from water control, p < 0.001. *Source:* Modified from Van Kampen et al. (2014a), with permission from Elsevier. The caption has been modified from the published article.

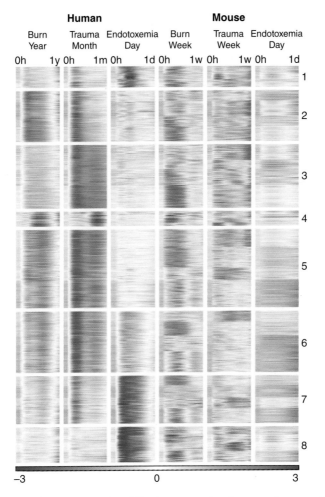

Figure 8.1 Illustration of genomic variation following trauma in mice versus humans, showing comparisons of the time-course gene changes for human burns, trauma, and endotoxin treatment and murine models of the same. K-means clustering of 4918 genes responsive to human systemic inflammation over time. Time interval for the human conditions: burns = up to 1 year; trauma = 1 month; endotoxemia = 1 day. Time intervals for mouse models: trauma and burns = 1 week; endotoxemia = 1 day (endotoxemia). *Source*: Redrawn from Seok et al. (2013).

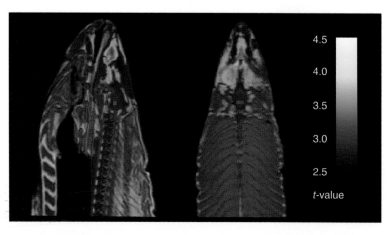

Figure 8.2 The "dead salmon" MRI and faux neural activity. *Source*: Bennett et al. (2009), under Creative Commons Attribution License.

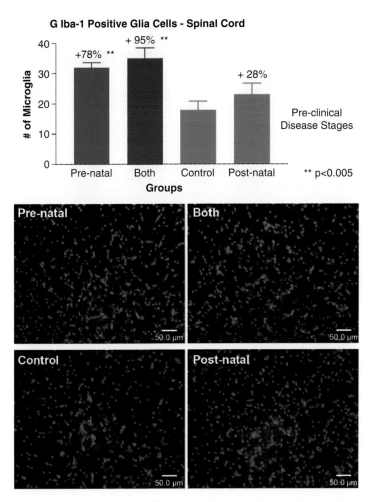

Figure 10.1 The FeBAD hypothesis in mice. Two types of toxic steryl glucoside together induced microglial proliferation in the lumbar spinal cord and striatum in groups of mice treated at prenatal, postnatal, or both prenatal and postnatal time points. Microglia expression was assayed in both the lumbar spinal cord and the striatum using an antibody against the ionized calcium-binding adaptor molecule 1 (Iba-1, red; nuclear counter stain (DAPI), blue; see color plates). Quantification of positively labeled cells was performed on the ventral horn of spinal cord sections. Student's t-test, $p < 0.05$; one way ANOVA, $p = 0.0028$; Tukey's for parental vs. control, $p < 0.05$; Tukey's for both vs. control, $p < 0.01$. Quantification was done under a light microscope using the 20× objective lens. The accompanying micrographs show representative data across the groups.*Source*: Banjo (2009).

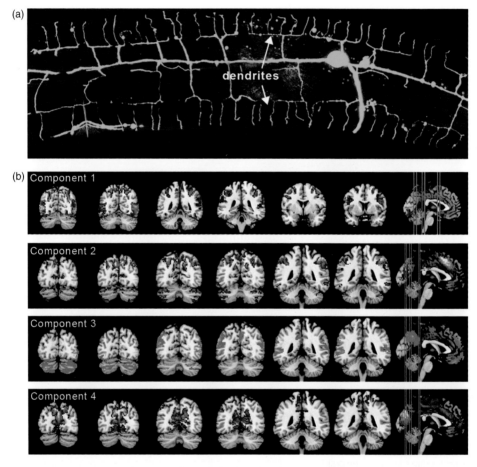

Figure 11.3 Neuronal lateralization of morphology and/or function from *C. elegans* to humans.
(a) Green fluorescent signal showing PVD neurons in *C. elegans* (see color plates). (b) Functional MRI images showing activated or deactivated brain regions involved in language and social tasks from the Human Connectome Project database. Blue areas indicate deactivated regions, while red areas indicate activated regions. The left and right hemispheres show asymmetry in activation and deactivation patterns.*Source*: (a) Adapted from Salzberg et al. (2013), with permission from Elsevier; (b) Dr. Todd Woodward, with permission.

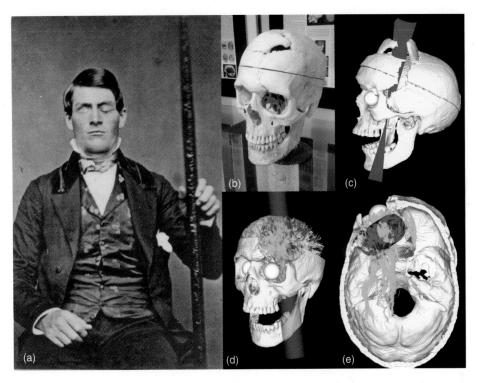

Figure 14.1 The CNS injuries of Phineas Gage. (a) Photograph of cased-daguerreotype studio portrait of brain-injury survivor Phineas P. Gage (1823–1860), shown holding the tamping rod that injured him. (b–e) Modeling the path of the tamping rod through the Gage skull and its effects on CNS structures (b) The skull of Phineas Gage on display at the Warren Anatomical Museum at Harvard Medical School. (c) Computed tomography (CT) image volumes of the individual pieces of bone dislodged by the tamping rod, the top of the cranium, and the mandible – reconstructed, spatially aligned, and manually segmented. (d) A rendering of the Gage skull with the best-fit rod trajectory and example fiber pathways in the left hemisphere intersected by the rod. (e) A view of the interior of the Gage skull showing the extent of fiber pathways intersected by the tamping rod in a sample subject (i.e., one having minimal spatial deformation to the Gage skull). *Source*: (a) Collection of Jack and Beverly Wilgus, under Creative Commons Attribution License; (b–e) Van Horn et al. (2012), under Creative Commons Attribution License.

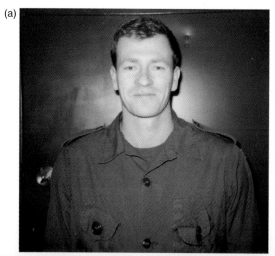

(a)

(b)

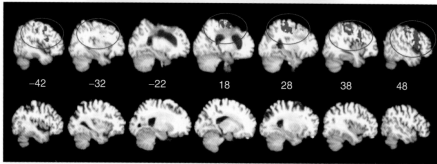

Figure 14.2 The CNS injuries of Trevor Greene. (a) Photograph of Lieutenant Trevor Greene, taken prior to his deployment to Afghanistan. (b) Sagittal view of mean lower-limb motor activation and mental-imagery activation on functional magnetic resonance imaging (fMRI), averaged across all time points (red; T1–T12, 33 months) (see color plates). Numbers indicate the x coordinate for each slice (Z > 2.3, pcorr < 0.05). *Source*: (a) Pierre Gazzola (https://www.flickr.com/photos/85013738@N00/), under Creative Commons Attribution License; (b) D'Arcy et al. (2012), with permission from Wolters Kluwer Health, Inc.

mouse dam at a stage of fetal development in which neurons in the lumbar spinal cord were differentiating. As with the Barlow et al. study, the pups were found to be more susceptible to a second subthreshold toxic dose of these steryl glucosides later in life, and, once again, males were more severely affected than females (Banjo, 2009; Banjo et al., 2009a,b) (Figure 10.1).

While there is a general paucity of other results in this area, these data from two different laboratories using quite different toxic agents suggest that toxin exposure in prenatal life may indeed be an important determinant of the emergence of a later neurological disease state. Indeed, this notion may not be surprising given the number of

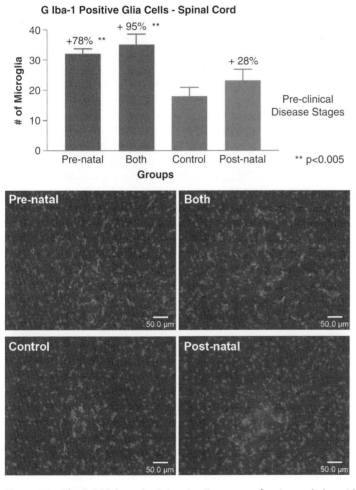

Figure 10.1 The FeBAD hypothesis in mice. Two types of toxic steryl glucoside together induced microglial proliferation in the lumbar spinal cord and striatum in groups of mice treated at prenatal, postnatal, or both prenatal and postnatal time points. Microglia expression was assayed in both the lumbar spinal cord and the striatum using an antibody against the ionized calcium-binding adaptor molecule 1 (Iba-1, red; nuclear counter stain (DAPI), blue). Quantification of positively labeled cells was performed on the ventral horn of spinal cord sections. Student's t-test, $p < 0.05$; one way ANOVA, $p = 0.0028$; Tukey's for parental vs. control, $p < 0.05$; Tukey's for both vs. control, $p < 0.01$. Quantification was done under a light microscope using the 20× objective lens. The accompanying micrographs show representative data across the groups. In this figure, only data from spinal cord is shown, but the results for striatum were qualitatively similar. *Source*: Banjo (2009). (See color plate section for the color representation of this figure.)

toxic molecules to which humans are exposed during fetal development. The list of such potential toxins is large, as cited in Chapter 6, and certainly includes such things as aluminum, various excitotoxins, bisphenols and other endocrine disrupters, agricultural toxic chemicals of various types, and a host of other molecules.

One still emerging area in which the FeBAD hypothesis may have the most weight in terms of neurological diseases is studies of ASD and schizophrenia. Atladóttir et al. (2010) reported significant increases in the numbers of ASD children born to mothers who had viral infections in the first trimester of pregnancy or bacterial infections in the second trimester. The second hit in such cases remains unknown, but it could be other forms of immune activation.

Patterson and various colleagues performed a series of animal studies to demonstrate ASD-like social outcomes in the offspring of pregnant mice exposed to influenza virus or given synthetic double-stranded RNA poly (I : C) to induce a pathogen-free immune response (Patterson, 2011; Malkova et al., 2012). Both types of stimulus provide examples of what has been termed "maternal immune activation" (MIA). Similar MIA-induced outcomes were seen with lipopolysaccharide (LPS) injections as a bacterial infection mimetic. In general, MIA in rodent models appears to be dependent on modulation by a subtype of nicotinic acetylcholine receptors (Wu et al., 2015).

These effects appear to be mediated by the cytokine interleukin 6 (IL-6) (Smith et al., 2007; Wei et al., 2012a), although other cytokines are also involved (Arrode-Brusés and Brusés, 2012), in a similar manner to those speculated to be involved in human ASD (Wei et al., 2011; Goines and Ashwood, 2012). The MIA outcomes did include some of the same pathological features as in ASD, including increased brain volume (Wei et al., 2012b) and brain regional specificity (Garay et al., 2012). As with ASD, the impact on males was higher than in females (Xuan and Hampson, 2014). The effects of such IL-6 activation appear to be permanent (Hsiao et al., 2012).

One fact that appears to be unavoidable is that aluminum salts as adjuvants are almost inevitably going to be involved in such reactions given their basic antigenicity and well-documented ability to do what adjuvants are supposed to do: hyperstimulate an immune response by increasing precisely the cytokines linked to MIA (Viezeliene et al., 2013).

Aluminum antigenicity is also likely to prove problematic from another perspective, in that accumulation of aluminum by any route into various CNS regions, or other organ systems, has the potential to trigger an antibody assault on those cells in which aluminum is already extant (Levy et al., 1998).

10.3   ASD as a Developmental Neurological Disorder

Autism and related disorders of the autism spectrum (i.e., Asperger's syndrome, pervasive developmental disorder not otherwise specified, Rett syndrome, etc.) are neurodevelopmental disorders characterized by dysfunctional immune function, stereotypic behaviors, and various degrees of impairment in social skills and verbal communication (i.e., delayed language acquisition and usage). In the United States, the average incidence, as of this writing, is 1 : 68 children, with the rates in males considerably higher than in females (Centers for Disease Control and Prevention, 2016).

Other neurological and medical conditions frequently co-occur with ASD, including mental retardation (30% of cases score mild to moderate; 40% score serious to profound retardation) (Fombonne, 1999, 2003) and epilepsy (40% of cases) (Tuchman and

Rapin, 2002). Comorbid behavioral and psychiatric conditions associated with the core symptoms include aggression, disruptive behaviors, hyperactivity, self-injury, sensory abnormalities, anxiety, depression, and sleep disturbances.

The most frequent non-neurological comorbidities associated with ASD are gastrointestinal (GI) abnormalities and underlying inflammation (Torrente et al., 2002; White, 2003; Balzola et al., 2005; Jass, 2005; Ashwood et al., 2006; Chen et al., 2010), feeding difficulties, and food sensitivities (Newschaffer et al., 2007).

ASD symptoms normally appear before 36 months of age. Regression or loss of skills occurs in 30% of affected children, usually at between 18 and 24 months of age (Rapin, 1997).

Abnormal neural connectivity is one of the key pathological features of the autistic brain. The term "connectivity" encompasses local connectivity within neural assemblies and long-range connectivity between brain regions. Similarly, there is also physical connectivity (hard-wiring), associated with synapses and tracts, and functional connectivity (soft-wiring), associated with neurotransmission (Belmonte et al., 2004). In the autistic brain, high local connectivity may develop in tandem with low long-range connectivity (Just et al., 2004), potentially as a result of widespread alterations in synapse elimination and/or formation and/or changes in inhibitory/excitatory synaptic ratios (Pettem et al., 2013).

As cited in Section 10.2, the potential role of immune dysfunctions in generating such anatomical features of ASD will be discussed in the next chapter. Overall, while the notion of immune system contributions to ASD remains controversial, the notion of immune system involvement in CNS development, at least in prenatal life, is now well established.

10.3.1 Etiology of ASD

The etiologies proposed for ASD show the same general range as those proposed for the well-known neurological disorders associated with aging, such as Parkinson's disease, ALS, and Alzheimer's disease (Figure 10.2). In brief, both genetic and environmental factors have been proposed.

To put ASD into a broader context of other neurological disorders and causality factors, it is useful to briefly recapitulate the general range of such potential factors in these diseases.

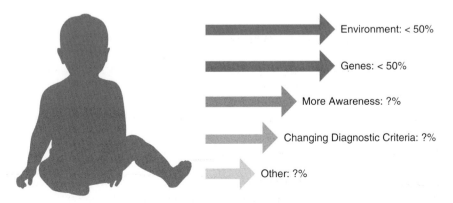

Environment: < 50%

Genes: < 50%

More Awareness: ?%

Changing Diagnostic Criteria: ?%

Other: ?%

Figure 10.2 Putative causal factors in ASD.

In ALS, it is clear that much of the literature of the last 20 years has focused preferentially on the search for genetic mutations leading to motor neuron loss, and the list of defective genes has grown larger over this period. As discussed, these include a number of variations in *SOD1*, *TARDBP*, *FUS*, *VEGF*, and *C9orf72*, all of which have added to the complexity of the polygenic picture without necessarily increasing the total percentage of ALS cases that are clearly gene mutation-derived. Overall, the various mutations may account for about 10% of all ALS, of which *mSOD1* may make up about 25% (or 2.5% of the total number of cases). Much the same general conclusions can be reached for the ratios of genetic to sporadic cases in Parkinson's and Alzheimer's diseases, as discussed previously.

None of this diminishes the potential role of susceptibility genes – mostly unknown – whose interactions with the various environmental toxicants are highly likely to be crucial to the development of these diseases. Yet, in spite of these conclusions, the dominance of a genetic causality perspective remains relatively firmly in place, for reasons already discussed.

This latter point has to be emphasized again, since the same perspective dominates much of the ASD field. For the same reasons given for ALS and the other diseases, this view is likely to be fundamentally flawed in that the incidence of ASD appears to show a significantly more dramatic temporal increase over the last few decades than that of the adult neurological diseases. It is thus equally likely, if not more so, that the changing rates of ASD do not reflect a primary genetic defect in the population of those affected.

To see just how valid a genetic etiology might be, it is nevertheless worthwhile to first examine the data that do exist. Studies have usually taken one of three approaches: (i) whole-genome sequencing, predicting the chromosomal localization for the disorder by scanning families with more than one affected member, especially twin studies (Smalley et al., 1988; Yuen et al., 2015); (ii) cytogenetic and molecular studies seeking *de novo* chromosomal anomalies and inherited mutations, including gene copy-number variations; and (iii) candidate genes studies examining the relationship between those genes known to be associated with abnormal brain development and the disorder phenotype.

Using these approaches, chromosomes 2q21–33, 3q25–27, 3p25, 4q32, 6q14–21, 7q22, 7q31–36, 11p12–13, and 17q11–21 have been shown to have some linkage to ASD (Freitag et al., 2010). Duplications, inherited maternally, on the 15q11-q13 region of chromosome 15 have been particularly associated with the spectrum (Cook et al., 1997). Deletions on chromosome 16p11 have also been shown to be associated with ASD, mental retardation, and other developmental disabilities (Kumar et al., 2008). Replicated copy-number variations from genome-wide studies have been found to be located on the following chromosomes: 1q21, 2p16.3 (*NRXN1*), 3p25–26 (*CNTN4*), 7q36.2 (*DPP6*), 15q11–13 (*UBE3A*, *OR4M2*, *OR4N4*), 16p11.2 (*MAPK3*, *MAZ*, *DOC2A*, *SEZ6L2*, *HIRIP3*, *IL6*), and 22q11.2 (Freitag et al., 2010). However, some of these variations have also been shown to be more common in patients with schizophrenia and mental retardation than controls, thus raising questions about their specificity to ASD.

Several studies have demonstrated that ASD reflects heterogeneous disorders whose etiology is linked with several rare monogenetic disorders, such as Fragile X syndrome and mutations in *TSC1/TSC2*, *LAMB1*, *CNTNAP2*, *PTEN*, *DHCR7*, *SHANK3*, *NLGN3/4*, or *RPL10* (Freitag et al., 2010). Synaptic cell adhesion and associated molecules, including neurexin 1, neuroligin 3 and 4, and SHANK3, which indicate glutamatergic abnormalities in ASD, have also been cited (Miles et al., 2005).

A large difference in concordance rates between monozygotic and dizygotic twins in several studies had led the heritability of ASD, or the proportion of liability attributable to genetic factors, to be estimated at about 90% (Folstein and Rutter, 1977; Steffenburg et al., 1989; Bailey et al., 1995). However, a more recent study of the same types of twins shows that genetic susceptibility to ASD is considerably lower (Hallmayer et al., 2011). In particular, environmental factors common to twins account for 55% of their risk of developing ASD, while genetic heritability explains only 37%.

A key problem with genetic investigations into ASD origins has been the lack of reproducibility and overlap in the various studies. Although 10 full genome screens have been reported to date (e.g., Lauritsen et al., 2005; Bacchelli and Maestrini, 2006; Klauck, 2006), and indeed have identified numerous regions of suggestive linkage, only a small subset of these linkages overlap across the various studies. Similarly, although more than 100 candidate ASD genes have been studied, there is no consistent replication of positive results. One investigator, speaking to reporters, described ASD patients as "snowflakes," with no two alike from a genetic perspective (Yuen et al., 2015).[2] The snowflake notion has been discussed previously in this book, in the context of some of the other neurological diseases.

What can be concluded from all this is that while there are some genetic associations, it is clear that the mode of inheritance of autism is not Mendelian but rather must reflect a polygenic, multifactorial etiology, with multiple gene–gene and/or gene–environment/toxin interactions (Pickles et al., 1995; Risch et al., 1999).

Some other hypotheses have been put forward to explain the changing rates of ASD, including the claim that the increase arises from a broadening of diagnostic criteria and/or a greater awareness of the disorder by the medical community and the public at large (e.g., see Hansen et al., 2015). This hypothesis basically states that the observed increase is, in reality, an artifact.

If these explanations for the change in ASD incidence are not correct, researchers are left with the most likely one left. This is, as already stated, that environmental factors are playing some role in a still unknown fraction of this spectrum of disorders. Many of these involve various triggers of autoimmune reactions. Included in this list is aluminum in various forms, including as a vaccine adjuvant, as cited in Chapter 6. As a side note, it is important at this juncture to recognize that the topic of ASD etiology is a distinctly contentious one, given that any mention of environmental factors raises the issue of vaccines. These aspects will be dealt with in greater detail in Chapter 11.

A complex gene–environment etiology for ASD is, in fact, supported by various newer studies, which appear to promote a model of ASD as a multisystem disorder with genetic influence, environmental contributors, and a distinct immune component (Pardo et al., 2005; Vargas et al., 2005; Theoharides and Zhang, 2011; Angelidou et al., 2012). In other words, the presumed combination of factors, both genetic and environmental, rather remarkably resembles the adult-onset neurological diseases discussed throughout this book.

Animal models of ASD are in accord with this interpretation, suggesting that genetic variation, rather than being strictly causal to the disorder, instead confers an altered vulnerability to exposure to environmental stressors (Hunter et al., 2010). In this regard, an epidemiological study of ASD that included a comparison amongst siblings suggested that individuals with ASD may react with less tolerance to environmental stressors than their siblings without the disorder (Glasson et al., 2004).

10.3.2 Juvenile Schizophrenia

A form of schizophrenia that occurs in childhood or adolescence is characterized as a chronic and relapsing psychotic disorder. Two types are described in the literature: very early-onset schizophrenia (VEOS, also known as childhood-onset schizophrenia), occurring in children younger than 13, with a prevalence of 1 in 10 000–30 000 (Werry, 1992), and early-onset schizophrenia (EOS, also known as adolescent-onset schizophrenia), occurring between 13 and 17 years of age, with a prevalence of about half that of the earlier form (Burd and Kerbeshian, 1987). Symptoms are categorized as positive or negative (e.g., what a patient has (hallucinations and delusions) or does not have (flat affects and lack of speech or concentrated thought)).

Diagnoses are based on the *Diagnostic and Statistical Manual of Mental Disorders*, 5th edition (DSM-5) (American Psychiatric Association, 2013), using the same criteria given for adult-onset schizophrenia and ASD, which require at least two of the following symptoms for 1 month, including at least one of the first three: delusion, hallucination, disorganized speech, grossly disorganized or catatonic behavior, and negative symptoms.

As with ASD, not to mention the adult-onset progressive neurological diseases, some combination of genetic susceptibilities and environmental triggers is likely to be responsible (Asarnow et al., 2001; reviewed in Asarnow and Forsyth, 2013). Some of the environmental factors that have been suggested to contribute to early-onset schizophrenia include obstetric complications (Rosso et al., 2000), prenatal infection (Brown and Derkits, 2010) of a presumably MIA type, untreated blood-type incompatibility (Brown and Derkits, 2010), regular cannabis use (Veen et al., 2004), and early childhood trauma (Arseneault et al., 2011). It seems likely that other environmental agents will be found, and it is more than plausible that some of these will be various of the toxins considered in other chapters, perhaps in a form of FeBAD-like multiple neurological hits.

The pathophysiology of the disorder includes brain structural abnormalities (Keshavan and Hogarty, 1999; Brent et al., 2013), including enlargement of the lateral ventricles (also found in the adult form) (Shenton et al., 2001), decreased brain mass, smaller frontal and temporal gray-matter volumes (Rapoport et al., 1999), decreased cerebral and thalamic volume, and white-matter abnormalities (Jacobsen et al., 1996; Shenton et al., 2001; Kumra et al., 2005).

The key points to take from this are that schizophrenia is a spectrum disorder, much like ASD, and that like the latter it in all probability arises from a complex interaction between genetic susceptibility and environmental factors. In regard to this last point, Sekar et al. (2016) have now provided a further genetic study of schizophrenia that implicates genes associated with major histocompatibility complex (MHC) proteins, notably complement component 4 (C4). These results add several interesting aspects to the search for the etiology of schizophrenia. First, they emphasize yet again the range of genetic contributors to the disease, reinforcing the notion that these are "snowflake"-like disorders, as discussed for ASD. Second, the observation that C4 genes are involved firmly adds schizophrenia to the list of those neurological disorders that may arise in part due to immune-system interactions (Chapter 11).

10.3.3 Juvenile-Onset Forms of ALS and Other Neurological Disorders

ALS can occur in relatively young adults as a result of certain genetic mutations, as cited in Table 5.2. It has also been reported following exposure to putative toxic factors, as in

ALS-PDC, including at least two cases that are apparently the result of vaccine adverse reactions (Huang et al., 2009). The latter come from a case study presented at a neurology meeting concerning two teenaged girls who developed ALS following vaccination against the human papilloma virus (HPV). The subsequent paper did not, however, note any correlation to the vaccine, but this omission seems to have been an editorial, rather than scientific, decision (senior author, C. Lomen-Hoerth, pers. comm.).

Early-onset forms of parkinsonism have also been reported for Guamanian PDC and following exposure to MPTP, both as cited previously.

10.4 Toxins and Developmental CNS Disorders

A number of toxic substances have been linked to developmental disorders, including ASD. These include toxic agricultural chemicals such as glyphosate (Seneff et al., 2012), various endocrine disrupters such as bisphenol-A (Kinch et al., 2015), and aluminum, all as cited in Chapter 6. In regard to a potential role for aluminum, the apparently epigenetic alterations in gene expression induced by this element may similarly suggest that a variety of environmental toxins can have similar epigenetic impacts. This area of research is currently not well explored.

10.5 Developmental versus Mature CNS Disorders

While the developing nervous system appears to have an enormous capacity for repair and restructuring (see Shaw and McEachern, 2001), such restructuring may also be the basis for some abnormal function, as in ASD.

Neuronal compensation for gene or environmental insults to the CNS will be limited by the type of insult and the stage at which they occur. Early gene defects, if not rapidly fatal, may be compensated for by the redundancy of function of other genes. Environmental toxin impacts, if they do not cross too many levels of organization within the CNS (i.e., from gene to cell, cell to circuit, etc.), may allow for neuronal compensation by unaffected cells or regions.

Neuronal plasticity is not, however, a simple process (Shaw and McEachern, 2001), nor one strictly linked to any one stage of neuronal development or age (see review by Anderson et al., 2011). For example, many of the events that are typically considered to be neuroplastic arise within a critical period as a result of altered sensory input, leading to anatomical and functional changes in the CNS. One example is that of ocular dominance plasticity, as previously discussed. Other forms of sensory reorganization can occur in adult animals – and, presumably, humans – under some circumstances.

Toxic molecules that can cause neuronal degeneration in adult animals and humans can do so at younger ages as well. In this context, it is important to distinguish between various forms of neuroplasticity in regard to recovery from injury and age. One type of neuroplasticity is termed "restitution" and describes how damaged neuronal pathways are in part restored. The other form is "substitution," in which some other part(s) of the brain take on the functions of those areas lost to the injury.

In both young and older CNS, compensatory mechanisms seem able to provide some system restoration, and it seems partially true that this can be more effective at certain, but not all, young ages than in adults. One example in which the young can more easily recover is after unilateral stroke.

The age-dependent nature of neuroplasticity, however, makes the picture considerably more complex. As Anderson et al. (2011) note, the vulnerability to disruption of early CNS developmental programs paradoxically makes the young CNS exhibit a greater capacity for neuroplasticity but a worse capacity for recovery. These authors describe a "recovery continuum," in which the variables contributing to the different levels of recovery include the following: the site, nature, and severity of the injury; genetic susceptibility factors; sex; and, most important of all, age at insult in relation to the stage of CNS development. These aspects may be very much part and parcel of what makes those putative etiological factors implicated in ASD discussed earlier particularly likely to impact younger, rather than older, individuals.

Perhaps one way to view the impact of toxic molecules across the lifespan is this: In young nervous systems, a neurotoxin can have two sorts of outcome: outright pathological consequences and circuit and system reorganizations. In mature nervous systems, the former prevails and compensatory mechanisms are less effective. In both immature and mature nervous systems, compensatory mechanisms that are ineffective may actually become part of the longer-term overall pathological outcomes.

A key determinant of the types of outcome produced in response to a nervous system insult is likely to arise from what some would consider an unexpected direction. This has been touched upon in previous chapters, and refers to the interactions of the nervous and immune systems across the lifespan. This topic is the subject of the next chapter.

Endnotes

1 Mary Temple Grandin, a person with autism, is a professor of animal science at Colorado State University. She has written extensively on her experiences with autism in relation to animals. The quote is from an interview on National Public Radio with Ira Flatow, January 20, 2006.

2 Comments by the study's senior author, Dr. Stephen Scherer, Centre for Applied Genomics, Hospital for Sick Children, Toronto. As quoted on CTV News (2015) Scherer said that, "We believe each child with autism is like a snowflake; one is unique from another. Surprisingly, our research found that in more cases than not, even siblings can have two different 'forms' of autism."

Part III

Interactions and Synergies in Neurological Disease

11

CNS–Immune System Interactions and Autoimmunity

"Interaction between the nervous and immune systems provides a physiological basis for psychosomatic medicine. In approximately 200 AD, the Greek author Galen wrote that melancholic women are more susceptible to breast cancer than sanguine women. Since then, a wealth of anecdotal evidence has convinced physicians of the importance of psychological factors in the prognosis of disease. This belief is now bolstered by substantial evidence that nervous system output can indeed modulate immune function. However, the interactions are not unidirectional. The immune system can also have powerful influences on the nervous system. This should not be surprising to anyone who has ever felt sick. Anomalies of immune system function can certainly cause diseases of the nervous system, and this may be manifest in psychiatric disease. It is clear that effective defense against infections requires a complex coordination of the activities of the nervous and immune systems, and that abnormalities in the relationships between the two systems can cause disease."

Dr. A.J. Dunn (1995)

From the Preface

7) The gene–toxin interactions leading to neurological diseases are not CNS-specific, but impact other organ systems as well. They may not be the cause of death or nervous system dysfunction, but ignoring these other organ impacts misses a number of crucial clues to disease etiology.

8) Still other organ systems are likely significantly involved in neurological diseases. A good example is the immune system, in which autoimmune reactions may be a primary player in the onset and progression of some neurological diseases. The immune system also plays important roles in normal neuronal development.

Neural Dynamics of Neurological Disease, First Edition. Christopher A. Shaw.
© 2017 John Wiley & Sons, Inc. Published 2017 by John Wiley & Sons, Inc.

11.1   Introduction

The twin aspects of immune interactions with the central nervous system (CNS) in development and health, as noted in the quote that opens this chapter, are only now coming into broader acceptance by both neuroscientists and immunologists. In the pages that follow, I will attempt to fill in more details of what is an expanding – and likely highly important – aspect of the interdependent functioning of both systems.

11.2   Immunity and the CNS, an Introduction to a Complex Topic

The two-directional interactions between the immune and nervous systems have been noted anecdotally for a considerable period of time. More recently, such interactions have been the subject of a rapidly growing body of research.

Needless to say, the amount of information now available is huge, and while I believe it quite important, it is not the main subject of this book. Nor can one do justice to such a large topic except to note some key features of the interactions of these two systems.

The first concerns the impact of the systems on one another during development. The second concerns the potential contribution of these interactions to both developmental CNS disorders and neurological diseases of later life.

The following sections will address some of the key pieces of evidence for interactions between the CNS and the immune system. As cited by Dunn (1995), these are the observations that:

- Alterations in immune function can be conditioned (and conditioning in the classical sense is a CNS function).
- Electrical stimulation/lesions to various regions in the CNS can alter immune responses.
- Stress alters immune responses.
- The activation of the immune system can be correlated with changing properties in neural cells.

Dunn also discusses what is a key point in the interactions between the two systems, namely that cytokines, common to both, can be considered as "immune-transmitters" whose actions are bidirectional. Similarly, some traditional neurotransmitters and various hormones can signal within both systems and bidirectionally, as well.

11.2.1   Innate versus Adaptive Immune Systems and their Roles in CNS Development

The innate ("natural") immune system is a nonspecific first line of defense against infectious diseases (Figure 11.1). It is composed of various cells and molecules that can recognize invading pathogens, and consists of eosinophils, monocytes, macrophages, natural killer cells, dendritic cells, Toll-like receptors, and complement system mediators (for a general overview, see Janeway et al., 1999). In this system, the first response to a given pathogen is relatively slow, but it becomes more rapid with a secondary exposure to the same entity.

In contrast, the adaptive immune system is specifically directed against invading pathogens (Figure 11.1). It contains highly specialized cells such as T (thymus-derived) and B lymphocyte (bone marrow-derived) cells, generating, respectively, cellular and

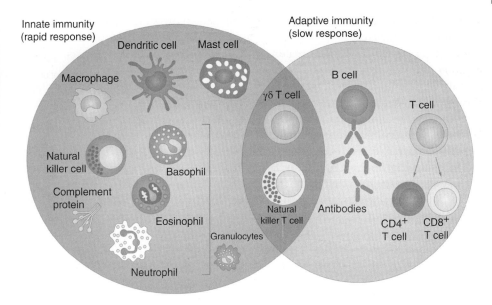

Figure 11.1 Innate versus adaptive immune responses. *Source*: Adapted from Dranoff (2004), with permission from Macmillan Publishers Ltd: [*Nature Reviews Cancer*].

humoral types of immune response. T cells, also termed T-helper, T4, or CD4 cells, are white blood cells that are essential for the adaptive immune response. "CD4" refers to a glycoprotein (cluster of differentiation 4) found on the surface of T cells and other cell types (e.g., monocytes, macrophages, and dendritic cells). T-helper cells do not themselves destroy invading pathogens as they have no phagocytic or cytotoxic capabilities, but they enable other cells such as CD8 killer cells to do so. Two types of T-helper cell are recognized, Th1 and Th2, each designed to eliminate different types of pathogen. Th1 cells produce interferon γ and act to activate the bactericidal actions of macrophages and induce B cells to make complement-fixing antibodies. These responses are the basis of cell-mediated immunity. The Th2 response involves the release of interleukin 5 (IL-5), acting to induce eosinophils to clear parasites. Th2 also produces IL-4, which facilitates B-cell isotype switching. In general, Th1 responses are usually directed against intracellular pathogens (viruses and bacteria), while Th2 responses act against extracellular bacteria, other pathogenic parasites, and toxins.

A second crucial aspect of the adaptive immune system, particularly in response to future pathogen responses, is the production of antibodies. Antibodies are immunoglobulins (Igs): large Y-shaped proteins produced by plasma cells. Igs come in a variety of isotypes: in placental mammals, there are five, termed IgA, IgD, IgE, IgG, and IgM. Ig isotypes are classified based on the various types of heavy chain making up the protein. For example, heavy-chain classes α, γ, δ, ε, and μ give rise to IgA, IgG, IgD, IgE, and IgM, respectively. These isotypes differ in their biological properties, functional locations, and ability to deal with different antigens. In brief, the main Ig is IgG, which, with its four variations, provides the majority of Ig-based immunity against invading pathogens. It is the only antibody capable of crossing the placenta. IgM is associated with B cell-mediated cellular immunity. IgD acts mainly as an antigen receptor on B cells that have not been exposed to antigens and activates basophils and mast cells to produce antimicrobial factors. IgE acts primarily as an antigen receptor on B cells that have not been exposed to antigens. Finally, IgA is found in mucosal membranes of the gut and the respiratory and urogenital tracts and acts to prevent colonization of these structures by pathogens.

Antibodies contain a variable region on the tip of the Y called a paratope. Each paratope can recognize a unique molecule of the pathogen, the antigen. In this way, an antibody can mark a pathogen or an infected cell to be attacked by other cells in the immune system or can serve to neutralize the pathogen. The so-called Fc region at the base of the Y allows it to communicate with other immune cells. The production of antibodies describes the primary function of the humoral immune system.

Antibodies are released by B cells, specifically differentiated B cells (B plasma cells). They can occur in two physical forms: a soluble form that is secreted from the cell and a membrane-bound form that is attached to the surface of the B cell (a B-cell receptor (BCR)). Soluble antibodies are released into the blood and tissue fluids. The BCR facilitates the activation of these cells and their differentiation into plasma cells or memory B cells. Both types of cell will remain in the body and remember that same antigen at a future presentation.

The response of the adaptive system is slower than that of the innate system, but is more potent and specific. Further, the memory of past pathogen exposure resides in the adaptive immune system. Unlike the innate immune system, adaptive immunity is found only in vertebrates.

When describing features of the innate immune system, it is necessary to consider the role of the "inflammasome." The inflammasome is an intracellular, multiprotein complex that controls the activation of proinflammatory caspases, primarily caspase-1. The complex generally has three main components: a cytosolic pattern-recognition receptor known as the nucleotide-binding oligomerization domain receptor (NOD)-like receptor (NLR), the enzyme caspase-1 (part of the apoptosis pathway), and an adaptor protein known as apoptosis-associated speck-like protein (ASC), which facilitates the interaction between the NLR and caspase-1 (see review by Walsh et al., 2014). The NLR subfamilies include NLRP3, the best-studied of this group.

The NLRP3 inflammasome is activated by various stimuli, including pathogenic signals (e.g., bacterial, fungal, viral) (Duncan et al., 2009; Ichinohe et al., 2009), endogenous danger signals (adenosine triphosphate (ATP), Aβ, uric acid crystals) (Mariathasan et al., 2006, Martinon et al., 2006; Halle et al., 2008), and environmental microparticles (e.g., silica crystals, aluminum salts) (Hornung et al., 2008). The latter are of obvious importance in consideration of the impact of aluminum salts used as adjuvants that may also gain ingress into the CNS.

NLRP3 activation is a two-step process. A first signal, such as the presence of microbial Toll-like receptor ligands, primes cells by producing pro-IL-1β expression. A second signal, such as ATP, activates caspase-1 and leads it to process pro-IL-1β and pro-IL-18 (Tschopp et al., 2002; Mariathasan et al., 2006; Halle et al., 2008).

The activation of NLRP3 is not completely understood, but three upstream mechanisms of activation have been proposed. These are ion fluxes (K^+ and other ions) (Petrilli et al., 2007), mitochondrial-derived reactive oxygen species (Zhou et al., 2011), and phagosome destabilization and the release of lysosomal enzymes (cathepsins) that digest proteins after cell death (Chu et al., 2009; Hoegen et al., 2011).

The effects of NLRP3 inflammasome activation within the CNS remain unknown in many cases, but recent evidence suggests it has a role in neurological diseases and, as already mentioned, in the context of adjuvant aluminum salts.

Some disease-specific molecules, such as Aβ, prion protein, and α-synuclein, have been reported to activate the NLRP3 inflammasome in microglia and macrophages (Halle et al., 2008; Codolo et al., 2013). In a transgenic mouse model of Alzheimer's disease, the knockout of NLRP3 or caspase-1 slowed memory loss and increased Aβ removal (Heneka et al., 2013). NLRP3 inflammasome loss in this model also skewed microglial cells to an M2 phenotype (see Section 11.2.2). In the mSOD1 model of ALS, NLRP3 does not seem to be required, although caspase-1 activation in microglia and the level of IL-1β secretion correlate with the amount of mSOD1 misfolding (Meissner et al., 2010). These last outcomes suggest that other inflammasome subtypes may be involved, or they may simply reflect yet another problem with the m*SOD1* model for ALS.

11.2.2 The Role of Microglia in Neurological Diseases

Another component part of the innate immune system as it specifically applies to the CNS concerns the action of microglia, the resident macrophages of the CNS. Microglia are activated in response to insult and disease, and are thus key components of the non-cell-autonomous aspects of neurological diseases.

Microglial activation, as cited in Section 11.2.1 and in various other places in this book, is widely considered to be part of the pathological sequence of events in neurodegeneration in the various neurological diseases.

In order to understand its roles, it is important to understand the types of microglial activation more generally. Activated microglia are broadly categorized into two different states: the standard activated M1 state and the alternatively activated M2 state. Generally, the M1 state promotes a neurotoxic T-cell response and is cytotoxic due to the secretion of reactive oxygen species and proinflammatory cytokines (e.g., IL-1, IL-6, and tumor necrosis factor alpha (TNF-α)) and because of a reduction in protective trophic factors (see Cherry et al., 2014, for review). These actions of M1 microglia serve to destroy foreign pathogens and polarize T cells to mount an adaptive immune response. The M2 microglial state produces high levels of anti-inflammatory cytokines and neurotrophic factors (IL-4, IL-10, IGF-1, CD200, and fractalkine) (Cherry et al., 2014). The M2 phenotype is generally associated with suppressing inflammation, conducting repairs, and restoring cellular and system homeostasis.

It is, however, increasingly clear that the activation states for microglia are more a spectrum of responses than two static conditions (Colton et al., 2006; Mosser and Edwards, 2008; Martinez and Gordon, 2014). In fact, these conditions are quite mutable. In this regard, various studies have shown that individual microglia can express both pro- and anti-inflammatory signatures at the same time (Fenn et al., 2014). Perhaps causal to this cellular diversity, the local microenvironment can supply both M1 and M2 cues simultaneously (Martinez and Gordon, 2014). In addition, there is now recognition that the M2 phenotype is not a single entity, but rather comprises various subtypes, including M2a, M2b, M2c, and Mox, each of which has unique features and functions that remain poorly characterized (Mosser and Edwards, 2008; David and Kroner, 2011).

Following injury to the CNS, microglia are recruited within the first hour and continue to accumulate for more than 1 month. Initially, the majority of these are of the M2 phenotype. However, within a week of the injury, the microglia transition to the M1 state (Hu et al., 2012; Wang et al., 2013). Other factors that play a role in the M2-to-M1 transition include the severity of injury and the location of origin of the microglia (e.g., white versus gray matter). Increasing age may also influence the microglial phenotype (Perego et al., 2011; Hu et al., 2012).

Microglial state transitions have also been shown to occur in neurodegenerative diseases, and their initial response may involve the release of neurotrophic factors and the maintenance of homeostasis. It is only when injured neurons appear to be beyond saving that microglia shift to their more destructive role. For example, in the m*SOD1* mouse model, microglia appear to switch from an M2 phenotype in the initially slow early phases of motor neuron dysfunction to an M1 expression. This shift may be one reason for the cascading failure that is so characteristic of this model, and indeed of ALS itself (Beers et al., 2011; Hooten et al., 2015). In Parkinson's disease, the presence of mutant α-synuclein has also been shown to switch the microglia into the M1 state (Rojanathammanee et al., 2011).

11.3 CNS–Immune System Interactions: More Detailed Considerations

The mechanisms by which peripheral (systemic) immune stimulation can impact responses in the CNS turn out to be fundamental for understanding not only the interactions between the CNS and the immune system, but also the roles such interactions play in the origins of some neurological, immune, and metabolic disorders.

As elaborated by Besedovsky and Rey (2007, 2008), such cross-talk is mediated by afferent signals transmitted by immune cytokines and other immune molecules, as well as efferent signals carried by hormones and neurotransmitters. Because the cross-talk between the CNS and the immune system occurs at multiple levels, it has been described by these investigators as the "immuno-neuro-endocrine" network. Two major functional systems involved in the network are the hypothalamic–pituitary–adrenal (HPA) axis and the sympathetic nervous system (SNS) (Elenkov et al., 2000), as discussed in Section 11.3.2.

Because the complex set of interactions that constitute the immuno-neuro-endocrine network play important roles in immune regulation, brain function, and maintenance of general brain-cell homeostasis, any disturbance of this delicately balanced network can result in pathological disease states affecting a range of CNS processes. These include general brain and immune functions, circadian rhythms, thermoregulation, glucose homeostasis, and a variety of other metabolic functions. In addition, neural activity itself can be dramatically altered in response to a variety of immune stimuli (Besedovsky and Rey, 2007, 2008).

A number of other observations have linked systemic immune stimulation to changes in behavior and nervous system pathology based on the common constellation of neurological outcomes associated with viral illnesses (e.g., influenza), including impairments in cognition, memory, learning and attention, social withdrawal, irritability, and depression. Research into so-called "sickness behavior" suggests that this condition is caused by elevations in proinflammatory cytokines such as IL-1β, IL-6, and TNF-α (Dantzer and Kelley, 2007), which cause both fever and, notably, alterations in the levels of key neurotransmitters (Dunn, 2006).

Tying these experimental observations to anatomical structures is the recent discovery of functional lymphatic vessels in the dural sinuses, which provide avenues for the exchange of fluid and immune cells between lymph nodes and the cerebrospinal fluid (Louveau et al., 2015).

11.3.1 Pathogen and Aluminum Activation of the Immune System in Relation to the CNS

Repeated administration of bacterial and viral antigenic protein fragments, many of which are adsorbed to adjuvant aluminum salts, is clearly analogous both in nature and timing to peripheral immune stimulation with microbial mimetics in experimental animals during early periods of developmental vulnerability. If administered during these periods (including early postnatal life), such potent immune stimuli can not only produce adverse neurodevelopmental outcomes in these animals, but can also permanently impair immune responses to subsequent immune challenges later in life (Boissé et al., 2004; Galic et al., 2009). Maternal immune activation (MIA) outcomes, some of which are linked to ASD, were presented in Chapter 10.

Many cytokines induced as part of an immune response, including those arising from adjuvants, can act as "endogenous pyrogens"; that is, they can induce a rapid-onset fever by acting directly on the hypothalamus, without the need for the formation of another cytokine (i.e., IL-1β, IL-6, TNF-α) (Dinarello, 1999; Conti et al., 2004; Besedovsky and Rey, 2007, 2008). While transient fever is an essential component of the early immune response to infection, a prolonged febrile response is a hallmark of many inflammatory and autoimmune diseases (Dinarello, 1999).

Fever-promoting cytokines produced in peripheral tissues by immune stimulation can enter the brain by way of the circumventricular organs (CVOs) (Dinarello, 1999). CVOs are structures in the brain with an extensive vasculature and are amongst the few sites devoid of protection by the blood–brain barrier. They provide one link between the CNS and peripheral blood flow, and thus are an integral part of neuroendocrine function. The absence of a blood–brain barrier to CVO molecule release allows the CVOs to provide an alternative means for the release of hormones and various peptides from the CNS into peripheral circulation. And, as already cited, the structural connections now demonstrated between the lymphatic system and the CNS only add to the potential for immune–CNS bidirectional ingress. In this context, persistent inflammation of the CNS appears to play a prominent role in neurodevelopmental and neurodegenerative disorders (Akiyama et al., 2000; Pardo et al., 2005; Vargas et al., 2005; Lukiw et al., 2012).

11.3.2 HPA–Immune System Interactions

IL-1β, the key proinflammatory cytokine, is released following NLPR3 inflammasome activation by aluminum adjuvants and exhibits multifactorial effects on the immune system (Li et al., 2007, 2008; Eisenbarth et al., 2008). IL-1β is also known to activate neurons in the central nucleus of the amygdala (Buller and Day, 2002). This nucleus plays a major role in the HPA-axis response to systemic immune stimulation (Xu et al., 1999). Abnormalities in the amygdala (Herbert et al., 2003; Munson et al., 2006) and alterations in cortisol levels indicative of a dysfunctional HPA axis are common in ASD children and may, in part, serve to explain the limited abilities of these children to react adequately to their social environment, as well as their tendency toward enhanced anxiety behaviors (Porges, 2005; Hamza et al., 2010b).

The HPA axis is not only crucial for regulating a broad array of psychological stress responses (Gunnar, 1992; Jansen et al., 2000; Davis and Granger, 2009; Gunnar et al., 2009), but also regulates neuro-immune stress arising from exposure to bacterial and/or viral stimuli.

From the preceding, it is clear that the HPA axis is one of the major pathways by which the CNS regulates the immune system (Wilder, 1995; Elenkov and Chrousos,

1999; Elenkov et al., 2000; Eskandari et al., 2003; Nadeau and Rivest, 2003). Alterations in HPA-axis regulation can lead either to excessive immune activation, and hence inflammatory and autoimmune disorders, or to excessive immune suppression, and thus increased susceptibility to infectious diseases. In this context, it is notable that many autoimmune/inflammatory conditions have been consistently linked to adjuvant administration and/or repetitive immunizations with antigenic components (Porges et al., 2005; Agmon-Levin et al., 2009; Tsumiyama et al., 2009; Tomljenovic and Shaw, 2012; Luján et al., 2013; Shaw et al., 2014b).

Cortisol, the main glucocorticoid hormone product of HPA activity, appears to have a crucial role in priming microglia toward a hyperactive and thus neurodegeneration-inducing M1 phenotype (Barrientos et al., 2012). In adult rats, prior sensitization of the microglia by cortisol potentiates the proinflammatory response to a peripheral immune challenge by lipopolysaccharide (LPS) and significantly augments the production of the inflammatory cytokines IL-1β, IL-6, and TNF-α in the brain (Frank et al., 2009). Some data link an aging-associated decline in CNS function to dysregulated cortisol homeostasis, which, when shifted toward higher cortisol levels, may predispose the aged brain to exaggerated proinflammatory responses to subsequent immune stimuli (Barrientos et al., 2012). Consistent with this view, elevated plasma cortisol levels highly correlate with glial reactivity in the brain, while in contrast adrenalectomy in aged animals reduces brain microgliosis (Landfield et al., 1981). Elevated exposure to glucocorticoids also induces excitotoxic levels of glutamate and reactive oxygen species, both outcomes capable of inducing neuronal degeneration (Sapolsky, 1993; Lee et al., 2002).

As cited in Chapter 3, glutamate is the major excitatory neurotransmitter in the mammalian brain, and is therefore crucial for normal brain development and function (Johnston, 1995; Griesmaier and Keller, 2012). However, excessive glutamate release is deleterious to neuronal viability and is thought to play a role in the pathophysiology of neurological diseases and neuropsychiatric disorders, including ASD (Blaylock and Strunecka, 2009; Griesmaier and Keller, 2012). In regard to ASD, children and adults with the disorder typically display higher serum levels of glutamate (Shinohe et al., 2006; Shimmura et al., 2011), as well as a specifically higher concentration of glutamate/glutamine in the amygdala and hippocampus (Purcell et al., 2001).

The higher levels of glutamate in ASD children find a direct correlate with the levels of glutamatergic receptors: at 2 years of age, the developing human brain contains more synaptic glutamate receptors than at birth, but the number of these receptors progressively declines over the next decade. The immature brain is thus likely to be more susceptible to excitotoxic insults than that of a young adult (Johnston, 1995). At the other end of the age spectrum, receptor subunit composition for various glutamate receptor subtypes also changes during life (Pickard et al., 2000), which may make the aged brain more susceptible to excitotoxic insults than that of younger adults, as cited in the previous chapter. Thus, the dynamics of glutamate levels and glutamate receptor characteristics across the life span makes neuronal vulnerability more pronounced in early and later life, albeit in different ways. In turn, this complex response pattern reflects the underlying complexity contributed by neural–immune–HPA interactions.

In regard to the point about glutamate-induced excitotoxicity, one of the most common therapeutic drugs used to treat ALS is riluzole (2-amino-6-trifluoromethoxy benzothiazole), whose main action is to decrease glutamate release (Bellingham, 2011), based on the notion that excitotoxicity is one of the causal events in the disease and leads directly to motor neuron degeneration. While the impact of riluzole on post clinical-diagnosis ALS is overall minor, the notion that the disease is at least a partial result of excessive glutamatergic activity seems well-founded.

In summary, given all of the data cited in this section, it becomes increasingly difficult to conclude that the CNS and immune systems do not interact to a considerable degree, both in development and in adulthood, as well as in health and disease.

11.4   Autoimmunity

Briefly stated, autoimmune disorders arise when an individual's own immune system generates antibodies that attack healthy tissues rather than the invading pathogens. Autoimmune reactions can also cause the abnormal growth of tissues and a variety of dysfunctional states. Examples of organ systems that can be affected include blood cells and vessels, connective tissues and joints, skin and muscles, the endocrine system, and, of particular interest in what follows, the nervous system.

Close to 100 autoimmune disorders are now recognized, with more added to the list every year. Well-known autoimmune disorders include systemic lupus erythematosus (SLE), celiac disease, rheumatoid arthritis, type 1 diabetes, and a host of other lesser-known disorders. In the CNS, autoimmune disorders include multiple sclerosis, Guillian–Barré, and myasthenia gravis.

Autoimmune disorders can have multisystem impacts, and individuals can have more than one such disorder at the same time. Likely examples of multisystem/multidisorder syndromes include fibromyalgia, chronic fatigue syndrome, and the emerging syndrome termed "autoimmune syndrome/inflammatory syndrome induced by adjuvants" ASIA. Gulf War Syndrome, which in many cases includes clearly negative impacts on the CNS (Deployment Health Working Group Research Subcommittee, 2001), likely also reflects a multisystem autoimmune disorder of the ASIA type. MMF is triggered by aluminum adjuvants and leads to clear changes in cortical function in the form of mild cognitive impairment (MCI). The observation that aluminum salts can themselves be antigenic lends support to the notion that MMF may have autoimmune as well as inflammatory features (Gherardi and Authier, 2012) and places it firmly within the ASIA spectrum of disorders.

It should be mentioned that the potential link between the various autoimmune/inflammatory CNS disorders and adjuvants, particularly aluminum adjuvants in vaccines, has led some investigators to question whether these disorders actually exist (Hawkes et al., 2015). Such views sometimes appear to reflect more the perceived need to provide continued public assurance about vaccine safety, rather than any actual reservations about whether such disorders are aluminum-induced and/or autoimmune in nature.

As already noted, aluminum is antigenic in its own right, and indeed it is typically added to vaccines as an adjuvant because it increases the antigenicity and long-term effectiveness of the primary antigen, usually some viral or bacterial protein fragment. The precise mechanisms of action of aluminum adjuvants are still being resolved almost 90 years after their introduction (Exley et al., 2010).

Whatever else one wishes to say about the role of aluminum adjuvants in autoimmune disorders, aluminum is distinctly not inert, nor are the cumulative amounts received necessarily trivial for CNS health, as detailed in Chapter 6. Indeed, as will become clearer in the present chapter, the interactions between the immune and nervous systems virtually ensure that adjuvant aluminum will impact both, even if the intent is only to modify the former.

Other explanations for autoimmunity include "molecular mimicry," in which viral or bacterial coat proteins or bacterial endotoxins have similar amino acid sequences to some part of neural cells. Such similar sequences may serve to provide a target epitope for antibodies produced against the pathogen (Levin et al., 2002). Guillan–Barré, for example, may follow various infectious diseases or vaccinations against the same diseases (Schonberger et al., 1979; Vellozzi et al., 2014).

Autoimmune disorders often display differences based on sex. For example, multiple sclerosis (Orton et al., 2006), MMF (Rigolet et al., 2014), and ASIA in general (Zafrir et al., 2012) appear much more often in women than in men (3.2 : 1; 7 : 3; 7 : 3, respectively). Many autoimmune disorders also show an age window; that is, a particular range of ages during which they are most likely to arise. The underlying reasons for both of these observations are unclear.

11.4.1 Bidirectional Role of Immune System–CNS Interactions and Autoimmunity during Neuronal Development

The mechanism by which peripheral immune stimulation affects responses in the brain is critical to understanding the potential role of the factors that may impact normal brain development. An important advance in understanding the function of the normal and the diseased brain comes from the recognition that there is extensive communication between the immune system and cells in the CNS, as cited earlier (see also Besedovsky and Rey, 2008, 2011) (Figure 11.2). As a result of this neuro-immune cross-talk, neural activity can be dramatically altered in response to a variety of immune stimuli (Barrientos et al., 2012), which lead to the *de novo* production of proinflammatory cytokines within the brain by activated microglia. In this regard, it is important to recall that repeated activation of once-resting microglia may induce an irreversible shift of the microglia from the neuroprotective M2 phenotype to the neurodegeneration-inducing M1 phenotype (Blaylock and Maroon, 2011; Blaylock, 2012).

Proinflammatory responses arising from peripheral immune stimuli early in postnatal life may be even more detrimental, because they result in an accumulation of proinflammatory cytokines and excitotoxic levels of glutamate within the brain, which can, in turn, promote inflammation and disrupt neural development (Ibi et al., 2009; Du et al., 2011).

Such immune stimuli can increase CNS vulnerability to subsequent immune insults, which can then permanently impair CNS function (Bilbo et al., 2005a,b; Spencer et al., 2007; Galic et al., 2008). For example, in rodents, peripheral immune stimuli with either bacterial antigens or viral mimetics within the first two postnatal weeks are sufficient to cause deficits in social interactions, altered responses to novel situations, anxiety-like behaviors, impairments in memory, long-lasting increases in seizure susceptibility, abnormal immune cytokine profiles, and increases in extracellular glutamate in the hippocampus (Spencer et al., 2005b; Ibi et al., 2009; Konat et al., 2011). All of these are features are observed to various degrees in ASD children (Tuchman and Rapin, 2002; Vargas et al., 2005; Newschaffer et al., 2007).

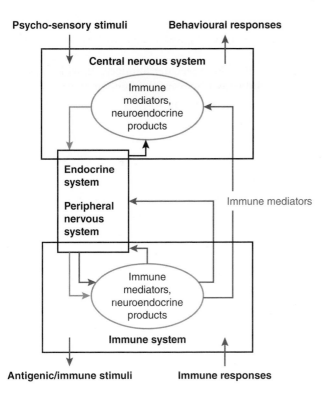

Figure 11.2 Bidirectional aspects of CNS–immune signaling. Schematic depicting the "immune–neuroendocrine" network, a multileveled dynamic network of interactions between the nervous, endocrine, and immune systems. The interactions within this network can be influenced by psycho-sensorial and immune stimuli. For example, immune cytokines released during activation of peripheral immune responses serve as afferent messengers from the immune system to the CNS, and can induce production of cytokines in the brain. In turn, CNS-derived cytokines can trigger neuroendocrine responses purposed to regulate the activity of immune cells and organs. Antigenic/immune stimuli can thus influence behavioral responses (i.e., "sickness behavior"). Likewise, psycho-sensorial stimuli can influence immune responses. The HPA axis is part of this network. The integrity of functional interactions between the neuroendocrine and the immune axis is an absolute prerequisite for homeostasis. *Source*: Adapted from Besedovsky and Rey (2007), with permission from Elsevier.

As will be discussed in Section 11.5.1, aluminum adjuvants have the capacity to induce the same types of outcomes. The similarities between these and MIA-like outcomes, as mentioned in Chapter 10, will be obvious.

11.4.2 Autoimmunity and Neurological Diseases

Autoimmunity may occur for a variety of reasons, amongst which is molecular mimicry, as cited above. Not only can antibodies target neurons, but they can target other neural cells as well, and in the process interfere with synaptic transmission (Whitney and McNamara, 1999). Both cell-mediated and humoral immune responses may also be involved, and may impact neurons and glial cells acting through cell-surface proteins.

The implications for both cell- and non-cell-autonomous mechanisms of neurodegeneration are obvious for the long-term outcomes leading to some neurological diseases (as discussed in Section 11.4.3 regarding ALS).

11.4.3 The Age-Related, Progressive Neurological Diseases and Autoimmunity

In regard to the neurological diseases that are the key focus of this book, autoimmune features appear in each, although the role and staging of autoimmunity in disease initiation and/or progression are not entirely delineated. It remains unclear whether the pathological outcomes of neurological diseases are caused by autoimmune reactions acting alone or in concert with other factors in a multiple-hit scenario, or whether the neurological disease outcome is permissive in allowing later autoimmunity to occur. The latter circumstance might arise by allowing greater immune cell ingress as pathological changes occur in the blood–brain barrier (see below). It is also possible that the two are separate, parallel events.

Evidence for a role of autoimmune reactions in ALS comes from several sources. Some older studies implicate antibodies to voltage-gated calcium channels in serum from sLAS patients that are toxic to neurons in cell-culture preparations (Appel et al., 1994; Smith et al., 1996).

Insofar as autoimmunity may be a factor in ALS, there are a number of suitable targets. These include both motor neurons and the supporting glial cells, leaving open the possibility that autoimmune reactions activating both cell-autonomous and non-cell-autonomous mechanisms are in play. In particular, dysfunctions in the innate immune cells of the CNS – the microglia – could have a clear role if driven into an M1 state.

In regard to autoimmunity in Parkinson's disease, some evidence exists for a type of two-hit process, in which the first hit is a toxin-mediated loss of blood–brain barrier function, and the second is an ingress of immune cells that act to destroy neurons in the SN (Monahan et al., 2008).

In the case of Alzheimer's disease, data for autoimmune contributions also exist. In keeping with the Parkinson's disease notion of a two-hit mechanism, in Alzheimer's disease there is direct evidence for compromised integrity of the blood–brain barrier and the presence of various Igs in blood vessels and neurons in patients' brains (Dahlström et al., 1990; D'Andrea, 2005; Theoharides et al., 2009).

11.5 Immune System Signaling Errors and Autoimmunity in ASD and Other Neurological Disorders

There is body of literature supporting the notion that abnormal activity of immune signaling (i.e., a form of failed biosemiosis) in the brain interferes with the establishment of appropriate neuronal circuitry during pre- and early postnatal life, thus potentially contributing to developmental abnormalities in the CNS (Boulanger, 2009; Garay and McAllister, 2010; Tomljenovic et al., 2014). Mice deficient in major histocompatibility complex (MHC) class I signaling and the complement cascade molecules (C1q and C3) exhibit defects in synaptic pruning in specific areas of the brain, as well as enhanced epileptic activity (Huh et al., 2000; Chu et al., 2010). Cerebellar Purkinje cells are a site of prominent MHC class I expression, suggesting that specifically timed changes in neuronal expression of this molecule may contribute to the disorder (Belmonte et al., 2004).

In ASD, an active neuroinflammatory process involving astrocytes is present in the cerebral cortex and the cerebellum, leading in the latter case to an extensive loss of cerebellar Purkinje cells (Vargas et al., 2005). Cytokine profiling shows that macrophage chemoattractant protein (MCP)-1 and tumor growth factor (TGF)-β1 derived from neuroglia are the most prevalent cytokines in ASD patient brains compared to their control counterparts. The cerebrospinal fluid derived from ASD patients likewise shows a unique proinflammatory profile of cytokines, including a marked increase in MCP-1.

These observations suggest that the ASD brain is a result of abnormal processes that arises from altered activity of the immune–neural pathways in the brain (Table 11.1). The observations of altered activity may be a manifestation of a form of signaling error, in this disorder. This notion ties into earlier discussions of biosemiosis and the impact of signaling errors in triggering neurological disorders of various types.

Other evidence in support of altered immune–neural pathways is the frequent finding of autoimmune manifestations, particularly those affecting the CNS, in ASD that are not limited to only a few nervous system antigens. Rather, the data show elevated levels of IgG, IgM, and IgA acting against nine different neuron-specific antigens found in the disorder (Vojdani et al., 2002). Additionally, significantly more ASD children show serum auto-antibodies in human brain, particularly in the cerebellum and cingulate gyrus, compared to their unaffected control siblings (Singer et al., 2006).

Immune system abnormalities in ASD are not confined to the nervous system, and considerable evidence points to a role of systemic immune-system dysregulation in the pathophysiology of ASD, which is likely to precede the inflammatory and autoimmune manifestations in the brain (Dietert and Dietert, 2008; Hertz-Picciotto et al., 2008). In addition to aberrant cytokine profiles, various studies have shown abnormal levels of blood lymphocytes, incomplete or partial activation of T cells following stimulation, and lower levels and decreased activity of circulating natural killer cells (Ashwood and van de Water, 2004; Ashwood et al., 2006, 2008, 2011).

11.5.1 Aluminum's Role in Immune-System Signaling Errors

Which factors might serve as triggers to abnormal immune function as it relates to the CNS in development or in adulthood? Chapter 6 details much of the information on aluminum toxicity in the context of neurological disease, including developmental disorders such as ASD. The MIA data cited in Chapter 10 further bolster this notion given aluminum's clearly demonstrated adjuvant, and thus immune-stimulating, actions.

As already noted, however, the subject of aluminum involvement in ASD remains highly controversial. In part, some of this controversy may arise from addressing developmental disorders in relation to a possible causal impact of this element. As noted in Chapter 6, a certain part of the medical community has discounted any deleterious role of aluminum for human health in general. More specifically, hesitation to accept a role for aluminum in ASD may arise because it is virtually impossible to avoid considering one major source of aluminum exposure: aluminum-adjuvanted pediatric vaccines.

So explosive is the potential impact of such a linkage that it often forces investigators to assert that aluminum could not be involved in ASD at all, in spite of the rather large literature on aluminum neurotoxicity cited here and in previous chapters. This position appears primarily to be an attempt to avoid any discussion of vaccine safety. From a strictly scientific perspective, albeit not necessarily from that of those concerned with

Table 11.1 Immune system role in ASD

Type of abnormality	Type of immune stimulus/ time of stimulation	Species	Outcome	Autism
Neurobehavioral	Poly I : C/early postnatal	Mouse, rat	Deficits in social interaction, increased anxiety (Ibi et al., 2009; Konat et al., 2011)	Impaired social skills, increased anxiety and stereotypic behavior (Theoharides et al., 2009)
	LPS/early postnatal	Rat	Altered responses to novel situations (i.e., reluctance to explore a novel object) (Spencer et al., 2005b)	Anxiety over novel situations, preference for routine (Jansen et al., 2000; White et al., 2012)
	Poly I : C/early postnatal	Mouse	Cognitive dysfunction (i.e., memory deficits) (Ibi et al., 2009)	Cognitive dysfunction and mental retardation (Fombonne, 1999; Newschaffer et al., 2007)
Neuroanatomical	Poly I : C/prenatal	Mouse	Compromised neurogenesis and abnormal formation of the cerebral cortex (Soumiya et al., 2011)	Abnormal neuronal morphology and cytoarchitecture of cerebral cortex (Herbert et al., 2003)
	Complete US pediatric vaccine schedule/postnatal, according to schedule	Monkey	Failure to undergo normal maturational changes in amygdala volume (Hewitson et al., 2010)	Impaired amygdala development (Herbert et al., 2003; Munson et al., 2006)
Neurochemical	Poly I : C/early postnatal	Mouse	Increased extracellular glutamate in the hippocampus (Ibi et al., 2009)	Increased glutamate in the amygdala–hippocampal region (Purcell et al., 2001)
	LPS/early postnatal	Rat	Increased seizure susceptibility (Galic et al., 2008)	Increased seizures and epilepsy (Ballaban-Gil & Tuchman, 2000; Tuchman & Rapin, 2002)
Immune	LPS/early postnatal	Rat	Abnormal cytokine profiles (Spencer et al., 2007)	Abnormal cytokine profiles (Pardo et al., 2005; Vargas et al., 2005; Ashwood et al., 2006, 2008; Molloy et al., 2006)
	Al-adjuvant/early adulthood	Mouse	Increased astrocyte and microglia reactivity (Bilbo et al., 2005a,b)	Increased astrocyte and microglia reactivity (Pardo et al., 2005; Vargas et al., 2005; Ashwood et al., 2006, 2008; Molloy et al., 2006)
	LPS/early postnatal	Rat	Exacerbation of inflammatory conditions (Spencer et al., 2007)	Immune hypersensitivity (Dietert and Dietert, 2008)

Note: Shared aspects between autism and abnormal neurobehavioral, neuroanatomical, neurochemical, and immune-system outcomes result from repeated peripheral immune stimulation by various stimuli during pre- and postnatal period.

reassuring the public about vaccine safety *per se*, this position would appear to be problematic.

In spite of such reservations, the available literature clearly shows that the neurotoxicity of aluminum in the CNS manifests itself in symptoms such as deficits in learning, memory, concentration, speech, and psychomotor control, as well as increased seizure activity and altered behavior (i.e., confusion, anxiety, repetitive behaviors, and sleep disturbances) (Tomljenovic, 2011). All of these are features of the overall spectrum of disorders included in ASD.

In regard to aluminum adjuvants, the prolonged hyperactivation of the immune system and chronic inflammation triggered by repeated exposure, combined with the unexpectedly long persistence of such adjuvants in the human body, are thought to be principal factors underlying the toxicity of these compounds. In regard to the latter point, one reason aluminum salts such as the hydroxide are so effective as adjuvants is the relative inability of the body to excrete or degrade them in comparison to aluminum derived through dietary exposure. This clearly demonstrated point from the literature is often overlooked or ignored when assessing vaccine safety, sometimes leading to spurious comparisons between the amounts of aluminum found in a standard vaccine and those in various food products or in the diet overall.

Over the last decade, *in vivo* studies in animal models and humans have indicated that aluminum adjuvants have an intrinsic ability to induce adverse neurological and immunoinflammatory outcomes (Petrik et al., 2007b; Couette et al., 2009; Li et al., 2009; Passeri et al., 2011). Some of these studies have led to the description of ASIA, which is known to comprise a wide spectrum of adjuvant-induced conditions characterized by a misregulated immune response (Meroni, 2011; Shoenfeld and Agmon-Levin, 2011). The ability of aluminum adjuvants to cross the blood–brain and blood–cerebrospinal fluid barriers (Shaw and Petrik, 2009; Khan et al., 2013; Luján et al., 2013) may in part explain the adverse manifestations following some vaccines which tend to be neurological in nature, with an underlying immuno-inflammatory component (Cohen and Shoenfeld, 1996; Sienkiewicz et al., 2012; Zafrir et al., 2012). Thus, as cited earlier in this chapter, aluminum's impact on the CNS is likely a component of the bidirectional aspects of CNS–immune interactions.

CNS damage has been directly linked to the immune-stimulatory properties of aluminum adjuvants in mice and sheep. In both cases, damage to the motor system was observed in both behavioral and cellular aspects. In particular, the sheep ASIA outcomes described by Luján et al. (2013) mimic in many aspects human neurological diseases linked to aluminum adjuvants.

In humans, one of the most thoroughly studied conditions linked to aluminum adjuvants is MMF combined with MCI. Patients diagnosed with MMF tend to be female (70%) and middle-aged at time of biopsy (median age 45 years), and to have received 1–17 intramuscular aluminum-adjuvanted vaccines (mean 5.3) in the 10 years before MMF detection (Gherardi and Authier, 2012). Clinical manifestations in MMF patients include diffuse myalgia, arthralgia, chronic fatigue, muscle weakness, and cognitive dysfunction. Overt cognitive alterations affecting memory and attention are manifested in over half of all cases. In addition to chronic fatigue syndrome, 15–20% of patients with MMF concurrently develop some type of autoimmune disease, the most frequent being a multiple sclerosis-like demyelinating disorder,

Hashimoto's thyroiditis, and diffuse dysimmune neuromuscular diseases (dermato-myositis, necrotizing autoimmune myopathy, myasthenia gravis, and inclusion body myositis).

The clinical significance of the MMF lesion at the site of injection was not fully understood until recently. The advent of *in vivo* animal tracer studies allowed investigators of the Gherardi group to follow adjuvant aluminum from the muscle to other sites in the body, making the pathway quite clear: Aluminum nanoparticles are transported to the draining lymph nodes by circulating macrophages and then into the brain (Khan et al., 2013). Once there, aluminum's unusual physical and biophysical properties and its ability to bind to and disrupt normal biochemical reactions render it capable of altering normal signaling (biosemiosis again) at every level of the CNS, and also of triggering autoimmune reactions through adjuvant action (see Shaw et al., 2014a,b,c for a general review) and through its own antigenicity.

The data for MMF cited here may suggest that some form of neurological or immune-system dysfunction could also arise in children, particular considering the potential body burden of aluminum that they can accumulate. While an adult MMF patient may have received up to 17 vaccines in the 10 years prior to diagnosis, the average child in the United States following the Centers for Disease Control and Prevention (CDC)'s vaccination schedule will receive the same number of aluminum-adjuvanted vaccines in their first 18 months of life (Tomljenovic and Shaw, 2011a,b). Early postnatal life in humans, as cited in Chapter 10, is a period of intense neurological development, during which the CNS are extremely vulnerable to neurotoxic and immunotoxic insults. It should be stressed in this context that toxins other than aluminum have also been proposed to be involved in ASD (Dietert and Dietert, 2008). This possibility does not diminish the potential impact of aluminum itself, however.

The ability of aluminum to adversely affect both the immune and the nervous system in an interactive manner make it a strong candidate risk factor for triggering developmental disorders such as ASD in which the two principal features are precisely those of neurological and immune-system signaling dysfunctions.

It should be clear by now that the etiology of ASD is not a simple process involving only genetic factors, but rather involves a multiple-hit type of etiology in which both immune- and nervous-system interactions play important roles. This notion is not particularly surprising given the existing literature on neurodegenerative diseases associated with aging (e.g., Parkinson's disease, ALS, and Alzheimer's disease), which often comes to many of the same conclusions.

11.6   Laterality and Autoimmunity in Neurological Diseases

While bilateral symmetry is a general rule in animals, it is not strictly observed at a more specific micro level. This can be seen in the nervous systems of very simple organisms such as *C. elegans*, in which various neural networks are generally symmetrical at a macroscopic level, but differ across the midline in specific branching patterns (Hobert et al., 2002). It can also be seen in humans in the broad similarity of structures at a macroscopic level, but with a more discreet pattern of functional laterality, as revealed by both cognitive-function tests and magnetic resonance imaging (MRI) (Figure 11.3).

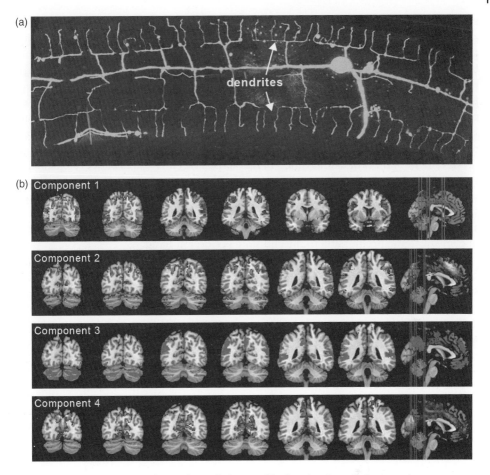

Figure 11.3 Neuronal lateralization of morphology and/or function from *C. elegans* to humans.
(a) Green fluorescent signal showing PVD neurons in *C. elegans*. (b) Functional MRI images showing
activated or deactivated brain regions involved in language and social tasks from the Human
Connectome Project database. Blue areas indicate deactivated regions, while red areas indicate
activated regions. The left and right hemispheres show asymmetry in activation and deactivation
patterns. *Source*: (a) Adapted from Salzberg et al. (2013), with permission from Elsevier; (b) Dr. Todd
Woodward, with permission. (See color plate section for the color representation of this figure.)

One indirect form of evidence for an autoimmune component in neurological diseases may arise from observation of initial laterality of motor deficits in both Parkinson's disease and ALS (Ahn et al., 2011; Assous et al., 2014; Devine et al., 2014; Zhang et al., 2014). The general observation in both diseases is that signs and symptoms often present initially on one side of the body, before becoming bilateral. This observation is so well known in Parkinson's disease that it figures as part of the transition in the Hoehn and Yahr Scale from Stage 1 to Stage 2 (see Chapter 2).

Although long known in both diseases, the phenomenon is not well studied in humans. However, in animal models of both diseases, a clear lateralized initial neuron loss has been demonstrated (Tabata, 2008; Van Kampen et al., 2014a,b).

Given that both Parkinson's disease and ALS have clear movement dysfunctions, such signs are likely to be easier to observe behaviorally than in neurological diseases such as Alzheimer's. In the latter, the impact on cognitive function is not going to reveal to simple observation an initial lateralization of deficits. However, considering the obviously asymmetric distribution of functions within cortical regions, it would not be surprising if the same sort of initial unilateral presentation of cognitive deficits, if not anatomical ones, did not also occur in Alzheimer's patients. There is some evidence that it in fact does so in precisely this manner, in that some impacts on cognition appear to be lateralized. Cortical atrophy is, however, described as asymmetrical rather than lateralized (Derflinger et al., 2011), but this may be a semantic distinction rather than a reflection of real differences in function versus pathology.

Overall, the subject of lateralization in relation to the early stages of neurological diseases so far seems to be an area of inquiry that has escaped detailed scrutiny. This is unfortunate, as it may offer insights into the progressive nature of these diseases and thus a potential future hope for halting the disease process before it has spread to both sides of the nervous system. It is, of course, clear that at the point when the diseases become bilateral, progression to the end state is closer at hand.

The initial laterality of dysfunction in neurological disease might arise in a variety of ways. These include relatively subtle neuroanatomical differences, including in the blood–brain barrier, which could act to render one side more susceptible to toxin or immune cell ingress. Since immune responses can occur bilaterally even when the insult is only unilateral (Kleinschnitz et al., 2005; Dubový et al., 2013), a two-hit type of process might be proposed in which an asymmetrical ingress of some toxic substance leads to a local inflammatory/immune response at the site of injury and at a similar point in the CNS across the midline. In a consideration of the human neurological diseases that appear to show lateralized initial deficits, this aspect might be viewed as one stage in

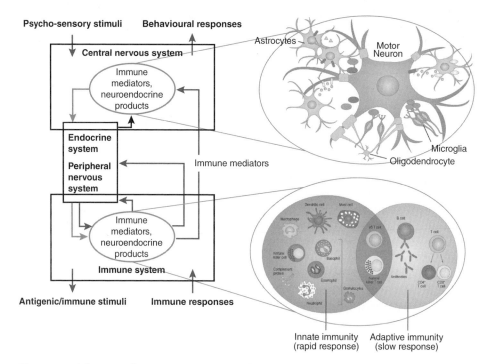

Figure 11.4 Schematic of a more "micro" version of immune–CNS interactions.

the overall progressive nature of each. In the context of a multiple-hit model, the notion that abnormal/toxic gene products and/or toxins could be exacerbated by the immune response might be plausible.

It may be mostly speculative at this point, but consider the following neurological disease-progression scenario: Some innate asymmetry in structural integrity in part of the blood–brain barrier exists in any individual's CNS. This asymmetry makes a particular part of the CNS more accessible to a systemic toxic compound. The local neural damage induced by the ingress of that toxin serves to activate a local immune response of microglial activation/cytokine release into surrounding areas. These areas then become vulnerable to further toxin ingress and exposure, and thus the process spreads to adjoining areas. The activation of the immune response across the midline weakens the blood–brain barrier on that side, inviting toxin ingress into the site. Such a mechanism might be termed a "toxin-induced immune push," with both factors needed for propagation in both lateral and bilateral compartments. The neural–immune interactions would in this case be a feed-forward mechanism, where each served to drive the other toward increasing neuronal destruction.

In a disease such as ALS, the immune response clearly becomes abnormal in that it serves to spread the damage by just such a feed-forward mechanism. In contrast, in an infectious disease such as polio, the immune response acts to halt the spread of motor-neuron damage by halting viral propagation.

11.7   Other System Disorders in Neurological Diseases: More Evidence for Autoimmunity?

As cited in Chapter 9, both developmental neurological disorders such as ASD and the age-related diseases such as Alzheimer's disease, ALS, and Parkinson's disease often show non-neuronal system abnormalities. There are several possible explanations for such findings. One could postulate that various toxic molecules impact various cell types throughout the body, but do so in different ways. The same might be said of the protein products of mutant genes. Another possibility is that such causal factors trigger, at least in part, an autoimmune reaction that serves, indirectly, to target other organ systems (Figure 11.7). This option might explain more parsimoniously how one toxin could have a multiplicity of effects throughout the body. I will consider such non-neuronal outcomes in more detail in Chapter 12.

11.8   Are There Infectious Disease Links to Neurological Diseases?

In regard to Parkinson's disease, evidence for an immune/autoimmune link is not extensive. Clearly, however, one form of parkinsonism can be induced by infection as a sequel to some cases of encephalitis (Bojinov, 1971; Ogata et al., 1997; Sacks, 1999), and this has led to speculation about a potential infectious etiology for the disease generally, either singly or in addition to a combination of other infectious agents, as in a form of the "infectious disease burden" mechanism (Sessa et al., 2014). To date, there have been few animal models of infectious disease-induced forms of parkinsonism.

There has been much speculation that ALS is caused by some form of infectious agent, such as the polio enterovirus. The rationale for this is that anterior horn motor neurons seem to be the primary target in both diseases (see discussion, see Chapter 14). Such speculation has been in the literature since the 1960s (for review, see Salazar-Grueso and Roos, 1994). Renewed interest in this hypothesis came about due to the finding of enterovirus nuclei acid sequences in ALS (see Ravits, 2005), but the overall conclusions remain controversial.

Retroviruses proposed as causal to ALS include the T-lymphotropic virus-1 (HTLV-1), human immunodeficiency virus (HIV), and human foamy virus (Viola et al., 1975; Salazar-Grueso and Roos, 1994; Hadlock et al., 2004). Amongst these, perhaps the best evidence is for HIV. However, whether the virus is causal to ALS or merely reflects a secondary aspect of HIV infection remains uncertain (Salazar-Grueso and Roos, 1994; Alfahad and Nath, 2013). Human endogenous retrovirus (HERV)-like sequences in the human genome have also been linked to ALS (Hadlock et al., 2004).

Still other potential infectious agents proposed for ALS include:

- West Nile virus, which presents with a poliomyelitis-like syndrome with an asymmetric lower-motor neuronopathy with or without meningoencephalitis (Leis et al., 2003).
- Hepatitis C, which can lead to a pure motor-axonal polyneuropathy (Costa et al., 2003).
- Prion disorders (e.g., Creutzfeldt–Jacob disease, Gerstmann–Straussler–Scheinker disease) with lower motor-neuron symptoms and signs, which occur in about 10% of cases (Worrall et al., 2000).
- Lyme disease (caused by spirochetal bacteria), which, in rare cases, presents as motor neuronopathy. Spirochetes have been cultured from ALS patients (Hemmer et al., 1997; Mattman, 2000; Koch, 2003), but the significance of this finding remains uncertain.
- Flavivirus (also termed Russian spring/summer encephalitis virus and Schu virus) with clinical and pathological features that resemble ALS (Müller and Schaltenbrand, 1979; Johnson and Brooks, 1984).
- Paramyxovirus (mumps), an adult history of which correlates with ALS development in about 20% of cases (Quick and Greer, 1967; Lehrich et al., 1974).

Animal models of ALS based on viral infection have also been employed. A prominent one has used the murine neurotropic leukemia virus (MuLV), also known as Cas-Br-E murine leukemia, in which animals developed a progressive hind-limb paralysis (Jolicoeur et al., 1983; Gardner, 1985). Another used age-dependent poliomyelitis (ADPM), a motor-neuron disease of mice, which showed degeneration of anterior-horn motor neurons, limb paralysis, and death by respiratory failure (Contag et al., 1989; Schlenker et al., 2001).

It would be premature to say that a viral or other infectious etiology has been ruled out for ALS. However, the actual extent to which infectious agents play a role in ALS remains controversial at best.

In regard to Alzheimer's disease, the notion of an infectious-disease etiology has not found any discernible support in the mainstream literature.

In summary, evidence for infectious-disease pathogens as etiological agents for neurological diseases remains varied and largely inconclusive, ranging from little or none in Alzheimer's disease to a range of potential viral agents in some cases of ALS.

The material presented in this chapter highlights the complex interaction between the nervous and immune systems and their further interactions with the endocrine system. These data set the background for a consideration of various forms of synergistic interactions leading to neurological diseases.

12

The Impact of Synergy of Factors in Neurological Disease

"The whole is greater than the sum of its parts."

Attributed to Aristotle

From the Preface

3) It is almost certain that gene defects/mutations alone will not explain most types of age-related neurological disease. Nor, for that matter, will obvious environmental stressors/toxins be found to be solely responsible in most cases. Hence, gene–toxin interactions are the likely source of most such diseases, acted upon by a number of other variables across the lifespan.

12.1 Introduction

Basically, Aristotle was right in that combined outcomes larger than the sum of their individual parts can be described as synergistic, regardless of the field of study. In pharmacology, for example, the concept of synergy tends to refer to drug interactions in which two (or more) drugs have a larger than additive effect on cells, organs, systems, or the entire individual. Additive effects are just that: a summation of the separate actions.

In pharmacology and other fields, it is often a lot more complicated than this, and a large number of effects are known, such as the antagonistic actions of drug combinations and a variety of other interactions (Jia et al., 2009).

12.2 Synergistic and Additive Effects in General and as Applied to CNS Diseases

In regard to the intersections of genes and toxins (or other environmental factors), there are a variety of types of both synergistic and additive effects to be considered. Genes can work synergistically with other genes or do so in an additive manner. Both can be termed "polygenetic" or "oligogenetic" (Figure 12.1). Similarly, the same sorts of synergistic and

Neural Dynamics of Neurological Disease, First Edition. Christopher A. Shaw.

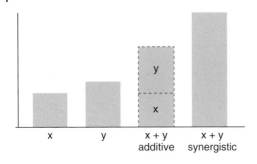

Figure 12.1 Additive versus synergistic effects.

additive impacts apply for toxin–toxin interactions, such as when combining various drugs.

Gene–environment interactions, also termed genotype–environment interactions, occur when some environmental factor impacts different genotypes in variable ways. In other words, the impact of an environmental factor will differ between groups sharing the same genotype and groups with different genotypes. At an individual level, this means that each person (apart from monozygotic twins, who are genetically identical to each other) is going to have a quite different genotype.

This gene–environment type of interaction is highly relevant when considering individual neurological disease manifestations in response to the same basic environmental factor(s). These may range from no effect at all to the expression of a fully developed neurological disease.

This last consideration ties in strongly with many of the themes developed in this book so far. First, with some clear exceptions, the vast majority of any of the age-related neurological diseases are not caused by single gene mutations, nor even by polygenetic mutations. Second, of the potential neurotoxins identified in the last decades, apart from some cases where humans or animals have been exposed to these toxins at extremely high concentrations, toxic substances singly or in combined presentations have not been shown to generate clear, large-scale neurological disease outcomes in human populations. The few exceptions are the clusters discussed in Chapter 3 and elsewhere.

Both of these statements are, of course, subject to future revision based on the probability that additional mutant genes or toxic substances are yet to be discovered and that either or both will be found to generate the various neurological disease spectrums. In the absence of such a future case, however, the current status is that most neurological diseases of the types considered here, at least the sporadic forms, cannot be attributable to any one factor, or to any obvious combination of factors of the same general type.

The ongoing, and still intensive, hunt for causal genes involved in Parkinson's disease, ALS, and Alzheimer's disease (and ASD as a neurodevelopmental disorder) is thus likely to end up with the same outcomes as the blind men and the elephant: each group doing the searching will see only one part of the overall picture and will interpret the whole based on this. It should be emphasized in the context of ALS-PDC that much the same experimental viewpoint prevails in the search for the causal factor.

One illustrative way to view neurological diseases that are not clearly of a purely genetic or toxin nature is to take some examples from other fields in which gene–environment (toxin) interactions are the key to expression of the disease phenotype. These examples are from the literature on alcohol, lactose, and gluten intolerances.

12.3   Gene–Environment (Toxin) Interactions in Non-neuronal Systems

The sometimes obsessive hunt for causal genes in neurological diseases tends to obscure the reality that the diseases considered in detail so far must necessarily arise from the sorts of gene–environment (toxin) interaction already discussed. By the same token, some of those looking for toxin etiologies often show a similar reductionist focus. What makes the situation unusual is that scientists coming from either perspective often actually do realize that gene–environment interactions will ultimately turn out to hold the answer to the origin of the age-related neurological diseases. It is therefore perhaps useful to consider in some detail the following examples from non-neuronal disorders.

While the detail of all of the following may seem to be overly redundant, my purpose here is to prove just how common such interactions may be and how they might shed light on gene–toxin interactions in neurological diseases.

12.3.1   Genetic Polymorphism and Alcoholism

The first example concerns so-called "alcohol use disorders" (AUDs), which are common and complex diseases with a strong genetic component. According to the World Health Organization (WHO), such disorders include approximately 3.3 million deaths per year worldwide (World Health Organization, 2014). In Canada, male cases are more common than females by almost a 3 : 1 ratio.

Alcoholism is the most severe form of AUD, with many genetic variants controlling alcohol use, initiation, metabolism, and psychological reinforcing behaviors (Quertemont, 2004).

In humans, more than 90% of ingested alcohol is eliminated and metabolized by the liver. Ethanol is first oxidized to acetaldehyde by the alcohol dehydrogenase (ADH) family of enzymes, and acetaldehyde is then oxidized to acetate by the mitochondrial enzyme aldehyde dehydrogenase (ALDH). The intermediate, acetaldehyde, is known to be a reactive and toxic molecule that causes aversive symptoms to alcohol, such as dizziness, nausea, and tachycardia.

ADH can be categorized into various classes based on structural similarities and kinetic properties (Edenberg, 2007). The class I enzymes, ADH1A, ADH1B, and ADH1C, contribute about 70% of total ethanol oxidization; the class II enzyme, ADH4, contributes about 30% (Hurley and Edenberg, 2012).

Amongst the many genes involved in alcohol metabolism, the ADH1B class 1, beta polypeptide (*ADH1B*), and ALDH 2 family (*ALDH2*) have the strongest effects on the risk for alcoholism and high levels of alcohol consumption (Hurley and Edenberg, 2012). The enzyme encoded by *ADH1B* has three known functional variants: *ADH1B*1* (reference allele), *ADH1B*2*, and *ADH1B*3*, which encode β1-ADH, β2-ADH, and β3-ADH, respectively. The ethanol metabolism rates for the β2-ADH and β3-ADH enzymes are approximately 30–40 times higher than for β1-ADH (Edenberg and Bosron, 2010). This fast reaction rate leads to a transient increase in levels of acetaldehyde in the liver and increases the risk of liver damage. However, due to aversive reactions, a greater ethanol metabolism rate decreases the risk of developing alcoholism. *ADH1B*1* is most frequently found in populations of European descent (allele frequency >95%). *ADH1B*2* is found at high frequency in East Asia, with over 90% of those of Chinese or Japanese descent carrying at least one copy of the allele. In comparison, its frequency is generally less than 5% in those of European/African descent (Thomasson et al., 1991; Osier et al., 2002). The *ADH1B*2* allele has been demonstrated to have a strong association with a lower maximum number of drinks likely to be consumed in a 24-hour period and a lower risk for alcoholism in those who carry it (Li et al., 2011; Bierut et al., 2012). The *ADH1B*3* allele is found most frequently in African populations, and has also been shown to have a protective effect against alcohol dependence (Li et al., 2011).

Alcohol dependence is a major cause of morbidity and mortality in Native North Americans. In a study that focused on Native people from California's southwest, approximately 6% were found to carry the *ADH1B*3* polymorphism, one of the protective alleles against alcoholism (Wall et al., 2003). Native Americans who carry the *ADH1B*2* allele are about one-third less likely to have a lifetime diagnosis of alcohol dependence than are those without it (Wall et al., 2003). The *ALDH1A1*2* allele was found in about 6% of the same group, and carriers were shown to have a significantly lower tolerance for alcohol consumption than those without it (Ehlers et al., 2004).

Amongst the many ALDH enzymes, ALDH2 has the largest influence on alcohol consumption. Individuals carrying at least one copy of the *ALDH2*2* allele display the "Asian flushing reaction" after consuming even a small amount of alcohol. Up to 40% of those of Chinese or Japanese descent carry at least one copy of this allele, which has a strong protective effect against alcohol abuse and dependence (Li et al., 2012).

In addition to the *ADH* and *ALDH* genes, genetic-linkage analyses and genome-wide association studies have successfully identified several other genes that affect alcohol dependence, including *GABRA2*, *CHRM2*, *PECR*, *KCNJ6*, *AUTS2*, and *IP11-HTR1A* (reviewed in Edenberg and Foroud, 2013).

Despite the protective effects of certain genetic variants, environmental factors, such as sociocultural context and environmental adversity, may override the effects of the protective alleles. For these reasons, the degree of importance of genetic influence on risk of AUD can vary in different populations and under different environmental circumstances (Young-Wolff et al., 2011), precisely as might be predictable from a gene–environment model.

12.3.2 Genetic Polymorphism and Lactose Intolerance

Lactase is the enzyme required for the digestion of lactose, a disaccharide sugar found in dairy products. In most humans, lactase activity declines significantly after weaning, and this reduction can lead to lactose intolerance (also known as lactase nonpersistence). Clinical symptoms include abdominal pain, flatus, and diarrhea.

Approximately 70% of the world's population develops lactase nonpersistence, although the distribution is highly variable amongst different ethnic groups and in different geographical areas. Northern Europeans, non-Native North Americans, and Australasians have the lowest rates, at between 5 and 15%; the frequency increases in Southern Europe and the Middle East, to about 50%; while in South America, Africa, and Asia, a very high frequency has been observed: over 90% in those of Chinese and Japanese descent and over 80% in some West African populations (Sahi, 1994; Swallow, 2003; Campbell et al., 2009).

Lactase is encoded by the *LCT* gene, located on chromosome 2. There is no polymorphism associated with lactase persistence (Boll et al., 1991). The wild-type *LCT* gene is characterized by lactase nonpersistence, while several single-nucleotide polymorphisms (SNPs) (located upstream of the 5' end of the *LCT* gene within the introns of the *MCM6* gene) have been associated with lactase persistence. The region containing these SNPs functions as a *cis*-acting element, stimulating the lactase gene promoter (Enattah et al., 2002; Olds and Sibley, 2003; Swallow, 2003).

A DNA variant, *C/T-13910* (rs4988235), has been identified as having the strongest association with changes in lactase activity (Enattah et al., 2002). This SNP is located 13.9 kb upstream of the *LCT* transcription initiation site. The original form, *C/C-13910*, is associated with low lactase activity, while the genotypes containing the mutant allele, *C/T-13910* and *T/T-13910*, are associated with high lactase activity. *In vitro* studies have shown that the *T-13910* allele has enhancer activity.

T-13910 occurs frequently in European populations and shows a high correlation with a lactase-persistence phenotype (Enattah et al., 2002). However, *T-13910* does not seem to be a good predictor of lactase persistence in non-European populations because the T allele is rarely found in sub-Saharan Africans even though these people show a high frequency of lactase persistence (Mulcare et al., 2004).

Recent studies have provided new insights into the genetic basis of lactose persistence in non-European populations. Three new SNPs have been reported that have a significant association with lactose persistence, including those found in East Africans (*C/G-13907* (rs 41525757), *T/G-13915* (rs 41380347), and *G/C-14010*) in the vicinity of *C/T-13910* (Tishkoff et al., 2007). The presence of a mutated allele has been shown to significantly enhance transcription of the *LCT* gene *in vitro* (Tishkoff et al., 2007). However, unlike the *T-13910* allele, these newly identified SNPs do not show increases in binding to the transcriptional enhancer protein OCT1, suggesting that an additional mechanism may play a role in causing lactase persistence (Ingram et al., 2007; Enattah et al., 2008).

12.3.3 Genetic Polymorphism and Gluten Intolerance

Gluten is the insoluble protein fraction of most grains used as food by humans. Its principal proteins are glutenin and gliadin. The latter contains large amounts of the amino acids proline and glutamine, which, for those sensitive to them, have been identified as the main aversive components of gluten.

There are three forms of adverse reaction to gluten intake: allergic (wheat allergy), autoimmune (celiac disease), and immune-mediated (gluten sensitivity) (Sapone et al., 2012).

In wheat allergy, the repeat sequences in the gluten peptides trigger the release of chemical mediators such as histamine (Tanabe, 2008). In celiac disease, ingestion of gluten causes the release of specific serologic autoantibodies such as serum anti-tissue transglutaminase and anti-endomysial antibodies, and elicits the gradual development of enteropathy (Sollid, 2000). Gluten sensitivity, a newer clinical entity, is characterized by gluten-induced intestinal distress without the involvement of allergic or autoimmune mechanisms (Volta and De Giorgio, 2012).

Amongst the three forms of gluten-related disorder, the pathogenesis of celiac disease has been most frequently associated with genetic predisposition.

Celiac disease affects approximately 1% of the population in the Western Hemisphere and, like alcoholism and lactose intolerance, is caused by a combination of genetic and environmental factors. Evidence for genetic factors include a significant increase in prevalence amongst first-degree relatives (10%) and monozygotic twins (75%) (Polanco et al., 1981; Sollid, 2000; Greco et al., 2002). Genetic linkage studies have shown that the disease is strongly related to the *HLA-DQ* genes, in which a majority of patients (80–95%) carry a variant of *DQ2* (alleles *DQA1*05/DQB1*02*) and others carry a variant of *DQ8* (alleles *DQA1*0301/DQB1*0302*) (Sollid et al., 1989). Individuals who carry double copies of *DQB1*02* (i.e., *DR3-DQ2* homozygous or *DR3-DQ2/DR7-DQ2* heterozygous) have a significantly increased risk for celiac disease (Sollid and Lie, 2005). Studies of the pathogenesis of celiac disease show that *DQ2* and *DQ8* possess superior binding affinities to gluten peptides, thus increasing the presentation of gluten to gluten-reactive CD4 T cells of the celiac intestinal mucosa (Lundin et al., 1993, 1994; Kim et al., 2004).

Although the presence of the *DQ2* or *DQ8* haplotype is necessary, it is not sufficient to cause celiac disease, and some estimates are that the effects attributable to *HLA* occur in only about half of those afflicted with celiac disease (Sollid and Lie, 2005). Moreover, *DQ2* is carried by approximately 30% of the general population without the disease, suggesting that *HLA* is not the only etiological factor.

Additional variants from non-*HLA* genes, such as polymorphisms of the *TNF* promoter (McManus et al., 1996) and *MIC* genes (Hüe et al., 2004), have been identified as celiac disease susceptibility genes. In addition, recent genome-wide association studies have pointed out 20–30 chromosomal regions that could potentially contain susceptibility genes (Rioux et al., 2004; van Heel et al., 2007; Dubois et al., 2010). There is relatively little consensus between these studies, however, suggesting that small effects are conferred by each of the non-*HLA* genes (Wolters and Wijmenga, 2008). These outcomes are in many ways reminiscent of the genetic studies of ASD discussed in previous chapters, and reinforce the notion of particular disease presentations being like individual "snowflakes."

The most important determinants of prevalence of celiac disease in any population are the frequency of *MHC-DQ* and exposure to dietary products that contain gluten. The prevalence of celiac disease is found to be much higher in populations with high frequencies of susceptibility genes. For example, the Saharawi population of Ara-Berber origin in Algeria has the highest prevalence of celiac disease in the world (5.6%), and this has been thought to be due to the high frequency of *HLA-DQ2* in this group combined with the use of gluten-containing grains as its staple food (Catassi et al., 1999). In contrast, celiac disease is rare in individuals of East Asian ancestry, for whom the frequency of *HLA-DQ2* is virtually zero and whose staple food is rice (Cummins and Roberts-Thomson, 2009). In populations from Western Europe, Northern and Western Africa, the Middle East, and Central Asia, the frequency of *HLA-DQ-2* is found to be more than 20% and the prevalence of the disease is approximately 1–2% (Malekzadeh et al., 2005; Cummins and Roberts-Thomson, 2009).

12.4 Gene–Environment (Toxin) Interactions in Neurological Disease

These examples of gene–environment interactions in non-neuronal systems are instructive in detailing how such interactions might determine the likelihood of any individual falling victim to one of the neurological diseases considered in this book.

Some efforts have been made in the direction of identifying similar interactions in neurological diseases. One example involves the putative link between both Parkinson's disease and ALS and exposure to agricultural chemicals. The paroxonase 1 gene (*PON1*), which codes for paraoxonase/arylesterase1 (PON1), an esterase that plays a key role in detoxifying various organophosphorus compounds, was examined in this regard

(Costa and Furlong, 2002). However, the outcomes from various epidemiological studies were not consistent with this interpretation.

In spite of the failure to link *PON1* definitively to these diseases, the fragmentary information extant from various human and animal studies continues to support a distinct role for various types of gene–environment and gene–toxin interaction.

Another example is the correlation between multiple sclerosis incidence rates and living in northern latitudes (Simpson et al., 2011). This correlation is too broad to be of much direct use, but it may tie into more specific biochemical co-factors such as the levels of vitamin D arising as a consequence of sun exposure. A third example comes from the sheep study cited in Chapters 6 and 11, in which sheep treated with vaccines containing aluminum adjuvants developed a motor-neuron disorder made worse by cold-weather conditions (Luján et al., 2013).

12.4.1 Summary of Gene–Toxin Interactions in Relation to Neurological Disease

As the examples of alcohol/lactose/gluten intolerance make clear, a particular molecule acting through genetic variations in individuals and populations can be deleterious to an organ system/organism. Alcohol is clearly a toxin in all cases, but the extent to which it can exercise its toxic potential depends on degradation. Lactase and gluten are not toxic *per se*, but they can have clearly detrimental effects (indeed, in the case of gluten intolerance and celiac disease, they can prove fatal (Ludvigsson et al., 2009)). Obviously, if one carries one of these susceptibility genes/polymorphisms but never consumes the molecule in question, then there is no consequence. It is only when both are present that the disease state arises.

Likewise, taking the view that neurotoxic molecules that can damage or kill neurons in various parts of the brain or spinal cord are present at low but ubiquitous levels, it follows that only those with the relevant genetic susceptibilities or genetic polymorphisms will be affected by them.

Viewed in this manner, the human population of any area can be viewed as being on an imaginary bell curve, with those with the relevant polymorphisms, who are thus most susceptible to the toxic molecule, on the right side (see Chapter 3). This fraction will be that part of the population that, in a particular time and place, is most likely to suffer neuronal damage.

The number of individuals so affected will not necessarily change except in four distinct circumstances: First, when the population increases, but the distribution of the polymorphisms remains the same. In this case, there will be an overall increase in prevalence without a change in incidence. Second, when the percentage of susceptible individuals increases, as on Guam. Such a population shift will have the effect of moving the percentage of those with the disease further to the right. Third, when the toxic molecule(s) increase dramatically in the context of a set percentage of genetic polymorphisms. In this case, the curve will also shift rightwards – and further increases in the molecule will shift it still further in the same direction. Fourth, when the latter two circumstances occur nearly simultaneously. This will cause a dramatic increase in the numbers affected. Whether such combinations account for the examples of neurological disease clusters discussed in Chapter 7 is unproven, but seems highly plausible.

12.5   Levels of Complexity in Gene–Toxin Interactions: Implications for Current and Future Therapeutics

The identification of genes causal to some forms of the various neurological diseases considered in Chapter 5 and elsewhere in this book has largely been derived from studies of disease expression in families. Within such families, the linkage to disease expression is almost certainly correct for those individuals expressing both the mutation and the disease, but by itself fails to account those who do not.

It is important to realize that families share more than just genes. They also share, in most cases, diet and exposure to potential toxins in the environment. Thus, while it may safely be said that mutations play a role in some individual cases of the various neurological diseases, they do not do so in the majority. Indeed, it almost seems as if the hunt for causal genes is beginning to reach asymptote toward whatever small percentage of the overall neurological disease cases actually exists. This last statement is likely to prove contentious for some in the field, especially those involved in the ongoing search for mutant genes in neurological disease.

Similarly, the hunt for causal, single, perhaps "universal" toxins acting to bring about neurological diseases may have run its course, in that most have already been identified. Further, these toxic substances have generally not been shown to be available to induce – or capable of inducing – the diseases in question in the majority of cases.

This does not imply that toxic substances still to be discovered are not involved in any current neurological diseases. Nor does it mean that such toxic molecules might not cause neurological diseases of the future. But, as noted in Chapter 3, the number of victims from the extant neurological disease clusters has not increased, and is likely even diminishing (as with ALS-PDC on Guam and Irian Jaya: see Chapter 7).

What it may mean, however, is this: the low-hanging fruit in neurological disease research has now been plucked. In addition, in both genetic and toxicity studies, overly reductionist perspectives and assumptions may have slowed progress in the field. Key examples of both include the 20-plus-year focus on mutant superoxide dismutase 1 (m*SOD1*) in ALS research (see Chapter 5) and the abysmal detours that the scientifically weak β-methyl amino alanine (BMAA) hypothesis (as cited in Chapters 6 and 7) has made in the hunt for environmental etiologies. Both might well be described as a form of "false flag" neurological disease research that, in the long run, may be seen as more of an impediment than a progress. Needless to say, these are not the sole negative examples for either genetic or toxin studies in the field.

The inevitable conclusion is that the origin of age-related neurological diseases will not turn out to be single gene mutations or single toxins alone. Rather, it will almost surely be a combination of both. Such diseases will increasingly be recognized as spectrum disorders with unique combinations of genetic, epigenetic, and environmental etiologies that operate through multiple-hit mechanisms to generate the disease phenotypes.

This view is, in fact, likely the most parsimonious way to view the various epidemiological studies such as those cited in Chapter 2. Taking all of these aspects into account may allow an individual's overall risk to be calculated, much as can be done for cardiovascular disease – but this can never be a precise neurological disease prognosis. At best, it may describe (as cardiovascular disease prognosis does) a percentage risk at a population level.

Finally, as discussed in Chapter 11, the systems-wide interactions between neural, immune, and likely endocrine dysfunctions may suggest that it really does not matter which system is the first impacted by genetic or toxic factors. Each will almost inevitably trigger the others in due course. Such reciprocal actions can be seem at a systems level in much the same way that excitotoxicity and oxidant stress are interactive at a cellular level.

There are clear implications of all of this for therapeutic approaches to neurological diseases. These will be fleshed out in Part IV, but they can be stated in brief as follows: The extreme range of genomic, proteomic, and metabolomic outcomes across the interacting systems in any individual case of neurological disease only becomes problematic when considering populations of affected individuals. If such studies are accurate, and if the considerations raised in this chapter apply, simplistic therapeutic approaches are not likely to be successful.

Part IV

Transition and Politics in Neurological Disease

13

The Current Status of Neurological Disease Treatments

"The backgrounded question is: how can we avoid factors that are known to increase biosemiotic entropy? Or putting the issue in a more positive form: how can we avoid increasing risks of injury in order to ensure and prolong health and well-being? From the clinical perspective, it is difficult to conceive of any higher goal than the prevention of injuries, disorders, diseases. Presumably, prevention is the higher goal in view of the fact that there would be no need for controlling diseases if they could be prevented in the first place. But how will prevention be possible if we do not understand etiology?"

Prof. John Oller[1]

From the Preface

9) Because of the complexity and interconnectedness of the CNS, damage at any level must necessarily cascade to other levels (e.g., cell to circuit, circuit to a particular region, etc.). So-called "cascading failures" will, at some point, trigger a total system collapse. Thus, after such a critical stage is reached, no effective therapy will be possible. For this reason, therapies designed to target late stages of disease, namely most at the "clinical" diagnosis stage, will inevitably fail and may simply exacerbate rather than relieve underlying pathological processes. The concepts from biosemiosis of the "true narrative representation" (TNR) apply here.

13.1   Introduction

As the quote that opens this chapter indicates, the ultimate treatment option for neurological diseases would be to avoid getting them in the first place. This is very much the rationale for vaccination to achieve immunity from infectious diseases, or the notions that diet and exercise can decrease the risk of cardiovascular diseases. In fact, while controversy still remains about the efficacy of various prophylactic approaches in medicine, few would dispute the key notion that it is better to prevent any of these diseases than to try to deal with the consequences after they have arisen. Such is not, of course, what is done in clinical attempts to treat neurological diseases. And, as Oller correctly notes, it is virtually impossible to prevent something when one does not know what causes it.

Neural Dynamics of Neurological Disease, First Edition. Christopher A. Shaw.

This is very much the situation in neurological disease research, a field rather unevenly divided into camps favoring a genetic etiology versus those looking at environmental/toxin factors. These perspectives have been fully discussed in Chapters 5–7. Only a small number of those working in the field are trying to look at the interface between genetics and environment, even though most would concede, albeit perhaps reluctantly, that this latter approach is actually correct and that most instances of the age-related neurological diseases arise from some combination of gene–environmental (toxin) impacts.

In many ways, in the absence of knowing the causal factors, the field has defaulted to seeking late-state treatments and "cures," whatever the latter word is actually taken to mean. This last point will be addressed in Chapter 16. Here, I want to focus on what has been done so far to address the clinical manifestations of neurological diseases, while in Chapter 14 I will begin to consider some novel potential avenues and their prospects for success.

13.2   Current Therapeutic Approaches to Treating Neurological Diseases

The current range of therapeutic options for central nervous system (CNS) diseases largely follows those for other illnesses, specifically the use of drugs designed to halt the disease process, surgical interventions of various kinds, the application of stem or fetal cell implantation to replace cells lost to the disease, and the replacement of defective genes in a "gene therapy" approach.

13.2.1   Drug Therapies

The outcomes of the various drug trials conducted in the last 20 years for the age-dependent neurological diseases have largely failed to show positive benefits. For ALS, over 50 randomized control trials (RCT), the putative "gold standard" of clinical trials, have been conducted. The tested drugs were designed to target putative mechanisms of motor neuron degeneration, including both cell-autonomous and non-cell-autonomous processes, as cited in previous chapters.

The list of drugs targeting the various mechanisms of neurodegeneration is extensive, including those presumed to act more or less selectively on genetic- or toxin-induced factors leading to excitotoxicity, oxidative stress, mitochondrial dysfunction, neuroinflammatory processes, proteinopathies, induced apoptosis and other forms of cell death, proteasome abnormalities, and so forth. Additionally, neurotrophic and growth factors have been used in attempts to overcome *whatever* the causal mechanism may actually be by providing support to neurons targeted in the disease (see Mitsumoto et al., 2014 for review; see also Table 13.1). Apart from riluzole administered to ALS patients, none of the drugs has shown any significant impacts on disease course, and even in the case of riluzole the beneficial effects are modest at best.

Riluzole appears to work primarily by inhibiting glutamate release (Cifra et al., 2013), but its overall impact seems to involve a number of mechanisms of action (Bellingham, 2011). This last may not be unexpected given that riluzole's use was predicated on the perhaps naïve notion that excess glutamate release leading to excitotoxicity was the primary feature of the disease process. While excess glutamate and excitotoxicity are doubtlessly involved at some level, the thought that halting a cascading failure by targeting one part of the late cascade was likely doomed to have only marginal outcomes.

Table 13.1 Recently completed Phase III randomized, placebo-controlled, double-blind, parallel-group clinical trials for Parkinson's disease (PD).

	Mechanism	Primary outcome	Study duration	Number of patients	Status
Safinamide (Borgohain et al., 2014)	MAO-B and glutamate release inhibitor	On time with no/or non-troublesome dyskinesia	24 weeks	669	Improvement in total On time, Off time, UPDRS Part III and CGI-C In the process of filing the marketing authorization application for Europe and the United States
Zonisamide (Murata et al., 2007)	MAO-B and glutamate release inhibitor	UPDRS part III	16 weeks	347	Reduction in UPDRS score Approved in Japan since 2009
Perampanel (Lees et al., 2012)	AMPA receptor antagonist	Off time	30 weeks (study 301) 20 weeks (study 302)	1514 (total for studies 301 and 302)	Unsuccessful: no improvement
Istradefylline (Mizuno et al., 2013)	Adenosine A$_{2A}$ receptor agonist	Off time	12 weeks	373 PD with motor complications	Reduction in OFF time Other Phase III trials showed efficacy Approved as an adjunctive treatment of Parkinson's disease
Preladenant (Stocchi et al., 2014)	Adenosine A$_{2A}$ receptor agonist	UPDRS parts II and III	52 weeks	1000 early Parkinson's disease	Unsuccessful: no evidence of efficacy

(Continued)

Table 13.1 (Continued)

	Mechanism	Primary outcome	Study duration	Number of patients	Status
IPX066 (Hauser et al., 2013)	Extended-release carbidopa-levadopa (1 : 4 ratio) formulation	OFF time	13 weeks	471	Reduction in Off time, but mean On time increased compared to immediate-release carbidopa-levodopa group
					Reduction in UPDRS scores and improvement in PGI, CGI scales
					Other Phase III trials showed efficacy
					FDA approval withheld
Sarizotan (Goetz et al., 2007a)	5-HT1$_A$ receptor agonist	ON time		398	Unsuccessful: no change in On time and increase in Off time
Pardoprunox (Sampaio et al., 2011)	5-HT1$_A$ receptor inverse agonist	UPDRS-motor	24 weeks	468 (Rembrandt study) 334 (Vermeer study)	Unsuccessful: no clear efficacy and poor tolerability
Perampanel (Lees et al., 2012)	AMPA receptor agonist	OFF time	30 weeks	763 PD with motor fluctuations	Unsuccessful: no difference in mean total daily Off time
			20 weeks	751 PD with motor fluctuations	

AMPA; CGI-C, clinical global impression of change; MAO-B, monoamine oxidase B; PD, PGI receptor, subtype 1A, patient global impression of improvement; UPDRS, Unified Parkinson's disease rating scale; 5-HT1$_A$, 5-hydroxytryptamine.

It is also worth considering that riluzole's multiple actions on neural cells make it likely to generate, at least in the long term, various unwanted side effects. This is a potential problem for all drug therapies, especially those in which the drug is supposed to target particular neuronal elements. When delivered systemically, however, given that drug effects can occur in various parts of the CNS and in other organ systems, the problem becomes greater.

As Mitsumoto noted, part of the problem overall with the ALS RCTs is that they were based on earlier animal studies with the very problematic mSOD1 model (see Chapter 8). Recent therapeutic approaches to mRNA inhibition (Williams et al., 2009; Koval et al., 2013) or the targeting of misfolded SOD1 (Liu et al., 2012) are based on the same models, and thus unlikely to fare much better in human trials.

In many other cases, poor study design, small initial sample sizes, and what might be termed the "Ioannidis" effect (i.e., the lack of reproducibility of many studies) seem to have contributed to the generalized lack of success.

Another factor is likely the time at which treatments typically begin. Leaving aside the problems with many animal models, *in vivo* studies can introduce the various drugs at any point, and earlier intervention will clearly have a better chance of success, at least in principle. In humans, of course, the drug cannot be introduced prior to disease diagnosis.

Parkinson's disease has fared somewhat better in drug-therapy approaches, but outcomes have been relatively static in recent years. L-DOPA, a dopamine precursor, does provide some initial symptomatic relief in many Parkinson's patients, but the effect is not long-lasting, and it eventually produces dyskinesias in those taking it (Marsden, 1994; Fox et al., 2008).

The basic premise with L-DOPA use is that as neurons in the SN degenerate, they become incapable of providing the neurotransmitter dopamine to activate neurons in the striatum. Thus, increasing dopamine by increasing synthesis to replace that lost to the disease process has been proposed as a solution. However, Parkinson's disease, as cited in Chapter 2, also shows non-dopaminergic outcomes during its course, so replacing dopamine could hardly impact these other affected cells or circuits in the CNS.

Other drug therapies have been less successful, at least in detailed RCTs. The problems cited for ALS apply here as well (see Table 13.2), including inadequate *in vivo* models that often bear only a cursory resemblance to the actual end-state human disease.

Alzheimer's disease drug therapeutic treatments are invariably failures, with the various acetyl cholinesterase inhibitors having marginal to nil positive outcomes. Table 13.3 summarizes these data.

Chapter 14 will discuss in more detail why the various attempts to treat neurological diseases of these types with drug therapies have routinely failed and why they will likely continue to fail.

13.2.2 Other Proposed Therapies for Alzheimer's Disease

A non-surgical procedure proposed in the recent literature involves the use of directed pulses of repeated scanning ultrasound to create egress pathways by producing a more permeable blood–brain barrier for some subtypes of soluble Aβ. The idea is that in so doing the molecule will exit the brain and thus lower the toxic burden that it presumably creates for neurons in the Alzheimer's disease brain (Leinenga and Götz, 2015). The study reports that the procedure does lower Aβ and improves cognitive performance. The technique reportedly also activates microglia, a stage of neurological disease that,

Table 13.2 Recently completed Phase III randomized, placebo-controlled, double-blind, parallel-group clinical trials for Alzheimer's disease (AD). *Source:* Modified from Mitsumoto et al. (2014).

	Mechanism	Primary outcome	Study duration	Number of patients	Status
Xaliproden (Meininger et al., 2004)	Neurotrophic factor	Survival VC < 50%	18 months	867 (study 1) 1210 (study 2)	Unsuccessful: no statistically significant improvement
Vitamin E (Graf et al., 2005)	Oxidative stress	Survival	18 months	160	Unsuccessful
Celecoxib (Cudkowicz et al., 2006)	Inflammation	MVIC slope	12 months	300	Unsuccessful
Pentoxifylline (Meininger et al., 2006)	PDE4B inhibitors and TNF inhibitors	Survival	18 months	400	Unsuccessful: survival worsened
Minocycline (Gordon et al., 2007)	Inflammation, apoptosis	ALSFRS-R slope	4 months lead-in 9 months	412	Unsuccessful: faster ALSFRS-R score deterioration; adverse effects with riluzole (Milane et al., 2009)
TCH346 (Miller et al., 2007)	Apoptosis	ALSFRS-R slope	16 week lead-in 24 weeks	591	Unsuccessful: more deaths at higher doses
IGF-1 (Sorenson et al., 2008)	Neurotrophic factor	MMT	24 months	330	Unsuccessful
Erythropoietin (Lauria et al., 2015)	Neuroprotective	Survival	12 months	208	Unsuccessful
Glatiramer (Meininger et al., 2009)	Inflammation	ALSFRS-R slope	>52 weeks	366	Unsuccessful

Drug (Study)	Target	Outcome	Duration	N	Result
Lithium (UKMND-LiCALS Study Group, 2013)	Autophagy	Survival	18 months	214	Unsuccessful
Talampanel (Pascuzzi et al., 2010)	Excitotoxicity	ALSFRS-R change	12 months	559	Unsuccessful: increased adverse effects. Phase 3 results available only as abstract
Ceftriaxone (Cudkowicz et al., 2014)	Excitotoxicity	Survival; ALSFRS-R change	>12 months	513	Unsuccessful
Dexpramipexole (Cudkowicz et al., 2013)	Mitochondria	Survival; ALSFRS-R	12 months	943	Unsuccessful. Post hoc analysis was done (Bozik et al., 2014)
Olesoxime (Lenglet et al., 2014)	Mitochondria	Survival	18 months	512	Unsuccessful

ALSFRS-R, amyotrophic lateral sclerosis functional rating scale-revised; MMT, manual muscle testing; MVIC, maximum voluntary isometric (muscle) contraction; PDE4B, phosphodiesterase 4B; TNF, tumor necrosis factor; VC, vital capacity.

Table 13.3 Drug Therapies: Alzheimer's disease. Recently completed Phase III randomized, placebo-controlled, double-blind, parallel-group clinical trials for ALS

	Mechanism	Primary outcome	Study duration	Number of patients	Status
Tarenflurbil (Green et al., 2009)	γ-secretase modulator	ADAS-cog and ADCS-ADL	18 months	1684 mild AD	Unsuccessful Another RCT in 900 subjects was interrupted New compounds (e.g., CHF5074, EVP-0962) are under development
Semagacestat (LY450139) (Doody et al., 2013)	γ-secretase inhibitor	ADAS-cog and ADCS-ADL	76 weeks	2600 mild–moderate AD	Unsuccessful: halted after interim analysis showing increased incidence of skin cancer and worsening of AD symptoms
Rosiglitazone (Gold et al., 2009)	B-secretase inhibitor	ADAS-cog and CIBIC+	Up to 1 year	~3800 mild–moderate	Unsuccessful: possible cardiac risks One out of three RCTs published results
Phenserine (Winblad et al., 2010)	Selective cholinesterase inhibitor	ADAS-cog and CIBIC	6 months	384 mild–moderate	Unsuccessful
Tramiprosate (Aisen et al., 2011)	Decreased Aβ aggregation or oligomerization	ADAS-cog and CDR-SB	18 months	1052 mild–moderate AD	Unsuccessful Another Phase III trial in Europe was interrupted
Bapineuzumab (Salloway et al., 2014)	Increased Aβ clearance, passive immunotherapy	ADAS-cog and DAD scale	78 weeks	1121 (APOE 4-carrier study) 1131 (non-carrier study)	Unsuccessful
Solanezumab (Doody et al., 2014)	Antiamyloid therapeutics: passive immunotherapy	ADAS-cog and ADCS-ADL	18 months	2000 mild–moderate AD	Unsuccessful, but a secondary analysis of mild AD patients pooled from two trials showed a significant effect on cognition (NCT01760005)
Flurizan (MPC-7869) (Myrexis, 2008)	Selective Aβ-42-lowering agent	ADAS-cog and ACDS-ADL	18 months	1684	Unsuccessful

Intervention	Mechanism	Outcome measures	Duration	Sample size	Result
Gammagard (Baxter, 2013)	IVIg	ADAS-cog and ADCS-ADL	18 months	390 mild–moderate	Unsuccessful. Trial data currently unpublished (NCT00818662)
Flebogamma (Instituto Grifols, 2015)	IVIg	ADAS-cog and ADCS-ADL: no results yet	14 months	350	Ongoing (NCT01561053). No published results
Valproate (Tariot et al., 2011)	Tau therapeutic	NPI, Quality of Life-AD, ADCS-CGIC, safety	24 months	313 moderate AD	Unsuccessful
Statins (Feldman et al., 2010; Sano et al., 2011)	HMG-CoA-reductase inhibitor	ADAS-cog	18 months	~1100 mild–moderate	Unsuccessful. Phase II trial ongoing to test potential as a preventive agent
Latrepirdine (PF-01913539 or dimebon) (Bharadwaj et al., 2013)	Stabilization of mitochondrial dysfunction	ADAS-cog and ADCS-ADL	12 months	1050	Unsuccessful. Results not published, and the study was not terminated due to the safety findings (Bharadwaj et al., 2013)
Xaliproden (Douillet and Orgogozo, 2009)	Serotonin antagonist with nerve growth factor effects	ADAS-cog and CDR	18 months	2761 mild–moderate	Unsuccessful
Omega-3 polyunsaturated fatty acids (Quinn et al., 2010)	ADAS-cog and CDR	ADAS-cog and CDR	18 months	295 mild–moderate	Unsuccessful

AD, Alzheimer's disease; ADAS-cog, Alzheimer's Disease Assessment Scale; ADCS-ADL, Alzheimer's Disease Cooperative Study – Activities of Daily Living Inventory; ADCS-CGIC: Alzheimer's Disease Cooperative Study – Clinical Global Impression of Change; CDR, clinical dementia rating; CIBIC, Clinician's Interview-Based Impression of Change; IVIg, intravenous immunoglobulin; DAD scale, Disability Assessment for Dementia scale; NPI, Neuropsychiatric Inventory.

as noted elsewhere, may have multiple outcomes. One clear problem with the notion so far is that it has only been tested on an animal model of Alzheimer's disease and so must be considered in the context of the problems with neurological disease *in vivo* models, as cited in Chapter 8.

A recent attempt to remove aluminum as a likely contributing factor in Alzheimer's disease involves the use of silicic acid. A pilot study by the Exley group in the United Kingdom has shown good tolerance for this compound, the removal of aluminum (as demonstrated by excretion through urine), and some improvement in cognitive scores in treated patients (Davenward et al., 2013). Since silicic acid is found in many forms of commercial mineral water, a successful larger-scale demonstration that something so simple and relatively inexpensive that could alter the course of Alzheimer's disease would be highly welcome in an otherwise fairly dismal therapeutic landscape.

13.2.3 Surgical Interventions

It should be obvious that replacing cells or circuits in neurological disease conditions is not going to be the same as replacing less dynamic parts of different organ systems (e.g., corneal transplants, hip replacements, etc). In this section, I will present the outcomes for the main neurological diseases in reverse order of least likely or to various levels of demonstrated success.

It should first be acknowledged that some recent case reports have noted successful surgical treatments for spinal cord injuries. In several publications, Tabakow et al. (2013, 2014) have described partial recovery of locomotion in a patient in whom mucosal olfactory ensheathing cells and nerve fibroblasts were removed from the olfactory mucosa and placed into the region of the spinal cord injury together with a sural nerve bridge.

This intervention for spinal cord trauma is encouraging, but preliminary. Further, how such treatments might be applied to the neurological diseases in question is not obvious.

In the case of ALS, while the apparent solution to motor neuron loss would be to replace motor neurons with either implanted fetal motor neurons or stem cells, the difficulties in such an approach are formidable. First, the cells would have to successfully integrate into the correct circuits. Why this may not be possible is the subject of the next chapter. A second problem, often apparently ignored in the field, is this: How do the replacement motor neurons find their way back to the muscles that they are expected to innervate in order to recreate a normal neuromuscular junction and thus normal motor function? As already mentioned, this is the subject of ongoing investigation in spinal cord injury and has not, as yet, been solved.

In Alzheimer's disease, the problem is multifaceted. In the disease, the circuits destroyed are widely scattered, as noted by Braak and Braak (1991). Where, then, to put the replacement neurons, and how might they correctly integrate into circuits in the various affected parts of the brain? This approach would no doubt be highly problematic and would be likely to induce as much pathology as it solves (Neill, 2001). This last consideration is perhaps the reason that neuron replacement therapies in Alzheimer's do not seem to be widely considered.

The application of various cell-replacement approaches in Parkinson's disease has shown the most success compared to ALS and Alzheimer's disease. In brief, the general strategy is to use grafts or fetal cells that are thought to produce dopamine in an attempt to replace dopamine in the nigro-striatal system. These cells are derived from various sources in humans, mostly the SN (Barker et al., 2013; Hallett et al., 2015). Other potential sources, including retinal pigment epithelial cells, have not been shown to produce sufficient dopamine (Gross et al., 2011).

In general, such cell-replacement approaches have had some success in Parkinson's patients, but the extent of the positive outcome very much depends on the clinic where they are carried out and the stage of the disease (Barker et al., 2013). However, given that Parkinson's disease involves the dysfunction of more than dopaminergic neural circuits, such therapies will not show efficacy against the cognitive and other dysfunctions that are typically manifested in the various disease stages.

With particular regard to potential stem cell therapies, the success in Parkinson's disease has been marginal (Luo et al., 2009; Ertelt et al., 2012), in spite of some potentially promising animal studies. Perhaps this failure of translation should not be unexpected, given that the *in vivo* studies involved the use of another problematic model, namely MPTP lesions in primates (Hallett et al., 2015). As Barker et al. (2013, p. 87) note, "…models of Parkinson's disease are poor imitators of the clinical disorder."

One approach to neural replacement is based on the observation that in some neurological disease conditions neurogenesis is diminished (Winner and Winkler, 2015). This outcome has also been found in animal models of neurological disease (Tabata et al., 2008). Such data may give rise to a possibly novel therapeutic approach whereby the loss of neurogenic potential is either halted or, conversely, enhanced in order to provide the basis for renewed neural circuitry. The potential for neurogenesis as a future therapeutic in neurological disease will be explored later in this chapter.

One relatively successful surgical approach to Parkinson's disease, used since the 1990s in over 100 000 Parkinson's patients, is deep-brain stimulation (DBS) (Benabid et al., 1987; Bronstein et al., 2011). DBS was approved by the US Food and Drug Administration (FDA) for Parkinson's disease treatment in 2002. It was later approved for the treatment of other neurological diseases, such as essential tremor (Benabid et al., 2009), dystonia, and obsessive–compulsive disorders (Denys and Mantione, 2009).

In DBS surgery, a microelectrode is introduced into part of the *globus palidus* or subthalamic nucleus, through which electrical stimulation can be applied. The goal is to change the electrical activity of the target brain regions in a controlled manner and thus alleviate some of the features of the disease. The exact mechanism by which DBS works remains unclear (Miocinovic et al., 2013), but it is presumed to involve changing electrical, chemical, and other neural network activity, particularly in the basal ganglia. Clinical trials of DBS have reported significant improvement in cardinal motor signs, including tremor, bradykinesia, and rigidity, with variable results for impairments in gait, balance, and speech (Deuschl et al., 2006; Okun et al., 2009; Weaver et al., 2009; Williams et al., 2010).

13.2.4 Prospects for Neurogenesis as a Treatment for Neurological Disease

Considerations that adult neurogenesis may be of use as a repair strategy for neurological diseases have been touted in recent years. The problems with this approach are several-fold. First, normal neurogenesis in the adult CNS is largely restricted to particular regions (e.g., retina, hippocampus, olfactory system, and subventricular zone). Secondly, such neurogenesis in normal development, along with aspects of synaptogenesis and synaptic plasticity, is controlled, in part, by some of the same proteins whose mutant forms are involved in neurological diseases (e.g., α-synuclein and huntingtin). Thus, encouraging neurogenesis in areas destroyed in the various neurological diseases (spinal and cortical motor neurons in ALS; SN in Parkinson's disease; cortex and hippocampus in Alzheimer's disease) may be extremely problematic. In part, this concern arises from the nature of neurogenesis which has been suggested to be a part of the actual pathological process in these diseases, rather than an attempt at system repair (Steiner et al., 2005; Winner et al., 2011).

13.2.5 Gene Therapy

Gene-therapy approaches have been considered for the various neurological disorders, based in part on gene-replacement attempts in diseases such as cystic fibrosis (Prickett and Jain, 2013). The general failure of the latter, as discussed in the next chapter, has apparently diminished the previous enthusiasm for such potential therapeutic applications to neurological diseases.

13.3 Summary

The general failure of neurological disease treatments to date in halting, let alone reversing, the signs and symptoms of these diseases should lead to an honest reappraisal that may be unpalatable to many victims of the diseases, their caregivers, their clinicians, and even basic researchers. Namely, if nothing has worked to date, the likelihood is that redoubling efforts in the same directions is not likely to succeed either.

Instead, if treatments are to prove efficacious, the field will almost certainly have to adopt novel strategies that have the following constraint: treatments will work better if given earlier rather than later. The reasons for this are likely obvious, but bear restating.

First, the earlier in the disease process an intervention takes place, the fewer the bifurcations that will have occurred in the disease cascade, and thus the fewer the potential side effects of targeting multiple degenerative events. The longer treatment is delayed, the greater the likelihood that additional parts of the affected cells, circuits, or even regions of the brain will have to be treated as well. At a genetic level, the longer the process goes on, the greater the chances for oligogenetic involvement (i.e., additional deleterious gene expression). The same consideration applies to the proteins affected, to various metabolic pathways, and so on.

At a neuronal subsystem level, as each of these diseases progress, additional parts of the CNS are affected: ALS and Parkinson's disease proceed from unilateral to bilateral presentations, and in addition move to regions of the relevant structures not initially impacted, let alone to regions of the CNS outside the primary target zones of the disease process. In regard to the latter, ALS and Parkinson's often also eventually show features of cognitive impairment as regions of the cortex and hippocampus are impacted. It should be remembered that prior to clinical disease onset, regions of the CNS not directly associated with the disease are also sometimes affected (e.g., olfactory regions in the brains of Parkinson's and Alzheimer's disease patients).

Second, the earlier therapies are used to target the disease process, the greater the likelihood that some of the neurons thought to be dead might still be alive, albeit dysfunctional. Some such neurons might perhaps be rescued and restored to normal, or relatively normal, function. This consideration makes the use of growth factors, especially if applied early, a better bet for success than the use of drugs designed solely to alter a single abnormal biochemical process. A case in point is the use of the neuroepithelial growth factor progranulin (PGRN).

Third, neural plasticity may always be operating, but in a disease state it may well become part of the pathological process, with aberrant connections and pathways being formed. These can become part of the overall problem (Shaw and McEachern, 2001), serving not only to further the overall dysfunction of the system, but also perhaps to inhibit any innate or therapeutic attempts at repair.

These considerations now lead to a more detailed discussion of where translational approaches may be able to go in dealing with neurological diseases. In brief, the field knows quite well what has not worked. It also knows what some proposed avenues are. Perhaps, therefore, it is time to totally rethink the problem based on the evidence at hand and not keep doing the things that do not work?

Endnote

1 Prof. John W. Oller is the Doris B. Hawthorne/LEQSF Professor in Communicative Disorders at the University of Louisiana at Lafayette. Personal communication.

14

The Future of Translational Research in Neurological Disease

> *Canst thou not minister to a mind diseased?*
> *Pluck from the memory a rooted sorrow,*
> *raze out the written troubles of the brain,*
> *and with some sweet oblivious antidote*
> *cleanse the stuffed bosom of that perilous stuff*
> *which weighs upon the heart.*
> William Shakespeare, *Macbeth*, Act 5, Scene 3

From the Preface

The material from the Preface cited in the previous chapter applies, but here also includes the notion of true narrative representations (TNRs) and the consequences of violating them.

14.1 Introduction

As cited in various previous chapters, the nervous system shows remarkable levels of "neuroplasticity," particularly early in life (Shaw and McEachern, 2001). Thus, sensory-map reorganizations and compensation for neuronal injuries occur more easily in young animals and humans than in those outside of some critical-period windows.

In various mammalian species, the early postnatal period is one of rapid neurogenesis and synaptogenesis, accompanied by neurotransmitter and receptor modifications and a host of other functional changes. All of these significantly alter brain morphology and function. To an extent, such changes occur in adult animals and humans as well. Neurogenesis appears to be more restricted in the areas of the central nervous system (CNS) and occurs at a much lower rate, but it still occurs (Winner and Winkler, 2015). And, needless to say, some sort of neuronal modification must obviously occur throughout life, as judged by the ability of animals and humans to learn, remember, and act on new information to guide behavior.

Neural Dynamics of Neurological Disease, First Edition. Christopher A. Shaw.
© 2017 John Wiley & Sons, Inc. Published 2017 by John Wiley & Sons, Inc.

14.2   Comparing Traumatic Brain Injury to Neurological Diseases

In addition to neurogenesis, neuronal and behavioral compensation for even dramatic CNS injuries remains extant in some circumstances. Two cases, described briefly in Chapter 1, serve to illustrate this point: one from the historical record and one of more recent vintage.

The first, a demi-classic in the neurology literature, concerns the case of Phineas Gage, an American railway worker who was catastrophically injured in 1848. Gage, 24 at the time of his accident, was preparing a demolition for the railway. A premature detonation blew a tamping rod, a 3 foot long/more than 13 pound metal pole with a pointed end, through his head. The rod entered under his jaw and exited at the top of his head, destroying the left frontal lobe. Gage was initially presumed dead, but within minutes of the injury he was walking and talking in spite of having lost considerable blood and an apparently major amount of brain matter from the exit wound.

Gage went on to what at the time appeared to be a nearly complete recovery. His speech and motor functions seemed to be almost on par with those he possessed before the accident. Remarkably, Gage appeared to have minimal cognitive deficits, although current means of neurological evaluation would no doubt have found more detailed dysfunctions (Figure 14.1). He did suffer, however, from increasingly debilitating seizures over the years until his death in 1860. Dr. John Martyn Harlow, a physician involved in Gage's care, wrote about the case (see Macmillan and Lena, 2010 for details).

Trevor Greene may be the Phineas Gage of the 21st century. Greene, a Canadian Army reserve officer, was posted to Afghanistan's Kandahar Province in 2006 as part of the Canadian military deployment to that country. Within weeks, he was struck in the head with an axe by a Taliban supporter during a meeting with village elders. The axe blow penetrated his skull and entered deep into his brain slightly off the sagittal plane, anteriorly from the frontal cortex and posteriorly to the parietal cortex along the central sulcus. The injury was thus to the right frontal and left parietal lobes, destroying both gray and white matter, the latter including part of the corpus callosum. In particular, the axe bisected the motor and pre-motor cortices.

The initial medical evaluation concluded that Greene would die of his injuries. When he did not, the expectation of attending neurologists was that he would be left in a permanent vegetative state. Greene went on to surprise his caregivers by gradually recovering verbal and considerable motor functions. After years of intensive physio- and speech therapy, Greene can now walk with assistance and speak coherently. He has written a book with his wife on the stages of his recovery to date.

Part of Greene's retraining and recovery seems to involve the use of a form of "neuroimaging," a technique partially developed by one of his later care providers, Dr. Ryan D'Arcy. The idea behind the technique is that the patient imagines the recovery taking place as he or she attempts to execute various motor tasks. According to D'Arcy, fMRI data support the recovery of brain circuitry in the context of recovery of function (D'Arcy et al., 2016) (Figure 14.2).

Overall, Greene seems to have recovered remarkably from what was an apparently devastating injury. How precisely such a recovery of function actually occurred in the case of Trevor Greene remains uncertain, but D'Arcy's explanation, supported by the current data, is as good a hypothesis as any. Indeed, these data and Greene's recovery offer considerable hope to those who have suffered various forms of traumatic brain injury (TBI).

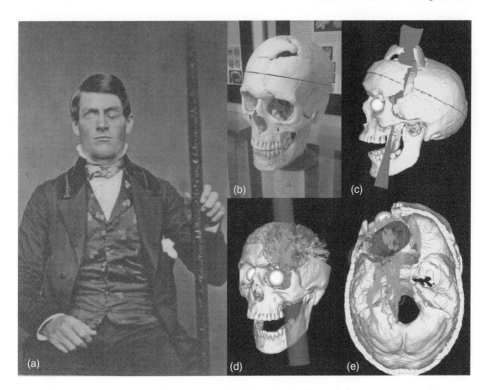

Figure 14.1 The CNS injuries of Phineas Gage. (a) Photograph of cased-daguerreotype studio portrait of brain-injury survivor Phineas P. Gage (1823–1860), shown holding the tamping rod that injured him. (b–e) Modeling the path of the tamping rod through the Gage skull and its effects on CNS structures (b) The skull of Phineas Gage on display at the Warren Anatomical Museum at Harvard Medical School. (c) Computed tomography (CT) image volumes of the individual pieces of bone dislodged by the tamping rod, the top of the cranium, and the mandible – reconstructed, spatially aligned, and manually segmented. (d) A rendering of the Gage skull with the best-fit rod trajectory and example fiber pathways in the left hemisphere intersected by the rod. (e) A view of the interior of the Gage skull showing the extent of fiber pathways intersected by the tamping rod in a sample subject (i.e., one having minimal spatial deformation to the Gage skull). *Source*: (a) Collection of Jack and Beverly Wilgus, under Creative Commons Attribution License; (b–e) Van Horn et al. (2012), under Creative Commons Attribution License. (See color plate section for the color representation of this figure.)

The Gage and Greene cases are remarkable and to some extent unusual, but are by no means totally unique. While TBI can be fatal, can induce comatose or vegetative states, or can leave the victim with permanent major disabilities, it does not always do so. In some large measure, the outcome depends on the precise nature of the neural destruction. Damage to respiratory centers in the brain stem, for example, is typically fatal unless the patient remains on constant artificial ventilation; cortical damage, however, can often be compensated for to some extent by other cortical areas, as when language returns after stroke (see Anderson et al., 2011). The key factors at play in such instances are the areas destroyed and the compensatory responses of the areas that remain.

Both Gage and Greene had dedicated caregivers working for their recovery, albeit nearly 150 years apart, with all that this time span entails for medical treatment. Added to this are factors such as age (both Gage and Greene were relatively young), health and general fitness, the undefinable contributions of spirit and determination, and likely a host of even less tangible factors.

(a)

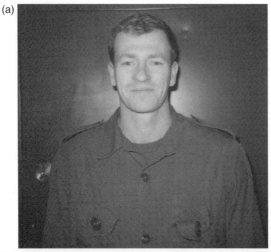

(b)

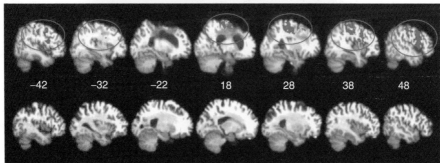

Figure 14.2 The CNS injuries of Trevor Greene. (a) Photograph of Lieutenant Trevor Greene, taken prior to his deployment to Afghanistan. (b) Sagittal view of mean lower-limb motor activation and mental-imagery activation on functional magnetic resonance imaging (fMRI), averaged across all time points (red; T1–T12, 33 months). Numbers indicate the x coordinate for each slice (Z > 2.3, pcorr < 0.05). *Source*: (a) Pierre Gazzola (https://www.flickr.com/photos/85013738@N00/), under Creative Commons Attribution License; (b) D'Arcy et al. (2016), with permission from Wolters Kluwer Health, Inc. (See color plate section for the color representation of this figure.)

So, as remarkable as the recoveries of Gage and Greene may be, the question that has to be raised is this: If people can show recovery from injuries as utterly devastating as these, why should they not be able to recover from the age-related neurological diseases, which cumulatively destroy far less of the CNS?

Part of the reason arises from the acute versus progressive nature of the respective injuries. In the cases of Gage and Greene, after the initial injury had occurred, other processes began. It should be noted that the neurological sequelae were not trivial and must have included some damage to sites near to the basic injury, potential infection, and the formation of scar tissues. Nevertheless, these injuries were, at some relatively early point, somewhat self-contained. As the initial injury responses abated, compensation by other CNS areas gradually filled in the functional gaps. In the case of Gage, the increasing number of seizures in the years after the accident speaks to some continuing deterioration.

In progressive neurological diseases, however, there is no respite. For reasons that are still not clear, neural damage in these diseases spreads and ultimately cascades. This cascading nature of neurological disorders does not allow new circuits to form around the damaged areas. The subsystem itself is damaged, even though the losses of the various cellular components may not all occur simultaneously.

Another potential reason for the recovery of Gage and Greene is that their cognitive abilities were not significantly impacted in the long term. Thus, both individuals could, once cognitively aware, participate in their own neural recovery. In contrast, in all of the neurological diseases in question (Parkinson's disease, ALS, Alzheimer's disease), general cognitive dysfunction occurs – indeed, it may begin sooner than the clinical diagnosis stage. Certainly, by the time of clinical diagnosis, or shortly thereafter, cognition has often been clearly been compromised. This leads to the obvious notion that earlier detection of the onset of any of these diseases could allow cognitive participation by the victims in some sort of compensatory rebuilding of neural circuits and functions.

One possible reason for the apparent anomaly between TBI and the progressive neurological diseases may lie in considerations of some recent theories about human consciousness. Koch (2012), citing his own work and that of his colleague, Dr. Giulio Tononi, describes what he terms the "theory of integrated information." The basic idea here is that a conscious experience is extremely "differentiated," and thus unique. A second feature of the theory is that a conscious state is highly "integrated," in that many areas of the cortex participate in it. The extent to which the system is synergistic with such integration is measured by the extent of consciousness, using the symbol φ. Koch writes that, "Maximizing φ is about finding the sweet spot between these two opposing tendencies" (2012, p. 129); that is, between differentiation and integration.

Finally, there is the issue of neural signaling itself, which ties in quite well with the notion of neural integrative functions. This is, once again, the concept of biosemiosis in the nervous system. I will address this further in Section 14.7, but it is hard to avoid speculation that, as damaged as the brain may be in TBI unlike in the neurological diseases, the non-damaged areas are biosemiotically intact. That is, they are able to send meaningful signals to the other non-damaged regions. In contrast, in neurological disease, the disease process makes the very signals themselves part of the overall problem.

This last point can perhaps be best understood in ALS, possibly the most catastrophic of the age-related neurological diseases, at least in terms of the speed of disease progression and the frankly fatal nature of the neuronal loss itself. There may be no better way to appreciate this dynamic than by comparing ALS to polio.

14.3 ALS and Polio: Comparing the Nature of Neural Degeneration and Progression in the Two Diseases

At end state in ALS, there has been significant loss of the α-motor neurons in the motor cortex, which provide the descending tracts, including the corticospinal tract, along with the motor neurons in the anterior horn of the spinal cord. The outcome is a progressive failure of various muscle groups controlling the limbs, the diaphragm, and others.

The key questions, as cited elsewhere in this book, are these: What causal factors and molecular process(es) lead to the loss of motor neurons? What are the underlying forms of neural damage? What makes the disease itself progressive?

The answer to the first remains unclear, but in most instances of sALS it is not a gene mutation/dysfunction and the resulting abnormal protein product. Just as certainly, it is not, in most cases, the outcome of an easily determined chronic toxicity.

As cited in other chapters, there are many clues, but no clear answers. In fact, many of the clues, while fascinating, do not necessarily translate into clear etiologies. For example, Weisskopf et al. (2005) conducted an epidemiological study that implicated *any* military service in the 20th century onwards as a risk factor for ALS. Other studies have noted that hyper-exercise seems to have a role. Still others have implicated various contact sports (Chiò et al., 2005, 2009; Abel, 2007).

From this short list, one could conclude that a range of factors might underlie the development of ALS: solvents, stress, other toxins, chronic head injuries, and so on. Clearly, not everyone who develops ALS has been exposed to all of these factors. What those who contemplate such things will almost certainly be left with is a huge range of gene–environment interactions that create ALS in unique ways in afflicted individuals.

The answer to the second question is becoming clearer all the time, and yet more extensive, as the myriad ways of damaging motor neurons are described by the emerging literature. As noted in various chapters, both cell-autonomous and non-cell-autonomous effects are involved in both sporadic and familial forms of the disease, and a number of these have been successfully modeled *in vivo*. For example, virtually any cellular organelle or process, if disrupted, will kill motor neurons in due course. Candidate targets are mitochondria, proteasomes, and the cell membrane itself – to name only a few of the major ones. On top of this, axonal transport malfunctions in either direction lead to alterations at the muscle end plate. A host of other sources of motor neuron degeneration have also been considered.

At the non-cell-autonomous level, there can be alterations in the supporting glial cells, including astrocytes (Vargas and Johnson, 2010), microglia (Brites and Vaz, 2014), and oligodendrocytes (Nonneman et al., 2014). Of course, if the mechanisms are non-cell-autonomous, at least in part, then many of the same sorts of events that go wrong in any individual motor neuron can go wrong in the glial cells as well. There is also every reason to believe that multiple cell-autonomous actions are involved in motor neuron death and that cell-autonomous and non-cell-autonomous dysfunctions overlap.

Overall, what one is left with is a quite large number of ways of destroying motor neurons and no particularly good way to decide whether some, many, or all of them are involved in ALS in any particular individual, let alone those within the ALS spectrum of motor neuron diseases (Figure 14.3). This conclusion raises serious problems for any

Continuum of Neurodegeneration

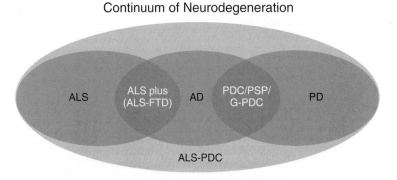

Figure 14.3 Schematic of a possible spectrum of neurological disease and fractal versions of the same.

therapy that relies on preventing one particular aspect of the disease process, unless the sequence of cascading events is precisely known.

Since the latter is not, in fact, the case, and is further unlikely to be known in the near future, the notion that multiple hits to any motor neuron must be addressed to prevent cell death can therefore rely only on a drug "cocktail," with the number of ingredients needed depending on the number of autonomous/non-autonomous processes that require remediation. Individual biochemical variations across the population are further going to make such therapeutics even more problematic.

It thus becomes ever less surprising that all drug-therapy trials to date have failed. Inadequate models do not help, either (see Scott et al., 2008; van der Worp et al., 2010; Mitsumoto et al., 2014; Zwiegers and Shaw, 2015). As cited in previous chapters, many of the same critiques apply to Parkinson's and Alzheimer's diseases, for both treatment paradigms and models.

In contrast to motor neuron death in ALS, that in polio (the paralysis associated with the disease is termed "poliomyelitis") is caused by an enterovirus of the *Picornaviridae* family.

Answers to the three questions posed for ALS seem to be a lot more tractable for polio. The virus enters the human subject through a fecal–oral route and reproduces in the intestines. In approximately 1–2% of those infected, it spreads to the CNS, where it targets motor neurons in the spinal cord, but does not affect upper motor neurons that contribute to the corticospinal tract. The virus capsid protein binds to the CD 155 receptor on the motor neuron surface to initiate the processes leading to cell death. The mechanisms of cell death appear to involve both necrosis and apoptosis. Those motor neurons that survive are often able to reinnervate de-innervated muscle fibers, creating larger-than-normal motor units that are nevertheless somewhat functional.

While the viral infection always has the same penultimate end state of dead anterior horn motor neurons, its progression is limited by the immune system, such that after the initial infectious period those motor neurons not destroyed remain unaffected and the motor dysfunctions cease to progress.

Following recovery from acute poliomyelitis, many of the deficits in motor function remain stable for years to decades. However, up to 78% of individuals post-disease experience a gradual loss of muscle strength, termed the "post-polio syndrome" (Ramlow et al., 1992).

Compared to ALS, polio is a simpler disease, in that one particular identified infectious agent causes damage to motor neurons and the infection is eventually brought under control by the immune system. There are, however, two caveats to this notion of simplicity: First, other viruses, as cited in Chapter 11, can cause motor neuron loss, and without examining antibody titers – especially for patients of the past – it is not possible to be certain that the polio virus was the causal factor. Second, in some measure, ALS may also involve either inflammatory or autoimmune processes, as discussed in Chapter 11.

Overall, a key difference seems to reside in whatever factor drives disease progression to involve those motor neurons not initially affected. As discussed in Chapter 11, given what the field now knows about CNS–immune bidirectional interactions, it is difficult to avoid speculation that the precise nature of such interactions is key. For example, in polio, the immune system acts as a negative-feedback brake to the further spread of motor neuron loss; in ALS, the toxin/gene product interactions with the immune system may operate more in a positive feed-forward manner to accelerate motor neuron loss.

14.4 Neurological Diseases as Spectrum Disorders: Implications for Therapy

The evidence presented thus far in the book reinforces the notion – one that is not particularly controversial – that ALS is a spectrum disorder in which etiologies, progression, and the involvement of other neural groups, not to mention other organ systems, are variable across the patient population.

This same conclusion is being reached in regard to the Parkinson's disease population, whether conventional idiopathic Parkinson's disease or the various parkinsonisms. It is difficult to imagine that the same would not apply to Alzheimer's disease as well. Neurological disorders such as ALS-PDC, PSP, and FTD lend themselves to an even wider spectrum that encompasses many of the overlapping sporadic age-related neurological diseases.

As with the ALS spectrum, a generalized "one size fits all" therapeutics approach is inevitably going to be a problem for any of these diseases at an individual level. While a case can be made that in each category a common point is reached in the disease process, the problem is that this stage is likely to be quite late in progression, when considerable damage to the various parts of the CNS has already occurred.

Therapeutic approaches, some of which were addressed in Chapter 13, would appear to be stuck between these two realities. In spite of this, the hope of effective treatment drives a number of researchers to keep seeking positive outcomes, and it is thus likely that a number of unsuccessful (and some potentially promising) clinical trials will be added to the list before this book is published. As an example, in ALS, the focus is likely to continue to be on drugs designed to block one of the myriad biochemical abnormalities arising in the disease.

A recent study using the mSOD1 model (itself problematic, as noted repeatedly in previous chapters) examined the potential of guanabenz and used in an inhibitor of endoplasmic reticulum stress, in the treatment of hypertension (Wang et al., 2014). The preliminary outcomes in the mSOD1 mice looks as if it has potential merit, as many such *in vivo* data studies initially do, but the eventual clinical outcome is likely to be disappointing (see, e.g., Mitsumoto et al., 2014).

An even more promising study, also using the mSOD model, is that conducted by Williams et al. (2016). In spite of the problematic nature of this model, these investigators may have come up with a potentially useful therapeutic for the mSOD1-fALS. In brief, they use the rapid-onset G93A transgenic to induce an ALS phenotype and then blocked its pathological expression, apparently permanently, with the copper complex CuATSM. The authors believe that this compound might also work in sALS, and they further claim some success using it in models of Parkinson's disease. Evidence for a common misfolded SOD in fALS and sALS is not convincing, as discussed in Chapter 5. Neither is it clear how the compound would serve to prevent the emergence of a Parkinson's disease phenotype, unless one were to postulate that all such neurological disorders arise from mitochondrial defects. In spite of such caveats, it remains possible, albeit not probable, that there may be some aspect of the CuATSM treatment that might serve to at least diminish motor neuron loss in ALS.

In addition, a variety of cell therapies are under development by various biotechnology companies, but data from early trials are thus far too preliminary to judge their potential future efficacy, in spite of the apparent enthusiasm with which they are viewed in some quarters (Goldstein, 2015).

In other studies, regulatory T-cell therapy has been recently proposed, based on the premise that autoimmune dysfunctions are involved in ALS, as indeed they may be (Beers et al., 2011).

At a gene level, attempts to manage mutations have turned to the possibility of using exon-skipping strategies to restore normal protein transcription (Dominov et al., 2014; Siva et al., 2014).

The successes of the various treatment regimes for ALS to date have actually been at a lower level than that found for "Lorenzo's oil," a mixture of glyceryl trioleate and glyceryl trierucate used as an oral remedy to treat a genetic disorder termed "X-linked adrenoleukodystrophy" (X-ALD). In X-ALD, the X-linked accumulation of saturated very-long-chain fatty acids (SVLCFAs) leads to a series of neurological disorders. Lorenzo's oil, named after the child whose parents first formulated it, does lower SVLCFAs and does prevent the emergence of the cerebral phenotype if administered prior to clinical onset, although detailed clinical trials are still lacking (Moser et al., 2007). Even with these shortcomings, most ALS clinicians would be only too delighted to have the equivalent of such a drug in their therapeutics arsenal.

14.4.1 Parkinson's and Alzheimer's Diseases

In Parkinson's disease, new drug trials are constantly ongoing, although success remains marginal (see Table 13.1). In Alzheimer's disease, attempts to control the level of Aβ are underway, both with continuations of the BACE1 work and with the use of ultrasound to mechanically disrupt Aβ deposits. Potential problems with these approaches are as discussed earlier in this chapter.

14.4.2 Progranulin as a Potential Therapeutic in Neurological Diseases

One fairly recent approach that may have some prospect of success involves the notion that in the various neurological diseases the neurons affected are not always destroyed by the time of clinical diagnosis. The perspective here is much like that in polio, namely that those motor neurons not initially destroyed can return to a functional state once the infection abates. These surviving neurons are then able to sprout and reinnervate muscles denervated by the loss of other motor neurons to the virus. If this held true, in principle, for ALS, then various trophic factors might serve to recover the damaged motor neurons and thus their function.

One such trophic factor is the evolutionarily ancient and conserved cysteine-rich protein, progranulin (PGRN), a secreted epithelial growth factor (Bateman and Bennett, 2009). PGRN appears to have a variety of cellular functions, including wound healing, cell proliferation, male-specific brain differentiation, regulation of tumorigenesis, and modulation of the inflammatory response (De Muynck and Van Damme, 2011). An 8 kb region located on chromosome 17q21 has become a subject of considerable interest for neurodegenerative diseases in light of evidence that PGRN may be important in the long-term survival of nerve cells (Ahmed et al., 2007; Cruts and Van Broeckhoven, 2008).

PGRN is derived from 13 exons and consists of 7.5 tandem repeats of a conserved 12-cysteinyl granulin motif (C-X_{5-6}-C-X_5-CC-X_8-CC-X_6-CC-X_5-CC-X_5-C-C-X_{5-6}-C (De Muynck and Van Damme, 2011). Proteolytic cleavage of full-length PGRN gives rise to several 6 kDa granulin (GRN) peptides, which are able to induce the same cellular actions. PGRN is expressed in multiple cell types, including mitotically-active epithelia, immune cells, microglia, and various types of neurons (He and Bateman, 2003; Ryan et al., 2009).

In animal models, including for TBI (Matzilevich et al., 2002), axotomy (Moisse et al., 2009), and, more recently, Parkinson's disease (Van Kampen et al., 2014a) and Alzheimer's disease (Minami et al., 2014), PGRN has shown some ability to preserve or restore CNS function. Some of these actions may be mediated by the activation of cell-survival signaling cascades such as of extracellular signal-regulated kinases and protein kinase B (Xu et al., 2011).

Some subtypes of at least one neurological disease, frontotemporal lobar degeneration (FTLD-U), appear to arise as a result of a haploinsufficiency in PGRN production, caused by as many as 60 mutations in the *PGRN* gene (Cruts et al., 2012; Petkau and Leavitt, 2014). Mutations in *PGRN* have not, however, been found to be a significant causal factor in most instances of either fALS or sALS (Petkau and Leavitt, 2014), although there is some evidence for a role in disease onset and long-term survival (Sleegers et al., 2008). The latter is a curious finding in that PGRN levels in humans and animal models actually increase during the disease course (Irwin et al., 2009; Philips et al., 2010). Much of this increase appears to reside in the microglia, a finding mirrored by the axotomy and Alzheimer's disease data. It is worth remembering that attempts to alter microglial phenotypes and functions are likely to prove to be complex in the dynamic process of neuronal degeneration. As promising as some of the *in vivo* data appear, especially in the Parkinson's and Alzheimer's disease models, it is important to remember the limitations of model systems in neurological diseases, as cited in Chapter 8.

14.5   Cystic Fibrosis and Gene Therapy

As cited in Chapter 13, gene-therapy approaches to neurological diseases seem to have faded away since the same strategies proved unsuccessful in a much simpler organ system – the lungs – in attempts to reverse the course of cystic fibrosis (CF), an autosomal-recessive disorder.

The gene responsible for CF is the cystic fibrosis transmembrane regulator (*CFTR*), which codes for a cAMP-regulated chloride channel on the apical surface of lung epithelial cells. There are almost 2000 known mutations to *CFTR*, which cause changes in ion and water transport in these cells, increase the binding of various pathogens, and cause increases in proinflammatory cytokines (Li and Naren, 2005).

Initially, the problem in CF was thought to be straightforward, given that the disease involves a single gene (Prickett and Jain, 2013). The idea was to treat the disease by modifying an individual's defective gene expression or by correcting the gene with a normal gene for the same function. After cloning the normal gene, different gene-transfer methods were tried, but all failed. Various explanations have been given for these failures, but a primary one appears to be the overall immune response to the inserted gene (Fischer and McCray, 2008; Griesenbach et al., 2011). Even drug therapies designed to control secretory processes have had only limited success, and even then only in a small percentage of CF patients (Ashlock and Olson, 2011).

If regulating lung physiology turns out to be such a difficult task, then how much more so is restoring neurons and neural function in the CNS?

14.6   Restoring CNS Function: What Is the Bottom Line?

The bottom line is that in order to restore function in a damaged CNS in Parkinson's disease, ALS, or Alzheimer's disease, some experimental/therapeutic conditions are going to have to be met. These include providing new cells, from whatever source, that display the correct complement of receptors and other surface molecules in order to correctly integrate and form functional connections in existing adult neural circuits. Notably, fetal or stem cells placed into an adult nervous system do not fit these categories without considerable modification of the microenvironment in which they are placed. Indeed, newer perspectives on cell doctrine suggest that without the control of both the replacement cells and the cellular microenvironment, success will not be likely and the possible side effects will not be trivial.

14.7   Biosemiosis (Part 3) and True Narrative Representations

One of the topics raised in several places in this book so far concerns the still-emerging field of biosemiotics, which deals with the nature of signals and their meanings in biological systems.

As noted, such signaling can occur at many levels in an organism: DNA through RNA to protein production, protein interactions and cascades to make functional cells, cell to cell in and between organs, and ultimately between one organism and another. A key aspect of such signaling was introduced by Oller and others (Gryder et al., 2013; Oller, 2013): the notion of the TNR, as cited previously.

The basic idea is that the sign (or sequence of signs), designated S, is mapped (π) on to an object, O (consisting of some actual material state of affairs in the physical world). The integrity of the relationship, $S \pi O$, is thus key to the functionality of the signal. Any error in S or π will tend to make the whole relation to O less sensible, tending toward a limit of uninterpretable nonsense.

Examples of disrupted outcomes can be found in gene mutations and/or RNA transcriptional errors in diseases such as cancer (Gryder et al., 2013), and it is reasonable to suppose that the same will hold for diseases of the nervous system as well. For example, genetic alterations at the DNA/RNA level will necessarily create nonsense TNRs that fail to correctly signal the type of protein to be synthesized, with subsequent consequences for cell function. Similarly, cells with nonsense TNRs for the signals they should send can only create aberrant signals to the next higher level, and so on.

Two key observations may be derived from these considerations. The first is that the extent to which a TNR is invalid is the extent to which the correct signal simply does not get sent to the next level and therefore the desired function breaks down, if it occurs at all. The second is that invalid signals may not only prevent some process from occurring correctly, but may also induce a pathological response.

I want now to consider two different cases in which invalid TNRs could provide downstream and long-term adverse outcomes. The first is the basis of the field of vaccinology, namely that the immune system can be fooled into launching an effective and long-lasting immune (ideally adaptive immune) signal on the basis of partial and/or incorrect information. (In the following, I will leave out the obvious social and other caveats, never mind benefits, of vaccine policy, as these are beyond the scope of the current argument.) The partial signal of a vaccine is typically contributed by a fragment of the disease pathogen, either viral or bacterial. The overtly false signal is also contributed to by adjuvants, particularly those containing aluminum. Since, as already documented, aluminum does not appear to have any biological role in *any* biota on earth, it cannot provide a valid TNR regardless of the apparent ability to provide a generalized activation to the immune system. This negative outcome is not aided by the partial signal provided by the antigenic fragment.

Given all of this, such an invalid TNR is unlikely to provide a correct long-term signal to the target system. Indeed, it appears that this is precisely the case in which vaccines using aluminum adjuvants tend to have limited or no ability to induce long-term adaptive immunity. The second consideration now applies: not only might the nonsense or semi-nonsense signal fail to give the response desired, but the cumulative weight of repeated nonsense signals may trigger adverse outcomes, for example in the nervous system with autoimmune reactions such as the ASIA syndrome (see Chapter 11). The larger the number of degraded signals produced, the greater the confusion in the immune system. As the latter increases, the possibility that something akin to an abnormal response will occur also increases. Given that the immune and nervous systems are intimately connected, as previously discussed, the potential for harm to the nervous system must inevitably increase. ASIA, as expressed in both the CNS and other systems, is thus perhaps not a random event, but rather a direct consequence of incorrect TNRs that may be time-, dose-, and frequency-dependent.

These relationships are depicted in graphical form in Figure 14.4, in which the y-axis plots a theoretical TNR from 0 to 100% (left axis) against the number of "nonsense" signals on the x-axis. Although the precise form of the relationship is not known, it is drawn here as a sigmoidal function. On the right side of the graph, the y-axis plots the induced pathological response that arises due to increasing level of false signals.

The second example involves hoped-for neurological disease therapeutics based on the use of stem cells or various forms of transplantation into a damaged nervous system. The current neurological disease literature is replete with attempts to restore neuronal function in various CNS disorders in this manner, but it may be worth considering,

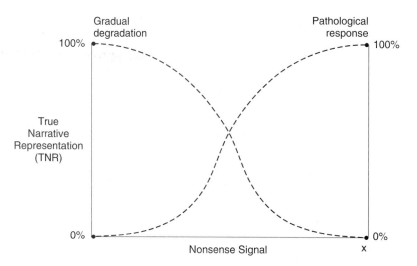

Figure 14.4 TNRs, dysfunction, and adverse outcomes.

based on biosemiotic principles, just what the outcomes are likely to be. Thus, while a stem cell can be made to differentiate under various conditions into any other form of mature cell, the conditions in the developing versus the adult nervous system differ wildly. Expecting that a stem cell will differentiate in all ways correctly in a damaged adult CNS would seem the perfect example of a false TNR in that while the signal may be there, the valid mapping conditions are not. Hence, the outcome is not likely to be correct. Further, as in the example of vaccines, failed TNRs of stem cells placed into an adult system may create conditions not for repair, but for further pathology. One Parkinson's disease funding organization has suggested such an outcome, and these concerns have been mirrored by more recent published literature (Luo et al., 2009; Ertelt et al., 2012).

These are only two of the many examples that can be contemplated. If correct, such considerations may set an upper limit on just how far some potential treatments can go before damaged messages becomes ineffective altogether.

What all of this indicates for future therapeutics is that attempts to fool the CNS with invalid TNRs may ultimately all be destined to fail. Indeed, the invalid TNRs may very well generate negative outcomes. If this is true, research in this area is a waste of precious funds that might be spent on prophylaxis or palliative care.

The development of a rational, rather than a sentimental, neurological disease policy that is effective in dealing with the realities of these diseases and the potential limits of some therapeutic approaches would seem warranted. Much of this argument will be described in greater detail in the next two chapters.

15

Defining the Limits for Neurological Disease Treatments

"God grant me the serenity to accept the things I cannot change; courage to change the things I can; and wisdom to know the difference."
Attributed to both St. Francis of Assisi and Reinhold Niebuhr[1]

From the Preface

12) Each of the sporadic/gene-susceptibility age-dependent neurological diseases represents not one entity but a spectrum of related disease states. Each case is therefore individual. Against such individual (and thus, unique) presentations, there can never be a generalized treatment. This applies particularly if treatment options are begun post-diagnosis. Effective treatments for neurological diseases, if they occur at all, can arise only from prophylaxis or the next-best option of extremely early-phase detection followed by strategic, targeted therapy. The only way to get to this stage is for governments and other entities to commit significant funds to providing a new perspective on such diseases. Essentially, this is a policy discussion, in which social priorities need to be carefully examined. Policy considerations are not the traditional role of scientists, but without the input of those doing the research, a policy re-evaluation will almost certainly not happen. Whether it does or does not is a choice. Needless to say, choices have consequences.

15.1 Introduction

It is important to acknowledge two issues before launching into the final chapters. The first will be apparent from the discussion in Chapter 8 about the limits to knowledge that can be derived from either observations of the neurological diseases themselves or the studies used to model them. These concerns apply to actually understanding the diseases in question, not to mention trying to successfully treat them.

The innate paradox here is the following: My conclusions in this book are drawn from data that may not, as per the critiques cited in Chapter 8, be correct, or at least correct in all respects. This problem has a solution, albeit a laborious one, in which converging lines of evidence from the scientific literature for the various conclusions are used. Space

Neural Dynamics of Neurological Disease, First Edition. Christopher A. Shaw.
© 2017 John Wiley & Sons, Inc. Published 2017 by John Wiley & Sons, Inc.

limitations prevent me from citing all of the relevant literature, both that which supports my perspective and that which opposes it. Nevertheless, readers need to be aware that this limitation exists and that it applies generally to the field as a whole, as well as to this book more specifically.

The second caveat is that in a lot of that which follows, I will make the claim that neurological disease treatments are destined, for the most part, to fail. However, declarations that something will never work or cannot be done, in general, are notoriously problematic and unreliable, as demonstrated repeatedly throughout history. In a variety of cases, the seemingly impossible has been decisively accomplished a short time later. This could occur here as well with future treatments for neurological diseases. Indeed, it is hard not to hope that such comes to pass.

15.2 The Complexity of the Human CNS versus One View of the Philosophy of Science

The preceding pages have tried to make the case that the nervous system of humans is a complex entity that is not well understood, not only in health, but perhaps especially in disease.

Consciousness itself is one of the key areas of normal human brain function, and the one that largely defines humans (Crick and Koch, 2003; Koch, 2012; Oizumi et al., 2014). It is also, in part, one of the fundamental aspects that are compromised by the age-related neurological diseases. In this context, a related issue from philosophy and conceptualizations about consciousness is whether a complex system that has consciousness can completely understand itself, or if only a higher-order consciousness can understand a lesser one. The view that the latter position is correct might be considered to fit within what some would term a "mysterianism" perspective (Nature Neuroscience Editorial, 2000). This perspective fits comfortably within the neurosciences of the present: the field still does not really completely understand simpler neural systems at all in their emergent behaviors, not even the very simplest ones. Such does not bode well for humans ever understanding their own higher brain functions, at least by using such brains alone.

It is certainly true to say that neuroscience has a lot to learn about how the human nervous system develops, how it changes developmentally and over a lifespan, and how it breaks down. In the context of the latter, would knowing how a nervous system breaks down allow clinicians to repair it to some semblance of normal, pre-disease-state function? And, depending on the level of damage, would making the system fully functional again give back the same, or a new, individual?

Since consciousness in one sense is very much tied to identity, the answer to the latter would seem to be "no." Taking an omelet and then reconstituting the DNA to get a new chicken would be an enormous technical challenge, but it is theoretically feasible. Replacing multiple neural circuits in a damaged human brain and expecting to get back the same individual is not.

Some of these conclusions, and those that follow, contradict a widespread view held by many scientists and lay persons alike that, "Given enough time, science can solve any problem." This viewpoint would appear to be more a statement of an almost religious nature than one derived from any particular body of evidence. And, the caveat of "given enough time" makes this hypothesis impossible to test and therefore falsify. The inability to falsify any hypothesis puts it into a realm outside that of the scientific method.

There are, of course, various examples of things that medical science has done remarkably well. In the developed countries, the general control of infectious diseases and changes in maternal childbirth mortality are but two examples.

From more of an engineering perspective, the now relatively widespread and largely successful use of *in vitro* fertilization (IVF) techniques is another prime example. Much progress has been made in the field of reproductive technology in general, where in recent years individuals infertile for a variety of reasons have been given the opportunity to have children. Leaving aside any bioethical issues, the success rate for various IVF therapies continues to rise, with better techniques available at each stage of the process.

The steps, as initially designed by Drs. Robert G. Edwards and Patrick Steptoe, who shared the Nobel Prize in 2010, are as follows: First, hormone therapies are used to stimulate the growth of ova in the follicles of the ovaries. Next, the ova are surgically removed and fertilized *in vitro* with partner or donor sperm. After 3–5 days of growth, an embryo is transplanted into the uterus. Extra embryos not needed at the time of the procedure can be crytoprotected for future use. Hormone therapy is then continued until the embryonic placenta begins to produce the hormones necessary to maintain the pregnancy.

The success rate for a live birth of the cumulative IVF procedures is highly dependent on the age of the mother and on the expertise of the IVF clinic, but can exceed 70%.

It should be noted that IVF is quite costly in many countries, and thus is a privilege largely reserved at present for the affluent few. Much the same financial consideration will apply to some of the proposed neurological disease therapies to be discussed in this chapter.

I have used the example of IVF as a prelude to a consideration of what neurological disease treatments would actually look like at different stages of the diseases in question. First, it should be noted that IVF has always been theoretically possible given the emergence of the appropriate technologies, and thus was essentially a question of applying these technologies as they become available. Neurological disease-state repairs pose very different problems, as I will show.

Before we consider these, however, I need to reiterate what is a key theme of this book: the likely individual nature of each case of neurological disease.

15.3 Examples of Unique Individuality: From Pilgrimages to Nature

The following may seem out of place in the context of a scientific assessment of neurological diseases, but I hope that readers will bear with me.

As cited in the Preface, in May and June of 2014, while this book was in progress, I walked the Camino Frances route of the Camino de Santiago with my wife and infant son. (In English, the translation is "The way of St. James.") This particular route begins in St. Jean Pied de Port, a small and very charming village in the French Basque region that abuts the foothills of the Pyrenees. It goes up and over the mountains into Spain, continues through the Spanish Basque region of Navarra and onward to the west through a number of other regions, before finally arriving some 800 km later in the Galacian city of Santiago de Compostella.

The Camino has been a major pilgrimage route for well over 1000 years, and although much has changed politically and socially in the countries it runs through, a large amount of the route itself remains relatively unchanged, at least in terms of the actual

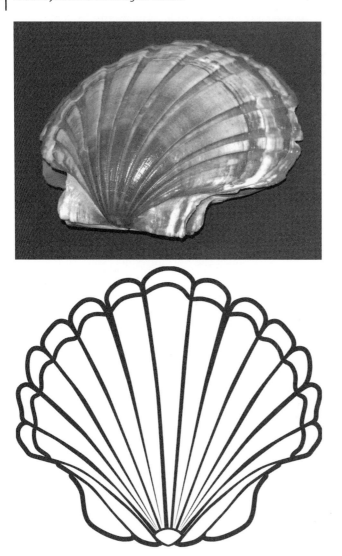

Figure 15.1 The scallop shell, the iconic symbol of the Camino de Santiago, carried by all peregrinos. (a) A real scallop shell. (b) A drawing of a similar shell.

locations. In some cases, former dirt tracks are now major roads, but the general geography is still more or less the same. Notably, the Camino Frances is only one of easily a dozen routes to Santiago, most of which begin in France, Spain, or Portugal. Others start further away, but later merge with one of those in Spain.

One explanation for the widely accepted symbol of the Camino, the scallop shell, is that the various ribs leading to the apex of the shell serve as a metaphor for the numerous paths to Santiago, the common spiritual and physical destination (Figure 15.1).

The male and female pilgrims ("peregrinos" in Spanish) of various ages who walk or bike the Camino come from a variety of countries, speak myriad languages, have wildly differing levels of physical fitness, vary in health status, may have past or current injuries, and so on. Some try to do the trek in 33 days or fewer. Others take much longer. Not all are actually on pilgrimage, although many are. Some walk the Camino for adventure or companionship, as a challenge, or even just for the exercise. The motive itself becomes one more variable in the individuality of the journey.

In addition to the personal factors of the peregrinos, weather, season, the state of the route, and a host of other constantly changing variables determine the path that they will take, and indeed determine whether they will finish at all.

From all of this, it rapidly becomes apparent that no two Caminos are ever the same, even if walked by the same person at different times. Thus, every individual very much "walks their own Camino." Why this is a relevant metaphor for neurological disease will, I hope, become clearer in the discussion that follows.

What should also have become apparent in the previous chapters are the following features of neurological diseases, at least those that are largely sporadic and age-related: First, in spite of considerable efforts, identifying causal etiological factors has proven remarkably difficult to do with any certainty. For example, the massive database search by Krewski (2014a,b), prepared for the NHCC/Public Health Agency of Canada, could, at best, rather vaguely hint at some environmental risk factors of Parkinson's disease, ALS, and Alzheimer's disease. It could neither establish with any certainty that these risk factors were actually involved, nor assign the proportion of those afflicted with any particular disease to any particular factor. Further, the study said nothing about synergistic interactions of various toxins (e.g., pesticides and aluminum), nor about toxin interactions with various susceptibility genes.

While there are individual cases in which some environmental factor may be causal, there is rarely certainty. High pesticide exposure on one farm might conceivably generate a parkinsonism in one member of a family, but it rarely does so in all members, who typically differ in age, sex, cumulative medical histories, comorbidities, and so on. Even on Guam at the height of the ALS-PDC epidemic, individual family pedigrees showed some members with PDC, some with ALS, some with both, and some with no neurological disease manifestation at all.

Similarly, the domoic acid poisoning in Eastern Canada did not uniformly affect those exposed to the toxin. Individual genetic polymorphisms such as those discussed in Chapter 12 and those relating to drug metabolism (Nebert et al., 1996), age, sex, and so on all affected susceptibility.

The reality is that apart from the clear examples of neurological disease clusters described in Chapter 3, there are no disease hotspots to be found anywhere else that can provide strong epidemiological evidence for particular toxins or toxin synergies. Conceivably, this could change in the face of some massive environmental toxin exposure, such as the dump of aluminum sulfate into the water supply in Camelford, England in 1988. However, even in that case, individual outcomes varied considerably and investigators struggled to provide anything beyond a plausible correlation with aluminum exposure to any of the cases of Alzheimer's that later occurred (Exley and Esiri, 2006). And, as noted, Guamanian ALS-PDC, once thought to be a clear example of a "geographical isolate" and a metaphorical Rosetta Stone for neurological disease, is hardly uniform in its presentation.

The lack of disease hotspots generally likely means that no toxic factor, alone or in synergy, is sufficiently concentrated to drive a significant number of people into a neurological disease state. This statement is qualified, however, since future Minimata Bay and domoic acid-type events are always possible, perhaps even likely, in an increasingly polluted world.

Second, even for the still relatively modest fraction of the age-related neurological diseases that have clear genetic etiologies, the presentation is not uniform in age of onset or progression. This is even true in Huntington's disease where the genetic component is well understood and affects only males. In animal models of all of these diseases, including Huntington's, the onset and progression of neural and behavioral deficits show considerable variations as well (see van Dellen et al., 2000 for an example from an *in vivo* model).

It might be that if researchers knew all of the potential toxins and all of the potential interactions with a range of susceptibility genes for each individual, they would be able to predict the likelihood of that individual developing the disease at some future date. However, this is not known for all the toxins in any locale, let alone the concentrations of these molecules. Nor do researchers know the vast range of potential interactions between toxins, and they have no idea at all about the even larger number of gene–toxin interactions that could conceivably arise. Finding these things out might be experimentally possible given sufficient financial resources and time, but it is quite unlikely to be achieved in any practical sense, for reasons to be discussed later.

None of this even touches upon the problem of individual microbiomes, which not only are highly individualistic, but have the capacity to influence CNS function and behavior (Hsiao et al., 2013; Sun and Chang, 2014). This field is rapidly evolving, and it seems increasingly likely that it will play a major role in the susceptibility of individuals to a range of factors. It might even contribute to some people developing one or more of the neurological diseases. The individual microbiome, like one's genome, is very much part and parcel of the haecceity of every human being.

A third issue is that the sporadic diseases are not uniform entities, but rather represent spectrums of disease. It is now widely recognized that Parkinson's disease and ALS are such spectrums, with individual manifestations showing some similarities in general type of end-state neurological damage, but not in presentation or rate of progression. Alzheimer's disease is almost certainly also a spectrum disorder, particularly when considered as one of the dementias.

A fourth key issue concerns the mechanisms of neural damage that lead to disease end state. As previous chapters have demonstrated, abundant evidence exists for a great variety of such events, including (but not limited to) oxidant stress, mitochondrial dysfunction, excitotoxicity, transcriptional errors, misfolded proteins, disrupted proteasome function, alterations in neuronal–glial interactions, and a host of others. Do they all occur in each case? Do they follow a particular time line, such that one leads to another in a cascade of events culminating in the end-state condition, or do these time lines vary? No one knows, and likely we cannot know from model systems. It is a safe bet that variations are considerable from individual to individual, but all cases still arrive at a final destination of neuronal loss and functional decline.

All of this, if correct, seems to lead to a somewhat unpalatable conclusion, at least for some researchers: Just as with journeys on the Camino, no two neurological disease manifestations, even in the "same" disease, are really fully the same. Thus, all cases of ALS do not arise, progress, and manifest in an identical manner. A similar conclusion applies to Parkinson's disease and Alzheimer's disease, as well. In other words, all humans walk their own Caminos of neurological health and sickness.

It may be worthwhile to consider this notion in relation to a species much simpler than humans: the oyster.

One thing that is not generally known amongst those not involved in oyster cultivation or the restaurant industry is that most commercial oysters in North America derive

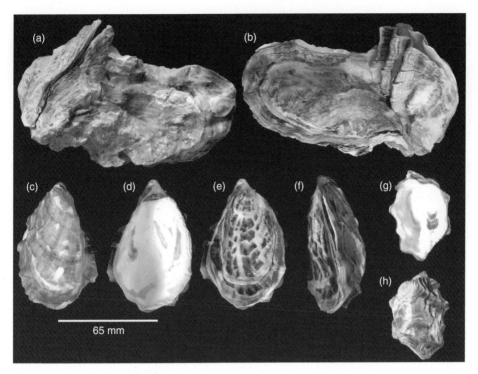

Figure 15.2 Morphological differences in varieties of oysters of the same species (*Crassostrea gigas*) in eastern North America. *Source*: Used with permission from Simon Grove (molluscsoftasmania.net).

from just three species. On the East Coast, there is the indigenous *Crassostrea virginica*. On the West Coast, there are transplanted *C. virginica*, the native *Ostrea lurida*, and the imported Pacific oyster, *Crassostrea gigas*. In spite of there being only one species on the Eastern Seaboard, the range of morphological and other characteristics found in *C. virginica* is huge. Similar morphological variations occur for all three species on the Pacific coast. In each case, the same species of oyster can vary considerably in size, texture, flavor, and so on, and these variations are determined by a range of factors, including local climate, water temperature, salinity, turbidity, currents, and a host of others (Brown and Hartwick, 1988; Miossec et al., 2009) (Figure 15.2).

If such variations hold for several species of oysters, then how could they not for a genetically more diverse population, such as humans, exposed to an even greater number of environmental factors?

The individual paths that any person follows from neurological health to disease depend on all of the factors considered in this section, including known and unknown toxin exposures over a lifetime, genetic susceptibilities, age, sex, comorbidities, stress, and so on.

While the incidences of the age-related neurological disorders appear to be increasing, there is no simple, or currently even feasible, means of determining whether any particular individual is going to fall victim to any of them. All that one can say with any certainty is that with increasing incidence comes a greater likelihood of developing one or more of them. Notably, this is a population prediction, not an individual one.

15.4   Therapeutic Windows for the Treatment of Neurological Diseases

The implications of the considerations raised in the previous section, in terms of prevention, early detection, and treatment, are likely to be far-reaching. First, unlike with infectious disease, the myriad causes of neurological disease cannot be prevented for all individuals. Nor can these factors be predicted with any certainty. Second, given the likely individual presentation of each disease, no general therapeutic is likely to work as a prophylactic measure in all cases. Third, post-clinical-diagnosis treatments will invariably fail. In this section, I will address each of these implications in turn.

15.4.1   Prevention

Prevention, of course, depends on knowing what to prevent, as per the Oller quote that opens Chapter 13. There are some very likely candidates for this list in the case of neurological disease: agricultural chemicals of various types, bioavailable aluminum and various heavy metals, endocrine-disrupting molecules, and various plastic-derived molecules, such as bisphenols, all derived from human activity; and toxic steryl glucosides and other toxins from nature. However, as already discussed, none of these can be the sole cause, and it would be remarkably difficult to assign even a percentage of those affected by neurological disease to any of these putative toxins. Further, needless to say, it would be both a social and a financial challenge to eliminate any of the molecules of human origin, although some would be easier to dispose of than others. For example, removing bioavailable aluminum from food products and vaccines would almost certainly help, but how much it would do so at a population level could not be known for years or decades, and in the absence of strong epidemiological data demonstrating a direct causal link, there would inevitably be extensive pushback from the aluminum industry, processed-food and pharmaceutical companies, and others.

15.4.2   Pre-clinical Treatment

Very early in the neurological disease time line, there may be windows in which halting the beginning of neural death cascades would stop the disease from progressing further (Figure 15.3), as there is in polio (Chapter 14).

A complication with early-phase treatment is how to identify the stage and underlying mechanisms of dysfunction. If every case is individual, then there will be some crucial step in which the cascading failure is beyond recovery. What that point of no return may be is not known, nor is it even definitively known if there is such a point. The crucial disease time points before this would have to be identified for each person before the onset of clinical markers of disease. It might be possible to do so with various biomarkers, ideally those found peripherally. For example, given that other organ systems are involved in all neurological diseases, it is possible to imagine that detecting early skin changes, for example in fibroblasts and keratocytes, would serve to identify pre-clinical ALS (Paré et al., 2015), while detecting early abnormalities in olfaction would have the same effect in Parkinson's and Alzheimer's diseases (Doty, 2012; Velayudhan, 2015). Indeed, the search for just such biomarkers is a subject of investigation in various laboratories and companies (see Shaw et al., 2007 for the former).

Alternatively, a general regime of treatment with molecules considered beneficial could be applied to everyone from early in life. For example, antioxidant molecules

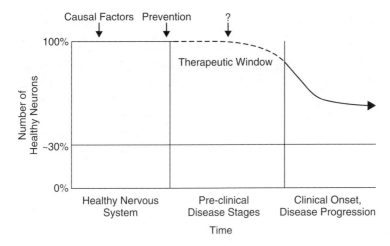

Figure 15.3 Schematic of the time line and therapeutic windows in neurological diseases.

could serve to combat free radicals, protective steryls could be used to block harmful ones, and so on. Various other considerations of the pre-clinical disease application of so-called "natural molecules" include the twin notions that prophylaxis is always going to be more successful than late-stage treatment and that various such molecules are less likely to have unexpected and deleterious side effects on the CNS or other organ systems (Amtul and Rahman, 2015). The application of ginsenosides in the *in vivo* model of Parkinson's disease presented by Van Kampen et al. (2014a) is at least as successful as any of the more recent pharmacological treatments and follows from a long, and often successful, history of treatments in humans in more of the so-called "traditional" pharmacologies. Much the same general strategy exists to diminish the population level of cardiovascular disease, so the idea has general merit.

15.4.3 Early-stage, Post-clinical Diagnosis and Treatment

Much of the discussion about prospects for treatment will necessarily hinge on what is meant by the term "cure." Although there is a very clear medical definition to be found in various dictionaries (e.g., the OED defines it as being to "relieve (a person or animal) of the symptoms of a disease or condition"), the reality is that there is no complete agreement even amongst medical practitioners on what a cure actually entails. If the aim in neurological disease is to restore the patient to a pre-morbid condition, before the loss of any neurons, altered neuronal–glial interactions, behavioral effects, and so on, then a cure is extremely unlikely. For one thing, the disease process(es) would have to be stopped completely, so that they could do no further damage. This would necessarily include halting secondary damage from cascading events. In the absence of knowledge about causal factors and the exact temporal phase and dimension of the cell-death cascades, this would become quite difficult, although perhaps not impossible. In cases where the exact causal factor could be identified and eliminated (e.g., with aluminum toxicity), one might have some hope of preventing some measure of future damage. Next, there would need to be some way to replace lost neurons and circuits, or at least reconnect circuits with surviving neurons. This, too, is not possible at present, and perhaps it never will be, given the very real theoretical constraints imposed by signaling theory, as cited in previous chapters, and as discussed further in the next subsection.

In regard to this latter point, it may be instructive to return to the differences between ALS and poliomyelitis. As discussed in Chapter 14, the damage inflicted by polio on motor neurons is limited by the immune response which stops the spread of the infection. It may be for this reason that polio is not typically bilateral in presentation, and thus spares many motor neurons. With polio, this is as close to a "cure" as is possible.

If ALS were also the result of some infectious process then the same might apply, in that stopping the pathological agent in some fashion might lead to the same sort of eventual partial recovery. If this were the case, however, then Koch's postulates could well apply and the identification of the infectious agent could lead to the means of preventing or stopping ALS's spread (e.g., by repairing and correctly activating immune function, rather than triggering autoimmunity, or by employing various antiviral or antibacterial treatments against identified pathogens). Once it was halted, as with polio, the surviving motor neurons might be able to reinnervate the muscles. It should be clear that the patient would not be returned to the pre-morbid state, but at least they would not get worse. For many – patients and physicians both – that would indeed be a cure.

While this would actually be a best-case scenario from a treatment perspective, the evidence for most cases of conventional ALS arising from an infectious disease etiology is not particularly persuasive. Even if such an etiology turns out to be correct for some fraction of ALS patients, the likelihood that all ALS arises in this fashion seems especially low.

Many of the general and specific considerations raised here also apply to Parkinson's disease. Given the propensity of nigral cells to sprout and reinnervate the striatum, halting the underlying causal agent and the progressive loss of neurons in the SN (which also usually begins unilaterally) might offer some hope that a partial recovery of function could be possible. As with ALS, there are proponents of an infectious disease etiology for Parkinson's disease (Chapter 11). Also as with ALS, however, the evidence is not generally compelling, and even if an infectious disease etiology could account for some fraction of sporadic disease, it would be highly unlikely to hold for all cases.

15.4.4   Post-clinical Treatment and its Caveats

Where the situation becomes most difficult, and indeed basically intractable, is with established neurological disease post clinical diagnosis. The notion of a cure, however defined, at this time point becomes increasingly difficult to imagine. At this stage, the affected part of the nervous system is undergoing a cascading failure. So many aspects of neuronal integrity and interaction are dysfunctional or dead, and so many crucial biochemical pathways have been disrupted, that the prospect that any drug, combination of drugs, or other treatment could address the myriad processes affected is hardly realistic.

This is a difficult thing for many in the medical community to accept as it seems to fly in the face of the philosophy-of-science viewpoint presented in Section 15.2. This view – that science can, given time, solve any problem – finds an intellectual niche in medicine with the corollary view that medicine will eventually find ways to treat all ailments, including all those of the nervous system.

I need to acknowledge that much of the following will face considerable criticism from various quarters, and this is perfectly understandable. For one thing, the current scientific/medical culture firmly holds that all questions are answerable, all problems solvable, and all medical conditions treatable given sufficient time and resources. A full critique of the philosophical underpinning to this view (not to mention the arguments against it) is outside the framework of this book.

In brief, however, those who hold the more "positive" view are well positioned within an established world perspective that holds that such beliefs have served humans well over the millennia, in that they are not only frequently correct, but also hopeful to the trajectory of the human endeavor.

A recent example of this sort of thinking comes from a decision by ALS Canada to shift much of its research program away from basic research toward translational studies. This was a somewhat unusual decision, given that ALS researchers still do not have many clues about its etiology, except amongst that small percentage of cases that have the gene-linked familial forms. Thus, almost without a doubt, a translational approach at this stage is doomed in advance to failure. Indeed, the last half-dozen clinical trials of various compounds have routinely failed to provide any benefit for ALS patients whatsoever (Mitsumoto et al., 2014). However, while this outcome is tragic for patients and their families, it is hardly unexpected.

Late-stage treatment is also likely to run into the limits set by theory. As discussed in various parts of this book, biosemiosis shows that incorrect signals cannot be used effectively, at least in the long term. Thus, stem cells put into an adult CNS are unlikely ever to connect correctly or, therefore, to function properly. In fact, as in Parkinson's disease, such an application may actually make the patient worse off (Piccini et al., 2005). The problem here is not that stem cells cannot be made to differentiate into the types of cell desired for treatment, but rather that any new cells will not really know what to do in the context in which they are placed. This is because the entire process of neuronal development is normally tightly scripted, both temporally and in terms of the myriad interactions with other types of cell (neurons and glia): a newly differentiated SN cell might be fine when placed into a developing CNS, where the clues are relevant, but it is going to end up without context in an adult nervous system. The problem is not solely that the signals sent and received by the new neurons are partial and likely even incorrect; rather, it is that the incorrect signals will at some point induce further inappropriate signals, which might induce more damage than benefit.

Of course, this speculation, based on concepts intrinsic to biosemiosis, may simply be wrong, or may not correctly represent the growing body of work in this field. However, the extent to which it is correct would seem to put quite strict – although not yet defined – limits on interventions such as those discussed in this chapter.

The dominant philosophical perspective has given rise to the hunt for genes and molecules, ideally few in number, that are the causal factors for neurological diseases. In essence, it reflects a kind of search for a neurological "Holy Grail" that is simple and pure: one gene and one toxin, and maybe some few interactions between the two. Once in hand, the eventual discovery will allow all sorts of medical miracles to emerge. Could this happen? Indeed it could. The history of science shows that it could. Is it ardently wished for by most? Yes, again, and I would be one such person: there could indeed be a dominant gene involved in even the sporadic forms of Parkinson's disease, ALS, and Alzheimer's disease; there could even be a few dominant toxins, or even a universal toxin. Is either of these possibilities likely, given the last few decades of neurological disease research and the material cited so far in this book? The answer is no, for all of the reasons given previously.

It is, however, undeniably true that many things once considered to be totally impossible to science or engineering have come to pass, often rapidly enough to embarrass those who doubted them.

None of this is to say that there are no possible solutions to the problems in neurological disease prevention, detection, treatment, or the various interrelated issues discussed in this chapter; rather, it is to point out that such solutions would have to address myriad other problems of various levels of complexity. These problems arise due to the lack of concrete etiologies for neurological diseases, the great likelihood of there being too many etiologies, as per the Camino example, and the seemingly intractable problems associated with trying to repair any part of an adult CNS at some stage of cascading failure.

Maybe the actual problem is less the need to find a neurological disease etiological Holy Grail, and more a question of having a clear understanding of what it is likely to contain, if it can be found.

Inevitably, the issue comes back to the notion of prophylaxis, as has worked relatively well for infectious diseases. Koch's postulates, often but not always valid, nevertheless lead to the notion that some pathogenic entity is causal to a particular disease state.

In brief, these postulates have four main clauses: First, the presumed infectious microorganism has to be found in high levels in those with the disease, and not in those without it. Second, the microorganism has to be isolatable from those who suffer from the disease. Third, the microorganism, when given to healthy subjects, should induce the disease. Fourth, the microorganism, when isolated from the secondarily infected host, should display the same identity as the original. Removing the source of the pathogen (sanitation, clean water, vaccination at a population level; Morrice et al., Scheduled 2017) and providing better nutrition have certainly changed the infectious disease incidence for a great variety of diseases, at least in developed countries. However, Koch's postulates do not apply to neurological diseases, however, or at least not to those sporadic ones for which the field has no clear causal factors.

Thus, it would be wise to stop hoping for single toxic molecules. However, a more general notion of prophylaxis could be employed, one that has already found considerable success in one area of modern health care: this is none other than the remarkable prophylaxis offered by modern dentistry. This subject will be explored in the next chapter.

Endnotes

1 St. Francis of Assisi, born Giovanni di Pietro di Bernardone (1181–1226), was an Italian Catholic friar and preacher. Karl Paul Reinhold Niebuhr (1892–1971) was an American theologian and ethicist.

16

The Politics and Economics of Neurological Disease

> *Each of us touches one place*
> *and understands the whole in that way.*
> *The palm and fingers feeling in the dark are*
> *how the senses explore the reality of the elephant.*
> *If each of us held a candle there,*
> *and if we went in together,*
> *we could see it.*
>
> Jalal ad-Din Rumi[1]

> *"Today you are You, that is truer than true. There is no one alive who is Youer than You."*
>
> Dr. Seuss[2]

From the Preface

12) Each of the sporadic/gene-susceptibility age-dependent neurological diseases represents not one entity but a spectrum of related disease states. Each case is therefore individual. Against such individual (and thus, unique) presentations, there can never be a generalized treatment. This applies particularly if treatment options are begun post-diagnosis. Effective treatments for neurological diseases, if they occur at all, can arise only from prophylaxis or the next-best option of extremely early-phase detection followed by strategic, targeted therapy. The only way to get to this stage is for governments and other entities to commit significant funds to providing a new perspective on such diseases. Essentially, this is a policy discussion, in which social priorities need to be carefully examined. Policy considerations are not the traditional role of scientists, but without the input of those doing the research, a policy re-evaluation will almost certainly not happen. Whether it does or does not is a choice. Needless to say, choices have consequences.

16.1 Introduction

In these last few pages, I hope to summarize where I think the field of neurological disease research is at present, what its current trajectory seems to be, and where instead it

Neural Dynamics of Neurological Disease, First Edition. Christopher A. Shaw.
© 2017 John Wiley & Sons, Inc. Published 2017 by John Wiley & Sons, Inc.

should be going. Much of that which follows is obviously going to be purely my opinion, my speculation, and, for some, my belief in the somewhat awkward notion that the choices faced are essentially political in nature.

16.2 The Problems with Single-Hit Models of Neurological Disease

A key problem in the search for neurological disease etiologies is that many scientists in the field approach the subject as if there is likely to be only one gene or one toxin responsible. In many ways, it is a zero-sum game, as one investigator's gene or toxin has to negate those of other researchers. Of course, such attitudes are not unique to the neurological disease research field.

Sometimes those inclined to this view are willing to admit a few other genes or molecules into the mix, but notably these are also considered to work in isolation. For example, from the "mutant genes cause ALS" perspective, variant (mSOD1), as cited in Chapter 5 and elsewhere, account for a fraction of all fALS (and a lower fraction of all ALS), but these mutations can exist quite happily alongside more newly discovered mutations, such as those for *C9orf72* and *FUS*, as long as the overall claims for other causal agents are not too extensive. Or, in other words, the fewer the causal factors the better, and genetic mutations and environmental toxins cannot both be found to be involved. The same mentality applies to many of those inhabiting the much less populous side of the research spectrum in which some toxic factor is considered to be key to disease origins.

To some extent, all of those trying to unlock the risk factors/etiologies for neurological diseases fall victim to this way of thinking. Indeed, it is far easier and more appealing than dealing with multiple, interacting factors. And, of course, it is vastly more fundable than the very complex experiments that would need to be done – if they were feasible at all – to examine toxin–toxin, gene–gene, or gene–toxin interactions.

In some ways, it is as if many neuroscientists are preconditioned by Koch's postulates on infectious disease; that is, that for each such disease there is one identifiable infectious agent – or, in this case, genetic or toxin equivalent – that is solely responsible. It remains of some historical interest that many of Koch's postulates have been shown to be incorrect or only partially true, but the perspective they promoted still seems to hold sway in the search for any neurological disease etiology.

What one might term the "Koch-postulate mentality" infects (pun maybe intended) neurological disease research to a remarkable degree, and perhaps nowhere is the problem more acute than in the ALS-PDC domain and in some of the expansions of this to the more conventional forms of Parkinson's disease, ALS, and Alzheimer's disease. Further, in no case is the problem more specifically problematic than when considering the variations of what is sometimes termed the "BMAA hypothesis." Indeed, were one to substitute the term "BMAA" for "microorganism," one would have an almost classical case of Koch postulate-like thinking at work.

As detailed in Chapter 7, the BMAA component of the ALS-PDC story has had an unusual pedigree even by the somewhat lax standards by which Koch-like postulates are applied to ALS-PDC and other neurological diseases. For one thing, the original observations that BMAA could induce neurodegeneration in a primate model of the disorder were neither consistent nor reproducible, nor did they even really generate a model that resembled the human disease either in neurological signs or in CNS pathologies.

The most recent iteration of the BMAA hypothesis, as introduced in Chapter 7, began with a fairly blatant misplotting of ecological field data to make the claim that the declining ALS-PDC disease timeline in the 20th century followed the decline of the fruit bat population on Guam (Cox and Sacks, 2002). In this instance, the purported association was assumed, rather than actual, but it was reported as the latter. These early papers by this particular group were promoted rather ostentatiously through the media – an unusual, but not necessarily unique approach.

As the fruit bat connection to the disorder began to seem less tenable, the story migrated away from BMAA in fruit bats to BMAA in cyanobacteria, the latter allegedly growing in the roots of the cycad as the obligate source of the molecule. However, cycads, at least those on Guam, are perfectly capable of generating BMAA without the need for the bacteria (Marler et al., 2010), which is not surprising given that BMAA is a fairly common plant-signaling molecule. This observation did not matter for those pursuing the hypothesis, since it had already migrated again.

In the most recent version of the hypothesis, BMAA is reported to be found anywhere that cyanobacteria grow; that is, in various waterways, oceans, and lakes (and even where they once may have grown, as in deserts). In lock step, the hypothesis has become ever more complex, in obvious violation of the Law of Parsimony (also termed Occam's Razor), eventually expanding to claim responsibility for the beaching of cetaceans as the latter consume fish laden with *Nostoc*. In regard to potential human victims, cyanobacteria-derived BMAA has been linked to a number of alleged clusters of ALS (Caller et al., 2012; Bradley et al., 2013). That these are not real clusters in the conventional sense ceased in some circles to matter once the notion was picked up by the media, which raised considerable alarm amongst those living next to lakes containing any level of cyanobacteria.

Somewhere in the trajectory of the BMAA story, the target shifted from Parkinson's and Alzheimer's disease, where it had originally been claimed to occur, to ALS. An ALS conference in Sydney, Australia in 2011 held a mini-symposium on ALS and cyanobacteria, which led various other investigators to follow up the notion that BMAA was the source of the disease.

Of course, a potentially valid etiology for any neurological disease does not have to originate in real (versus faux) data, and indeed, as recent publications have shown, BMAA may have some odd role to play as a contributing factor in some forms of neurodegenerative disease (Dunlop et al., 2013). However, many of the existing data consist of remarkably weak experimental outcomes (see de Munck et al., 2013), which suggest that a certain momentum has been achieved out of all proportion to what these data actually show. It is worth noting that the work has now come full circle back to Koch's postulates, in that some investigators are now proposing that ALS arises, in part, from colonization of the human gastrointestinal (GI) tract by cyanobacteria, which then release BMAA. The fact that these data are not yet published makes this claim uncertain at best. It would be vastly more effective and informative to apply instead the Hill criteria (see Chapter 5), by which the BMAA hypothesis would almost surely fail. However, relatively few scientists in the field seem conversant with the application of these criteria, and it appears that those favoring this hypothesis have not considered applying them.

All of this illustrates that a synergy of a number of factors can greatly influence any given field regardless of the quality of the data. Such outcomes will inevitably lead to significant hazards in the search for the true underlying nature of the same. This example also shows just how eager the scientific community is to pursue the view that neurological disease arises from simple versus complex and interactive causal factors. All of this, once again, shows that it is far more appealing for there to be one causal gene or one causal toxin, in keeping with the legacy of Koch's postulates.

The point of all this is that this line of speculation, based on very few actual experimental data, has damaged the search for toxins that might actually be involved in ALS-PDC and related diseases elsewhere. In brief, the more outlandish the claims, the more suspect the entire subject of toxins in ALS-PDC overall has seemed to become for a more general scientific audience. This is not to say that researchers should not follow whatever lines of evidence they think hold the most promise or that such research should not be funded, but rather that doing such studies, and in particular doing them badly, has a consequence for others working in the field.

Somewhat less obviously, Koch-postulate thinking in genetic studies has had much the same effect, even if the actual experiments were performed far more rigorously. For example, Deng et al. (2011) examined some 40 individuals from five families who had some form of ALS and identified a mutation in *UBQLN2*, a gene that codes for an ubiquitin-like protein, ubilquilin2. The mutation is X-linked and dominantly inherited, and its neurological outcomes include both ALS and ALS-dementia of the FTD type. The results implicated proteasome malfunction in these disorders. A follow-up paper using a transgene model expressing the mutation gave primarily hippocampal neuron pathologies, but not those of motor neurons (Gorrie et al., 2014). The authors went on to try to link mutant *C9orf72*-associated ALS and dementia with FTD.

Thus, even studies done well, as in this example, can still have the same cumulative effect on the field as a whole if they serve to reinforce the single-hit mentality.

16.3 Summarizing the Main Themes by Chapter

With the previous section in mind as a form of cautionary principle, it is worth revisiting the key themes developed in the book so far before considering some different approaches to neurological diseases, their origins, and their treatments:

- The nervous system of humans is an exceedingly complex entity. The same is true of the nervous systems of other vertebrate species, but arguably that of humans is the most complex and dynamic that we know about (so far). Although all organ systems in humans and other animals show age-related deterioration, the nervous system is acutely sensitive to such changes since neurons in older humans and animals are not widely regenerated.
- There are a number of neurological diseases in humans, but three of the most devastating are those typically associated with aging: Parkinson's disease, in which neurons in the nigro-striatal system die, leading to increasing movement disorders, but which also shows a cognitive-loss component; ALS, in which there is a loss of motor neurons and a loss of motor function, but which also often shows a cognitive decline; and Alzheimer's disease, in which the loss of neurons in the cortex and hippocampus affects memory and cognition. Alzheimer's and Parkinson's diseases have a relatively high prevalence for neurological diseases, and the overall numbers appear to be larger than in years past, not necessarily solely due to a larger aging population. ALS has a much lower prevalence, but it may be increasing overall.

- The cumulative costs of these diseases alone are daunting for patients, their families, and the medical system as a whole. As prevalence changes, the costs become even more of a societal burden (Alzheimer's Society of Canada, 2010; Hyman, 2012). If incidence is also increasing, the problems are compounded. These latter conclusions have been made in relation to Alzheimer's disease, but apply to the others as well.

- Although each of these diseases appears to be uniquely different from the others, there are considerable levels of similarity between them all. Additionally, each alone is not a simple disease with one set of stereotypic features, but rather seems to reflect a spectrum of disorders. There exist a few clusters of each, suggesting genetically or environmentally determined "hot spots," but such clusters are quite few in number. The lack of more clusters generally suggests that causal factors are relatively ubiquitously distributed, albeit at relatively low levels –too low, at least, to create acute disease manifestations.

- The human nervous system, being highly complex, is highly prone to disruption, which can lead in time to a "cascading failure."

- Early-onset forms of these neurological diseases are typically familial and of genetic origin. Most cases of all three, however, do not have a clearly identified genetic component. Much effort has been devoted to bringing the majority of the sporadic cases of each into a genetics-based framework. This effort has largely not succeeded.

- The study of environmental toxins has shown some correspondence with the identified neurological disease clusters, but, as before, the relative lack of clusters leads to the conclusion that the toxins studied so far are not the active principals in all cases. The interaction of gene–environmental (toxin) factors leading to neurological diseases seems most likely to be the source of most neurological diseases of the types considered here.

- The disappearing neurological spectrum disorder, ALS-PDC of Guam, highlights this last point. ALS-PDC is the main large-scale, definitive neurological disease cluster for ALS, parkinsonism, and Alzheimer's-like dementia. It is a true geographic isolate, as proposed by Kurland. As of this writing, no clear genetic etiologies have been identified, in spite of intensive efforts to do so. Similarly, in spite of considerable work done to isolate toxic influences over almost 60 years, no unambiguously causal toxins have been confirmed.

- ALS-PDC represents a clear example of a unique combination of genes and environment in which neither is dominant, but when both are combined within a particular time window the observed cluster of neurological disease is created. When this combination of factors evolved, the individual disease manifestations began to decline. The same decline occurred with the neurological disease cluster in Irian Jaya.

- Attempts to understand neurological diseases, to identify etiologies, and to design treatment options are inherently limited. Observationally, they are limited by the nature of the disease processes and thus the inability of scientists to peer into pre-clinical disease stages. Experimentally, they are limited by the nature of model systems, whose inadequacies become quite apparent in any real-world application. The apparent inaccuracy of much of the scientific literature in addition the so-called "decline effect" make evaluations of existing data problematic, albeit perhaps not impossible.

- The neurological diseases discussed here are progressive, meaning that they become worse over time. The stages in this progression are not known with any accuracy. Post-clinical timelines tell researchers little or nothing about pre-clinical phases.

Model systems, as already mentioned, cannot be used with any particular accuracy, or at least they have not been so used to date.

- Developmental disorders of the CNS, such as ASD, reflect more a form of pathological plasticity than the overt pathology of adult-onset neurological diseases such as ALS and the others. The latter, however, may have their origins early in life, long before the appearance of adult-onset signs and symptoms.

- The links between the immune and nervous systems in health and disease are pronounced. In particular, the immune system is intimately involved in both neuronal development and CNS disorders (e.g., ASD). The immune system may also become part of the cascade of events driving neuronal loss in neurological diseases through autoimmune reactions.

- Many factors thus influence the origin and progression of neurological diseases. Given the large numbers of potential factors involved, it becomes ever harder to think of these diseases as arising from a single factor, or even from a small set of causal factors. The spectrum nature of each of the diseases suggests that every individual case of any of them is unique, not only in presentation and progression, but also in origins, interactions, and so on. The only thing that such diseases clearly share between them is their end states.

- Treatment outcomes for any of the neurological diseases considered here have, to date, been highly varied. Some Parkinson's disease treatments have demonstrated limited success in controlling some aspects of the disease, primarily movement disorders. These, however, are not "cures" in the conventional medical meaning of the word. No such success has been apparent with any treatment for ALS or Alzheimer's disease.

- Emerging treatment strategies seem to be largely variations on those considered so far. Given the spectrum nature of the diseases, their individual presentations, and the stage at which treatment can be realistically initiated, these strategies are not likely to fare any better than those that have failed previously.

- These considerations set a limit on the prospective treatment options for neurological diseases at an individual level.

This last statement goes against both the current fixation on attempting to cure complex diseases after they have become established and the mentality that each disease can be reduced to some simple collection of genes or toxins, as discussed in Section 16.2. One conclusion that tends to arise from this view is that if the grant-funding agencies and non-governmental organizations (NGOs) provide a lot more money to keep doing the same things that have been done so far, viable treatment options will suddenly come into focus. This conclusion is worth considering in more detail in the next section.

16.4 Can the Amount of Money Spent Change these Outcomes for Neurological Disease Treatment?

The argument that more funding will change disease treatment success is both a "motherhood" statement and, at the same time, an unlikely outcome if the overall direction of the funded research does not change in lock step.

First, as discussed in the previous chapter, the notion of a cure really does not apply to the neurological diseases considered so far. Second, more money spent on animal models or treatment strategies that have already failed is not likely to enable them to work any better in the future. For example, the m*SOD1* model for ALS did not suffer from a lack of funding over the last 20 years; quite arguably, it took in the vast bulk of ALS research dollars. In spite of this, no useful therapeutics arose from this model (see Mitsumoto et al., 2014). Spending 10 or 100 times the amount already spent would not have changed this outcome, although it may be that the eventual conclusion that the model was inadequate might have been appreciated much earlier.

Similarly, the constraints imposed by the inability to detect any of these neurological diseases at onset, dependent as they are on the numbers of those afflicted, would not necessarily be lifted by spending more money. It might be that more funding would have led to a more rapid and complete compilation of etiological factors, and this list might have then helped researchers arrive more quickly at the conclusion that each case is individual. However, in terms of curing the diseases, more funds would not have accelerated the process.

The relatively costly Neurological Health Charities Canada (NHCC) project described in Chapter 2 spent about 25 million taxpayer dollars and came up with remarkably little in terms of clearly identified risk factors for neurological diseases (Public Health Agency of Canada, 2015). In hindsight, this was not due to any lack of dedication amongst the separate organizations that began the project or the directing staff members. Nor was it even due to any shortcomings in the scientific abilities of those who ran the various studies. Rather, the end result – a lack of clearly defined risk factors – simply emphasizes one of the key themes of this book, namely that the neurological diseases in question are spectrum disorders in which each individual's outcomes depends on unique interactions across a lifespan. Here, as elsewhere, more funds would not necessarily have changed this outcome, but the realization might have come about much sooner.

Funding in general remains an endless problem for those involved in neurological disease research, as in other disciplines. National granting agencies in the United States and Canada provide funds for relatively few of the applications that are submitted. More specialized funding entities based on the particular disease have the same problems and face, in addition, a continuing need to balance basic research funding with the need for money for translational research and patient care. And, as cited earlier, the funds that do get allocated for research tend to be given to the same sorts of studies that have already failed to produce tangible results for patients (see, for example, a recent major grant to the Broad Institute, 2014). It is as if doing more of the same, but with more money, as per the recent "Ice Bucket Challenge," will make all the difference.

The Ice Bucket Challenge, to date, has generated nearly $100 million in the United States and a proportionate-to-population amount in Canada. Certainly, for an "orphan" neurological disease such as ALS, this is an amazing windfall, and the enthusiasm within the ALS community, amongst researchers, clinicians, and patients, is palpable and completely understandable.

A somewhat more sober reflection on what this means in the long-term is warranted, however. First, as a social media/marketing phenomenon, the Ice Bucket Challenge was brilliantly conceived and executed, albeit it was neither conceived nor executed by the ALS organizations themselves. Second, there is no doubt that other disease charities will now strive to duplicate such "challenges" in the future, and they no doubt wish they had come up with the notion for their "own" diseases in the first place. However, the aptly termed phenomenon of "donor fatigue" is real, and it seems likely based on past experience that the ALS community may have achieved a "one-off" effect. To go beyond this in future years, researchers would have to demonstrate that the \$100 million raised made a tangible benefit in curing the disease. As this is not likely to happen, donors will move on to other causes and ALS funding will return to its pre-2014 levels, at best.

It may be instructive in regard to this last point that questions to the ALS Association of the United States and ALS Canada about how the money would be spent elicited only vague replies. This may be because the influx of funding was still so new. It is a safe bet, however, that both organizations will do what they have usually done and put the new funds into administration, patient care, and, lastly, research. The first is understandable, the second laudable, but the third is problematic if research funding is allocated as it typically is. If the trend toward putting research funds into "translational" treatments before the etiologies or progression of the disease are understood continues, then this will simply be moving the field along the same path that has failed in the past. As a sidebar, it seems highly likely that whatever funds are allotted for basic research will go to the newer genetic models, while the benign neglect of environmental etiologies and gene–toxin interactions continues.

Time alone will tell, but if this is the best that comes out of the Ice Bucket Challenge funding, then the outcome is fairly predictable. And, it should come as no surprise.

In 2012, Dr. Steven Hyman, the director of Harvard's Broad Institute, gave a plenary address at a Society for Neuroscience (SfN) meeting in which he raised a number of key points in regard to future treatments for neurological diseases, particularly Alzheimer's disease. In regard to the latter alone, Hyman expressed concerns that the costs to the medical system as a whole of an increasing level of Alzheimer's disease in the aging population of the United States were going to bankrupt the system. At the same time, Hyman noted shrinking funding from national granting agencies and further observed that one major alternative source of funding, the pharmaceutical industry, was pulling out of the research stream. Hyman's suggestion was that philanthropy might pick up the slack, perhaps combined with private-sector investors interested in both philanthropy *and* profit. It is not clear how likely this is to happen.

To put the challenges facing neurological disease treatments into a broader context, the outcomes from other fields might be helpful. In cancer research, vast sums have been invested in seeking genetic etiologies. Some linkages have been found, but not for most cancers, nor for most cancer patients (Ledford, 2015). Toxic substances were also considered, but they have not, at least in any simple manner, been able to account for most cancers of most kinds, and again not for all patients. In response, some of the newer views emerging in oncology are at variance with both gene- and toxin-hunt strategies. Some researchers now postulate that the number of stem cell divisions (Tomasetti and Vogelstein, 2015) and karyotic speciation (Duesberg et al., 2011) are the factors that give rise to cancers, in a sort of random "bad luck" model of the various forms.

Thus, cancers, like neurological diseases, are remarkably individualistic. Some aspects of haecceity make some individuals more prone to these outcomes (e.g., genetic background, exposure to toxins, epigenetic modifications, age, etc.), but in both categories of diseases there is little likelihood of ever finding a unitary etiology. As in the previous chapter, each Camino, as walked by each individual, is different.

16.4.1 Problems of Haecceity and Quiddity

What are the problems posed by individuality for treatment in neurological diseases? How do issues that arise from considerations of biological signaling figure into this?

A key theme espoused in this book turns on the notions of haecceity and quiddity: basically, the uniqueness and essence of a thing, respectively – in this case, that of each human being. Such considerations apply not only to each human generally, but also to the deterioration of that most complex part of humans, the CNS. Just as no two individuals are ever identical in all morphological or psychological features, regardless of genome, even in monozygotic twins, so will no two individuals ever respond to the myriad neural stressors in the same way, over the same time frame, or even necessarily at an end state. Neurological disease haecceity is thus a more formal conceptualization of the Camino metaphor presented in various places in this book.

A countervailing view to such haecceity and my contention that neurological disease damage cannot be undone after the earliest stages hinges on the notion that, given enough time and sufficient money, science can solve every issue that might arise in human affairs. This includes repairing a damaged nervous system, regardless of stage. Such faith in a future science is akin to the faith of various religions: it is impossible to refute, given that the time line upon which the statement relies appears to be endless. One can indeed imagine, in some distant future, that science will have progressed to the point where it can do things now considered impossible. It is currently difficult to conceive of taking an omelet and reconstituting a viable egg, leading to a chicken. Nevertheless, if one could recover the heat-denatured DNA, anneal the DNA and put it back together into chromosomes, and insert it into the nucleus of a chicken ovum in place of the ovum's initial DNA, then one might succeed in getting a viable chick. The question then becomes this: Why would one bother to do so from a practical perspective, apart from the ability to demonstrate that it could be done, theoretically and experimentally?

In some measure, the same problem can be posed in regard to a damaged human nervous system, particularly one in which cognitive function is impaired in part or in whole. Could one replace damaged neural cells and circuits and make them functionally "normal" again? Perhaps. Given, however, the reality of rising health care costs, this seems to be a highly unlikely outcome, except perhaps for the very richest amongst us. Even so – even given such riches – the likely insurmountable problems are those of haecceity and quiddity: that is, those things that make you "you," your memories and thoughts, all sculpted by experience, are the ones now compromised by the neuronal damage. Putting replacement cells or circuits back into a neurologically compromised individual does not make them the person they once were – it makes them someone different. This may not necessarily be a terrible thing, but if is not the same person being replaced, the question is the same as in the chicken analogy: Why would one bother to do so, and at what cost?

16.4.2 Problems Posed by Biosemiosis (Part 4)

As cited throughout the book, biosemiotics, or signaling in biological systems, is a new field, amalgamating the concepts derived from semiotics in linguistics and philosophy and applying them to biological systems. Examples include the signaling that occurs from genome to protein expression, in which the genetic information coded in DNA is considered to be the "signal," the various transcriptional machinery of RNA the "translation" of that signal, and the proteins thus formed the "object." As described by various authors (Oller, 2013, 2014; Gryder et al., 2013), the success or the health of the system exists when the signaling is successfully applied. Another way of stating it is as Oller has done in describing the successful transmission of information as a TNR. When signaling fails, the system is propelled toward a state of entropy.

In the gene–protein example, there are many stages in which such failures can occur, with the impacts larger the earlier they occur. For example, mutations in a gene will lead to the transcriptional machinery – the RNA – transcribing an erroneous signal, which when translated will generate a protein that may not perform its normal function. During transcription, the RNA may provide alternative versions of the end-stage protein, and errors here may also have deleterious consequences. Such potential signaling errors carry forward from the proteins to cellular function, from cellular function to systems at higher levels of organization, and so on. Thus, failures at lower levels can lead progressively to more complicated dysfunctions at higher levels.

It is conceptually relatively easy to imagine how biosemiotic errors in a pathway from genes to proteins can arise (e.g., in diseases such as cancer) and lead to system dysfunction. The conceptualization, however, becomes significantly more complex when dealing with a system which by definition is a signaling device (e.g., the nervous system). In this case, genetic errors can transition to different states – percolate in chaos theory – to protein dysfunction or abnormal polymorphisms, onwards to cellular alterations, to circuit breakdowns leading to neural system crashes, and finally to errors in overall CNS function and behavior. In other words, there are multiple nested levels of organization in which biosemiotics errors can bifurcate repeatedly.

Viewed in this way, it should not be surprising that genetic errors can induce neurological diseases, as indeed they do in some early-onset cases, as described in previous chapters. Perhaps it is surprising that they do not do so more often. The answer to why this is not the case may lie in the following considerations: Those genetic disorders in signaling, or in altered RNA transcription in some disorders, are routinely catastrophic in the familial forms of the diseases. In other words, the familial forms are heading inexorably toward a tipping point beyond which cascading failures set in motion the inevitable slide toward complete system failure much earlier in the disease process. The non-familial forms are not so destined, perhaps because of error-correcting functions at all levels from genes to systems and the innate redundancy of many neural systems.

While not much may be done about genetic defects leading to neurological diseases, in the sporadic forms the key to neurological disease treatment is likely to lie in prophylaxis. An example of how this might work has already been demonstrated in another field, as mentioned in Chapter 15 and discussed in the following section.

16.5 General Considerations for the Future of Neurological Disease Research

As detailed in Chapter 8 regarding model systems studies of neurological diseases, any effect, especially in small populations, is going to be impacted by a range of variables, some known and controlled for, others not. Some of the latter may not even be known, or may be considered inconsequential. These variables, however, are unlikely to be truly inconsequential, especially in small populations, where their impact may be greater than in larger populations, such as in humans generally. Small populations of experimental animals, or small populations of humans in various circumstances, may thus tend to temporarily exaggerate impacts of various presumed causal factors for neurological (or other) diseases and thus give results that are basically misleading. This outcome can occur in spite of adequate power analyses and regardless of how significant any current measurements may seem to be.

As in the studies of Ioannidis (2005) and others (which may also, perhaps, be subject to the "decline effect"), the implications of the ratio of accurate and valid research versus that which is not, data that can be reproduced versus that which cannot, and so on, have major consequences in the search for understanding and treatment. Thus, much of what the field thinks it knows about the nature of neurological diseases, the models of these diseases, and the potential for therapeutic benefits is at present extremely tenuous.

These points are amply illustrated by contemplating the goal of identifying risk factors for disease origin or progression. That this has not been attainable for the sporadic forms of the diseases is clear from the preceding pages. This goal may not even be completely feasible for the familial forms, since these too may depend in some measure on co-factors for the severity and rate of progression. As a practical case in point, the recent risk-factor analysis conducted for the NHCC/Public Health Agency of Canada (PHAC) listed a variety of factors linked to Parkinson's disease, ALS, Alzheimer's disease, and others. In spite of this, at the end of the study, the conclusions were remarkable vague. For example, exposure to agricultural chemicals came up in relation to each of the three age-related progressive neurological diseases, but it was not concluded that such toxic exposure alone caused them. The same conclusion – or lack thereof – could be reached from the broader scientific literature for exposure to aluminum, heavy metals such as lead and cadmium, various so-called "excitotoxins," metabolism-disrupting agents, estrogen mimetics, nicotinamide compounds, toxic steryl compounds, solvents, and a host of others. In each of these cases, researchers had, or could create, animal models that showed some or most of the neurological phenotype of the respective diseases. But to do so, they were typically forced to use toxin concentrations likely higher than those to which humans might normally be exposed, in order to overcome the more constricted time period of a model study.

Of course, these concerns do not mean that the individual chemical agents are not involved, merely that they are unlikely to be solely involved when it comes to human susceptibility to develop any of the neurological diseases.

This last point is very much the polar opposite to the perspective argued by various investigators cited at the beginning of this chapter: that there is some form of universal toxin that will provide the key etiology to any, or all, of the neurological diseases. This view is unlikely for weakly neurotoxic substances such as BMAA, and almost as unlikely for more powerful neurotoxins such as aluminum. The reason for this is simple: When dealing with a human population, even one as geographically isolated as Guam's Chamorro population once was, the range of exposures to any single or collection of toxins is going to be subject to a huge range of variables. A partial list of these variables includes geography in the modern age (relatively few individuals in Western society live their whole lives in one locale), the levels of the putative toxins at each locale, the amount of time spent at each locale, the age at which exposure occurred (from fetal life to old age), individual genetic makeup, polymorphisms within that same makeup of biochemistry, and sex.

This conclusion is in contrast to that of modern medicine, which is often focused on late-stage cures. If rather than a single causal factor – either a toxin or a gene – for the majority of cases of any such disease, each case were itself a form of geographical and biochemical "isolate" unique to the individual, then cures at any stage, if feasible, would be equally uniquely individualistic.

One way to look at this is to consider some forms from nature, such as the scallop shell (see Chapter 15), in which there are multiple, but finite, paths to the apex or point of origin. Perhaps an even better example might be the major and minor branches of a tree, which all ultimately lead to the trunk. If the trunk represents the expression of a given disease, then each branch represents a particular way to get to that same final destination. In the case of neurological disease, each branch leads eventually to dead SN neurons in Parkinson's disease, dead motor neurons in ALS, dead cortical and hippocampal neurons in Alzheimer's disease, and so on. Each disease is thus a spectrum of subdiseases, each with its own particular collection of etiologies and synergies.

This view may not, of course, be correct, and many in the field will continue to hope for single, or at least manageable, levels of causality. Thus, the BMAA proponents, and others like them pursuing other toxins, not to mention those seeking universal genetic causalities, may turn out to be correct, although the zero-sum-game mentality still applies and all will not be satisfied.

If there were one "bad" toxin doing one or a range of deleterious things, then the obvious solution would be to avoid it in the first place and/or remove it in some fashion once it is inside the CNS. Similarly, a mutant gene might be subject to correction by way of some futuristic gene therapy or by targeting the harmful downstream products of gene expression either early in life once the gene is detected, or later in life once the disease has begun to express. If, however, there are not universal toxins or genes, then there will be some nearly impossible challenges to the prevention of the neurological diseases. First, each individual case comes to the end stage uniquely, and thus there is no single way to avoid the constellation of toxins/susceptibility genes that lead to it. An individual might avoid aluminum exposure over a lifespan, for example, but how are they to avoid all of the toxins that might equally contribute to neuronal loss? Removing one particular source of toxicity is likely to provide only an individual, rather than a population change in risk factors. Even if one were to avoid all the risk factors – and the economic implications of doing so would be daunting – there would still be some prospect that some individuals would get the various diseases. In other words, reducing all identifiable risk factors could propel the population toward zero instances of such diseases without actually reaching zero. This may be the best that can be done.

In regard to treatment, in the early stages, individual forms of each disease would require individual, personalized treatment based on the disease-inducing factors. This would likely be challenging not to mention expensive. In later stages, where the various branches come together, one would face the very fact of late-stage neurological disease, namely the reality of cascading failures in which multiple dysfunctions are all extant and thus not treatable with any combination of therapeutics.

The field may be left with the uncomfortable circumstance, at least in the view of Western medicine and social philosophy, that the age-dependent neurological diseases are, in general, not subject to simple prophylaxis, generalized early detection, or, especially, effective treatment at late stages.

Based on current preconceptions and training, such notions are very difficult for many in the field of neurological disease research or treatment – let alone the lay public – to accept. Western medicine is, after all, a very "can-do" sort of enterprise, and Western science has firmly inculcated the notion that the scientific method will, eventually, solve any sort of problem that might arise. One sees similar views at play in other disciplines, such as climate change or Mars colonization. In medicine, this viewpoint persists in cancer treatment, which indeed has had some success in some forms of cancer over the last few decades (unlike neurological disease treatment, in which progress is modest to non-existent).

This view of science and medicine is quite dominant at present, and it would be difficult to argue that such viewpoints do not hold sway at the National Institutes of Health (NIH) and various other major and minor funding entities. Indeed, one would be hard pressed to get a grant from any of them if the initial premise proposed was that some sort of cure to any of the subject diseases was not plausible.

The answer here, in my view, is not going to arise from blind faith in the mysterious power of the scientific method over undefined time spans, or from endless attempts to tackle the same problems in the same way, but rather from a completely different approach. This would almost surely be one of semi-personalized medicine, in which the field recognizes that (i) any individual and population measures need to be prophylactic in order to be most effective; (ii) any case of neurological disease is going to be unique to the individual, due to the nearly endless variations afforded by individual genetic makeup, susceptibility factors, environment, microbiome, immune interactions, and so on; (iii) as such, each case has its own set of causal factors and time line for progression; and (iv) each case needs to be solved, if it can be solved, by addressing it at an individual level. A schematized way of looking at this is provided in Figure 16.1.

Given the current way of thinking about neurological diseases, it is difficult to conceive of any form of personalized neurology that might be used to address them, perhaps because so little is still known about the intersection of genetic, environmental, and other factors or the progression from onset to clinical diagnosis. As already discussed, attempts to force all forms of any of these diseases into the same genetic or environmental etiologies have slowed rather than accelerated progress.

The "one-size-fits-all" mentality so dominant in the world of vaccinology is just as prevalent in neurology, where most research dollars are spent on finding the "causes" (singular) and the "cures" (also mostly singular). The fact that this approach has been remarkably unsuccessful to date seems to have little impact on overall thinking in the field, since the counter to arguments pointing out this obvious defect is to fall back on future science as a panacea. In other words, rather than attempting anything new, scientists often firmly hold on to dogmatic statements of faith.

Faith sometimes translates into effective measures, and much of the preceding should be considered in the light of a proverb attributed to the Chinese that, "The person who says it cannot be done should not interrupt the person doing it." The obvious response to this is that those "doing it" should get on with it. I ardently hope they will do so, and in this way prove my arguments wrong.

In spite of the hope contained in this proverb, faith alone does not help in seeking a long-range strategy for neurological diseases, unless coupled to something more practical. One does not have to leave the health community to find a practical example of the success of prophylaxis and personalized medicine: that example comes from modern dentistry.

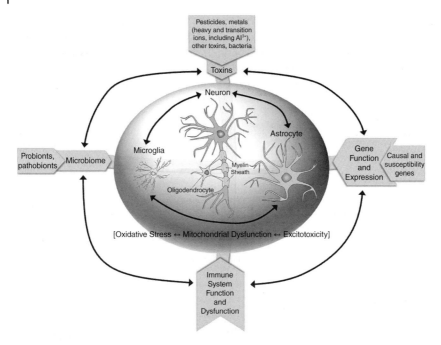

Figure 16.1 Schematization of some of the likely interactive elements leading to the age-related neurodegenerative diseases. The elements shown to be involved include *toxins* of various sorts (metals such as aluminum, various industrial molecules, pesticides either from nature or of human manufacture, bacterial toxins and metabolites, etc.), *genes* (genetic defects and polymorphisms, either as causal to neurodegeneration or as susceptibility factors for other stressors), the *microbiome* (pro- and pathobionts, and their ability to detoxify or release toxins), and *immune system* function and dysfunction. The available evidence suggests interactions between each of these elements. In turn, all impact the neuronal microenvironment, which includes not only neurons, but also supporting astrocytes, microglia, and oligodendrocytes. In this scheme, the initiation of neuronal dysfunction can be precipitated by any of these key elements. Given their interactions, perturbing any one of them will eventually affect the others. This scheme is not intended to be exclusive of other factors that may play a role in neuronal degeneration, such as age and sex.

16.6   The Advent of Modern Dentistry and Dental Prophylaxis

In most Western countries up until the 20th century, dentistry was a sub-branch of various other professions. For example, barbers were often those who did the routine removal of diseased teeth.

In fact, for much of recorded human history, oral hygiene was largely not practiced. Until the 20th century, few people, at least in the West, cleaned their teeth at all. The resulting dental caries and gingivitis were not treatable and the downstream consequence was that most adults would have lost some, if not all, of their teeth by what we now consider middle age. Indeed, tooth loss was considered to be a normal part of aging. As well, before the advent of modern sterile surgical techniques and antibiotics, impacted wisdom teeth were often a death sentence.

The realization that this state of affairs was not inevitable was quite long in coming. As the modern dental profession emerged, it became clear that the loss of teeth could be prevented by a combination of population and individual measures. At the population end, there were education campaigns designed to teach people to care for their teeth from early life onwards. In addition, governments at various levels took measures to prevent some putative causal factors. Dentistry now understands the factors leading to both caries and gingivitis much better (a case where Koch's postulates often do apply), and, in the developed countries, with advanced medical care and government and insurance programs to pay for the same, dentistry now routinely controls the underlying causes of tooth loss from early in life.

Community water fluoridation and fluoride self-care products have conventionally been credited as a strong control measure against dental caries (Jones et al., 2005), notwithstanding concerns about fluoride in general, and in particular as a CNS toxin at higher concentrations. However, a massive recent analysis of the exiting literature by Cochrane Collaboration researchers has cast doubt on the assertion that fluoride in community water supplies has anything whatsoever to do with reduced levels of cavities (Iheozor-Ejiofor et al., 2015). This last example illustrates, yet again, how widely held assumptions in the medical field, regardless of the subject, should never be assumed to be either "proven" or beyond question in place of further evaluation and research.

Regardless of the eventual status of the data on water fluoridation, the use of a common vector, in this case water, to prevent tooth decay was at least an attempt to apply a preventative measure to dental health, much like the use of vaccination to protect against various infectious diseases.

At the individual level, in many countries, regular, personalized dental care providing early cavity removal and cleaning, as well as regular check-ups, is now the norm for much of the population (Burt, 1978; Sakki et al., 1994; Garcia and Sohn, 2012). In addition, the advent of prophylactic dental treatments has reduced various secondary ailments associated with caries and gingivitis (Sheiham, 2005). With such measures firmly established in the richer nations, the loss of teeth with aging has become a far less frequent event for most people.

Thus, a relatively simple set of procedures, applied early and throughout life, has markedly changed the aging process in relation to dentition, and with this the very quality of life (Figure 16.2). It should be noted, however, that these changes in dental health come at a cost. In the developed countries with universal health care, most

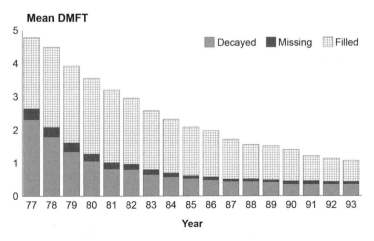

Figure 16.2 Dental prophylaxis at work. Mean decayed/missing/filled teeth (DMFT) components in 12-year-old children in Australia from 1977 to 1993. *Source*: Davies et al. (1997) and used with permission from John Wiley & Sons, Inc.

people have access to such treatments. In less developed countries and those without universal health care, such prophylaxis is available only for those wealthy enough to afford it.

Another example of attempted prophylaxis comes from vaccinology, which uses various vaccine formulations in an effort to combat infectious diseases before they arise. Notably, there seem to be significant problems with fundamental theory in this field, and distinct problems in practice (e.g., the use of aluminum adjuvants, as detailed in Chapters 6 and 11). Nevertheless, the prevention of infectious diseases has often been successfully accomplished in vaccinology (Morrice et al., Scheduled 2017), as it has in dentistry.

Overall, the strategic direction established by dentistry is one that neurology could well emulate: while teeth and neurons are obviously quite different things, the principles applied to preserving the former could almost as easily be applied to the latter.

16.7 Addressing Neurological Diseases at the Individual and Population Levels

These principles would be the following. First, identify the major causal factors that induce neurological disease at a population level and take whatever steps are required to remove them from the human biosphere. A good example would be removing aluminum from any product that could cause ionic aluminum to become bioavailable and gain access to the human body. There are numerous toxins that could be dealt with in the same manner. While these measures might never eliminate all cases of neurological disease, they would surely diminish the numbers of victims in the future. This is not really all that difficult to imagine, nor impossible to do.

Would it cost a lot of money? Almost certainly it would, but hardly as much as the increasing rates of neurological disease do in terms of the financial and other impacts on individuals, families, and society.

The choice is actually pretty straightforward. The field can keep doing what it now does and keep failing, or it can adopt the quite logical, and successful, example from dentistry, and at least have some preventative effect on long-term neurological health at a population level.

16.7.1 Prophylaxis as a Medical Strategy for Neurological Disease Prevention

A strong stream in neurological disease therapy research has been in attempts to correct neurological diseases through the physical replacement of lost cells or the reinitiation of processes leading to such cells being born anew in the CNS. These have not worked out as well as was hoped, as detailed in Chapters 13 and 14.

This is not the case for many non-neuronal disorders, where organ-transplant surgeries, along with the necessary immunosuppression, have worked well for a variety of ailments. Successful treatments have included corneal transplants and hip replacements, which have now become routine. These may indeed be "stop-gap" measures. However, in the context of the projected lifespans of the individuals usually involved, the time frame may be appropriate. For example, a hip replacement may last for 10–20 years. If the expected lifespan of the patient is the same, then the problem is mostly solved.

Replacement strategies for neural circuits, however, are limited by the problems of biosemiosis cited in previous chapters. In their absence, is there an alternative for neurological diseases? Could a form of long-term "neurological hygiene" be applied to prevent, or at least diminish, the incidence of neurological diseases? How would such practices be applied to sporadic neurological diseases in the absence of clearly identified causal factors?

Admittedly, given the complexity of the human nervous system, the spectrum nature of the diseases, and the range of variability for contributing factors, such personalized neurology would be a lot more difficult to realize than that of personalized dental care. In this regard, it is certainly true that the individual collection of risk factors in neurological diseases might stymie the prevention of all such cases. Nevertheless, the identification of the major risk factors and their elimination almost certainly would diminish the current trend toward increased prevalence and maybe incidence. Societies could choose, for example, to limit the bioavailability of chemicals such as aluminum compounds salts and various toxic agricultural chemicals, not to mention a host of other likely neurotoxic culprits.

16.7.2 The "Politics" of Neurological Disease

It must be noted that such social decisions are essentially political in nature: Enough people would have to demand this outcome and then convince politicians in the notionally democratic counties to make the necessary laws. All of this would be subject to an almost certain pushback from various industries and their lobby groups. To aid in the fight against such lobbying efforts, scientists involved in the relevant research would have to become more publicly outspoken.

And all would have to accept that removing such molecules from the modern world would come with certain economic costs and a likely change in modern life.

Many people are already making choices at an individual level to minimize exposure to neurotoxic compounds, but there is a limit to the amount of protection that an individual choice may afford when surrounded by a badly polluted environment.

This returns the discussion to the previous point that such choices are realistically made at a societal level and are, ultimately, the only real solution. We may be prepared to accept an ALS rate of 3 per 100 000 or an Alzheimer's rate of 20–30 per 100 000 as the cost of maintaining the industrial world as it is, but if the rates are really increasing, then there will inevitably come a time when the price of the current way of doing "business" will no longer be worth the societal and monetary costs. When that point will be reached remains uncertain, but that such a point *will* be reached, with the eventual bankruptcy of every modern medical system, seems to be increasingly apparent. The projected time for this dire outcome, as cited by Hyman (2012), is not all that far away, and certainly within the lifespan of many of those reading this book. It will be an unavoidable conclusion that the failure to make this decision now means that society may have to accept several more generations in which many people succumb to neurological diseases that might have been prevented.

This is a choice.

The second part of the prophylaxis option, just as for dentistry, is to provide for early treatment to prevent neurological diseases from progressing to the point of system collapse. Such a treatment regime would require a form of very personalized medicine to screen everyone across the lifespan for biomarkers of neurological disease of whatever nature, biochemical or behavioral. Such a program would come with enormous costs, of course, but, as before, these costs would likely be far less than the current and projected costs of neurological diseases. Just as dentistry now routinely prevents tooth loss in most of the developed countries, similar measures in neurological disease prophylaxis might, in much the same manner, diminish individual CNS damage and thus population levels of neurological disease. The overall goal here would be to make neurology as mundane, at least in regard to the age-related neurological diseases, as dentistry now is for dental health.

This, too, is a choice.

16.7.3 The Role of Scientists in the Politics of Neurological Disease Prophylaxis

It is relatively rare in this day and age that basic – or even applied – scientists become involved in active advocacy or politics to fight for policy shifts relating to the implications of their work. There are clear exceptions, such as physicists concerned with nuclear war and the various advocacy groups for different professions, such as the American Medical Association (AMA) and various neurological disease organizations. Nonetheless, it is unusual for individual scientists to take such advocacy positions. Part of the reason is that many working scientists tend to view policy decisions as someone else's problem or jurisdiction. Part of this inaction involves the traditional "ivory tower" sort of perspective, in which science is considered to be above, or at least beyond, such practical considerations.

Generally, there are also very cogent reasons for not getting directly involved. Scientists in industry usually cannot do so. Nor, usually, can those working for governments. Scientists at universities will find themselves under various constraints at different phases of their careers: graduate students and postdoctoral fellows are too junior and vulnerable in general; new faculty members tend to be too busy fighting for grants and tenure, and certainly do not need to add anything to their promotion "packages" that might be considered too controversial or that would put their university or their grant agency on the spot. Those scientists who do speak out on policy issues tend to be the older, tenured faculty members who are more secure professionally and financially. But even in such cases, holding grants and keeping tenure or one's laboratory space tend to be interrelated realities. Getting placed on an unfavorable list with a grant agency for anything that could be construed as a negative critique of that agency's policies is hardly a career-advancing move.

All of these are perfectly valid reasons for individual scientists to leave policy considerations to those in the regulatory agencies, government, and various professional bodies and get on with what they do, or think they do, best.

However, I would argue that a number of emerging factors make this stance less feasible, and indeed less defensible, than it was in the past. One of these is basic morality combined with economics; the other is self-defense.

From the societal "greater good" perspective, consider the following: Neurological diseases currently cost the economy many billions of dollars per year in the United States alone, as cited in Chapter 2. Dementias and their subset, Alzheimer's disease,, make up the vast bulk of this cost. This situation is not going to get better on its own. Indeed, every projection is that it will get much worse.

Everyone with one of the major neurological diseases is subtracted from being a functional member of the economy. Each takes out additional persons as care givers. The social and economic costs, which are now astonishing, will become even more so in the coming decades, and ultimately, may bankrupt the health care system. The only way of preventing this given the current way of doing things is for a country to abandon those afflicted, which is, in essence, a form of moral bankruptcy. The same series of outcomes will occur in every "developed" country.

In regard to self-defense, most of those reading this book know someone with a major neurological disease. Inevitably, all will know more persons so afflicted. These diseases will affect our families, and they may just as likely strike us down as well. Indeed, it is a virtual certainty that amongst the readers of this book are many who will succumb to such diseases in the future.

Social morality, economic wellbeing, and basic self-defense, pure and simple, would call upon us all as scientists to take leading roles in fighting for policy changes and the funding to realize such changes.

Scientists are not supposed to be social revolutionaries, but if they are not, then choices all too often get left to those less informed – or to politicians, often the least informed. The will to take action can accomplish the unexpected, even the near miraculous. To quote from Hannah Arendt's essay, "What is Freedom?" (Arendt, 2006):

> History, in contradistinction to nature, is full of events; here the miracle of acci-dent and infinite probability occurs so frequently that is seems strange to speak of miracles at all. But the reason for this frequency is merely that historical pro-cesses are created and constantly interrupted by human initiative, by the *initium* man is insofar as he is an acting being. Hence it is not in the least superstitious, it is even a counsel of realism to look for the unforeseeable and unpredictable, to be prepared for and to expect "miracles" in the political realm [...]
> in the realm of human affairs, we know the author of the "miracles." It is men who perform them – men who because they have received the twofold gift of freedom and action can establish a reality of their own.[3]

The notion that "everything is politics" is often overstated in political/activist circles, but at its core it has merit, at least in the public sphere. If, in a free society, our discussions and debates about social directions eventually instruct policy, then taking part in the same and failing to take part are both political decisions. The difference is that the latter, unlike the former, cannot deliver miracles.

Many scientists fall into the latter category in that however "political" they may be in the normative range of politics as defined by participation in the electoral process, they often fail to engage in "politics" in the sense of advocacy in their own field. For example, advocating for a change in social policy in regard to preventing or treating neurological diseases is often considered to be too political. Yet many are completely comfortable letting special interest groups (e.g., the SfN and NHCC) advocate such change when it comes to securing funding for research. The subject of funding, however, is intrinsically part of the discussion of prevention/treatment.

It is as if being an advocate for a new way of approaching neurological disease would somehow be an unfair use of specialized training and insight. The consequence of scien-tists not being political as advocates for change, however, is that the politicians and the pharmaceutical industry, who may or may not listen to the lay public, are left to decide policy. Of course, what is remarkably ironic about all of this is that the politicians making the financial decisions are just as likely to succumb, or have family members succumb, to neurological diseases.

The *status quo* mentality thus leads to the current outcome: In the effort to com-bat neurological diseases, there are no effective treatments and little funding to come up with any. Various NGOs plead with Congress (or Parliament in Canada, or what-ever national assembly), and sometimes a few financial crumbs fall from the table to advance research. Yet, as funding for armaments and armies tends to rise, the so-called "paylines" for research shrink.

One wonders what a poll asking a simple question on financial priorities would show. For example, suppose one posed the question, "Considering the possibility that you or someone you know will get Alzheimer's disease, would you rather put more money for research into the NIH or have more jet fighters?" Given the incredible financial and thus political power of the defense lobby to sway public opinion in the United States, it could be that Americans would opt for the latter. However, Canadians asked a similar question in a Canadian context surely would not, and I would bet most people of other countries would not, either.

All of this puts the subject of preventing or treating neurological disease in a rather odd predicament. In a nutshell, enormous progress could be made in reducing neurological disease incidence if the national priority were to do so, existing monies could accomplish this if they were allocated to this purpose in a new strategic manner, and most people would likely support doing so. In addition, it would, in the short and medium terms, be more financially prudent to do so than to have government or individuals pay for such measures. This is much like the frequently made financial observation that it is cheaper to house the homeless than to pay for the minimal social services they use if left on the streets. In spite of all of this, such policy shifts have not, to date, happened. As social or medical policy, this is remarkably short-sighted. One thus has to wonder why the situation does not change. The most obvious answer is that special interests do not want it to, or maybe that those in power simply want other things much more.

In a free society, this can be changed. And, arguably, those who know the most about neurological diseases should be the ones leading the discussion. If more scientists became actively – rather than passively – political, their political "activism" would inevitably serve to instruct the lay public. That lay public, in turn, would have the scientific resources to make the politicians do, with the public's own money, what most people might come to see as a priority.

If this were to happen, it seems there could be only two possible outcomes: Either we live in real democratic countries, which, when sufficiently motivated by the public, would make politicians choose public, rather than private, priorities. Or, we do not live in democratic countries, and the *status quo* will prevail into the future.

It will be interesting in the decades to come to see which of these outcomes occurs.

Perhaps, in the end, it is not really a question of whether these choices will be made or not, but when they will have to be made.

Endnotes

1 Jalal ad-Din Muhammad Rumi (1207–1273) was a poet, jurist, Islamic scholar, theologian, and Sufi mystic.
2 Theodor Seuss Geisel (1904–1991) was an American writer known for his numerous children's books. From *Happy Birthday to You!*
3 Hannah Arendt (1906–1975) was a German Jewish political theorist and one of the most influential political philosophers of the 20th century.

Glossary

akinesia Complete lack of movement.

aluminum The 13th element in the periodic table. Aluminum is the third most common element in the earth's crust after oxygen and silicon, and the most common metal. In nature, it is mostly complexed with silicate compounds. The aluminum ion (Al^{+3}) is a cellular toxin and, in particular, a neurotoxin. Aluminum compounds find widespread use in a range of industrial and medical applications. Aluminum has been linked epidemiologically and experimentally to neurological diseases/disorders of various kinds.

Alzheimer's disease A disease involving the loss of neurons in the brain, primarily in the cortex and hippocampus, which are concerned with learning and memory. Hallmark pathological features, seen post mortem, are the presence of amyloid beta (Aβ) protein plaques and neurofibrillary tangles (NFTs). Alzheimer's disease is progressive and is the most common of the age-related neurological diseases. Treatment options are limited in effectiveness, although newer therapies offer some potential promise.

amyloid beta (Aβ) A protein deposit associated with neuron degeneration. Amyloid is found in the brains of individuals with Alzheimer's disease in the form of dense insoluble protein blobs called "plaques."

amyloid precursor protein (APP) A protein found in various organs, including the brain, heart, kidneys, lungs, spleen, and intestines. The normal function of APP in the body is unknown. In Alzheimer's disease, APP is abnormally processed and converted to amyloid beta (Aβ) protein – the protein deposited in amyloid plaques.

amyotrophic lateral sclerosis–parkinsonism dementia complex (ALS-PDC) The neurological disease spectrum of Guam and other locations in the Western Pacific. ALS-PDC describes diseases that range from ALS to a form of parkinsonism with dementia, as well as a combination of the two. There is also a form of Alzheimer's-like disease. ALS-PDC has been linked epidemiologically to the consumption and other uses of the seeds of the cycad (*C. micronesica* K. D. Hill).

amyotropic lateral sclerosis (ALS) Also known as Lou Gehrig's disease. One of the motor neuron diseases that destroy lower and/or upper motor neurons. It is typically fatal within 3–5 years from clinical diagnosis. Signs include the progressive loss of motor functions leading to respiratory failure. There are both sporadic and familial forms, the former making up the vast majority of all cases. A loss of cognitive function may also occur. There are currently no viable treatment options.

antibody A type of immunoglobulin (Ig): a large Y-shaped protein produced by plasma cells. Igs come in a variety of isotypes, classified based on the type of heavy

Neural Dynamics of Neurological Disease, First Edition. Christopher A. Shaw.
© 2017 John Wiley & Sons, Inc. Published 2017 by John Wiley & Sons, Inc.

chain they are made of: heavy-chain classes named, alphabetically, α, γ, δ, ε, and μ give rise to IgA, IgG, IgD, IgE, and IgM, respectively. These isotypes differ in their biological properties.

apoprotein E (APOE) A class of apolipoprotein produced by the liver and in macrophages. It mediates cholesterol metabolism through one of three main isoforms (2, 3, and 4). In the central nervous system (CNS), it is produced by astrocytes and transports cholesterol to neurons by way of APOE receptors. *APOE*, the gene coding for APOE, is found on chromosome 19 and consists of four exons and three introns. *APOE* transcription is regulated by the Liver X receptor, which is involved in cholesterol, glucose, and fatty acid homeostasis. The *APOE4* isoform is linked to ALS and Alzheimer's disease.

apoptosis A form of programmed cell death that occurs either as a controlled event during development or as the result of instructions from other cells in various disease states. An example of the latter is microglial-induced apoptosis of neurons in neurological diseases. Apoptosis is distinct from necrosis, a form of cell death induced by injury. Necroptosis has features of both.

astrocyte A specialized support cell in the nervous system. Astrocytes regulate concentrations of potassium ions and serve as storage sites for some amino acids such as glutamate. During development, certain types of astrocytes guide neuronal axons to their correct locations in the nervous system. In neurological diseases, astrocytes are altered into an "activated" form that may be part of the pathological process of neuronal degeneration.

ataxia The complete loss of the control of movement.

autoimmune/inflammatory syndrome induced by adjuvants (ASIA) A syndrome involving adjuvant-induced autoimmune reactions that can impact any organ system, often with multiple systems abnormalities present. Aluminum vaccine adjuvants are considered a key contributor to ASIA. One clear example is that of MMF.

autoimmunity Immune cell-mediated destruction of the body's other cells/tissues. Autoimmunity is not well understood, but there appear to be numerous types, affecting various organs. The number of potential triggers for autoimmune reactions is extensive, and may include aluminum adjuvants.

β-methyl amino-L-alanine (BMAA) A weak excitotoxin found in cycad and other plants as a free amino acid. It appears to activate both AMPA and NMDA glutamatergic receptors. BMAA appears to have signaling roles in plants. It has been implicated in ALS-PDC and other neurological diseases by various investigators.

β-oxalylamino-l-alanine (BOAA) An excitotoxin associated with lathyrism. BOAA activates glutamatergic AMPA receptors.

biosemiosis An emerging discipline that is concerned with biological signaling. The term "biosemiosis" comes from a combination of "biology" (life) and "semiotics" (meaning).

blood–brain barrier The collection of cells and membranes that prevents ingress of certain substances into the brain.

bodig A neurological disease of Guam that combines features of Parkinson's with those of Alzheimer's disease. Formally termed parkinsonism dementia complex (PDC).

bradykinesia Slowness of voluntary movements.

butterfly effect The notion from chaos theory that small perturbations can have larger long-term consequences. The lay metaphor is that a butterfly flapping its wings in the Amazon may, depending on various other circumstances, lead to a hurricane in New York.

Camino de Santiago Literally, "the way (or path) of Saint James," an ancient pilgrimage route that ends in the Spanish Galician city of Santiago de Compostella. There are various routes to Santiago. One of the most common is the 800 km Camino Frances, which begins in the French Basque city of St. Jean Pied de Port and runs over the Pyrenees and westward through northern Spain.

cascading failure The triggering by some deleterious event of further such events, leading to a system collapse.

cell doctrine A fundamental basis of modern biology that holds that cells are the basic structural and functional units of all living organisms.

Chamorro A person of the indigenous population of Guam and others of the southern Marianas Islands.

chaos theory The study of nonlinear dynamics. In chaos theory, an apparent lack of order in a system still obeys particular laws or rules. Originally described by Dr. Edward Lorenz, a meteorologist, the key concepts are that even complex systems have an underlying order and that even small or simple events can lead to complex outcomes. The latter is sometimes termed "sensitive dependence on initial conditions."

chorea Movements of any part of the body that seems to be "dance-like."

complex system (and complex adaptive system and behavior) A difficult-to-define concept in which a number of different systems share common features, including multiple interactive elements and a "sensitive dependence on initial conditions." A complex adaptive system is one that can "learn" and thus change its behavior.

cortex The outer layer of the brain, consisting of five or six main layers of cells. Cortical areas include those for the primary senses (e.g., vision and audition) and those termed "association areas" (the sites of most cognitive abilities in humans and other higher mammals). Alzheimer's disease destroys neurons in various regions of the cortex, leading to memory loss and the loss of other cognitive functions. Note that there are various sublayers within the layers of cortex, primarily in primates and humans.

cycad An ancient order of plants that are often mistakenly considered to be of the palm family, but are in fact gymnosperms. Various orders and species of cycads exist around the world. Those on Guam are of the species *Cycas micronesica* K.D. Hill. Consumption or medicinal use of the seeds of the cycad on Guam and elsewhere has been implicated in ALS-PDC of the Western Pacific.

decline effect The loss of previous statistical significance in experimental data.

domoic acid A kainite receptor agonist arising from some forms of phytoplankton. Kainate receptors are one of three primary types of ionotropic glutamate receptors. The Eastern Canadian cluster of neurological outcomes followed the consumption of mussels that had bioaccumulated domoic acid.

dysarthria A motor speech disorder resulting from neurological injury to the motor component of speech production. Dysarthria is characterized by a poor articulation of phonemes, leading to impairments in various aspects of vocal communication.

dyskinesia In general, difficulty in performing voluntary movements. Dyskinesias are involuntary, often hyperkinetic movements that may not be purposeful and are not fully controllable by the person affected. In the case of Parkinson's disease, these can include the inability to initiate or stop a movement.

dysphagia Difficulty in swallowing.

dystonia Spasms of individual muscles or groups of voluntary muscles of various types. Dystonias can be sustained or intermittent, sudden or slow, and painful or painless.

emergent properties Basically, outcomes that exceed the sum of their parts. The behavior of an ant colony versus that of an individual ant or collection of ants represents an emergent property of this type of social insect.

epigenetics The study of changes in the phenotype or of when environmental or other external events alter gene function and expression without altering DNA.

etiology In medical terms, the cause of any given aliment.

fadang Flour made from the seeds of the cycad *Cycas micronesica* K.D. Hill on Guam.

familial ALS (fALS) The early-onset form of ALS, most commonly linked to gene mutations. Key amongst these are *C9orf72* and m*SOD1*. It is notable that all of the fALS mutations combined do not account for more than 10% of all ALS patients.

fasciculation A muscle twitch (e.g. a small, involuntary muscle contraction and relaxation).

festination In Parkinson's disease, an involuntary gait feature in which the patient takes short, accelerating steps. Typically, the trunk is flexed forward and the legs are flexed stiffly at the hips and knees.

fetal basis of adult disease (FeBAD) The hypothesis that prenatal events predispose an individual to later – perhaps much later – postnatal illnesses.

Framingham study A longitudinal study of thousands of people designed to elicit risk factors and the nature of the progression of cardiovascular disease in the United States. The initial study was begun in the 1940s and has continued with the offspring of the original participants and their grandchildren.

free radical An ion with one or more unpaired electrons. Free radicals are highly reactive with cellular membrane components such as lipids, proteins, and DNA, and are thus very damaging. They are thought to be a major factor in neurodegeneration, although the stage at which they participate in neuronal loss is not known.

frontotemporal dementia (FTD) A group of disorders produced by progressive nerve cell loss in the frontal or temporal lobes of the brain. A form of FTD is found in ALS, in which cognitive function is highly compromised. This is often termed "ALS-FTD."

gene A discrete sequence of DNA that encodes instructions for making a specific protein. The protein, in turn, does a specific task and thus affects the functions of a given cell. The protein is considered to be the product of the gene. Gregor Mendel (1822–1884), an Augustinian friar, is widely considered to be the founder of genetics.

glia Support cells of the nervous system, consisting of three main types: astrocytes, microglia, and oligodendrocytes (all of which have functional or cellular subtypes). Astrocytes surround and provide various support functions to neurons, for example by controlling the concentrations of various ions and some neurotransmitters. Microglia act as scavenger cells of the nervous system, serving much the same function as macrophages in the immune system; initially, when acting in a supporting role, they provide growth factors such as progranulin to injured neurons. Oligodendrocytes provide insulation along the axons of neurons, without which electrical signal propagation would fail. Schwann cells are a specialized type of oligodendrocyte that insulate the axons of neurons which form nerves projecting to the peripheral muscles. Other oligodendrocytes insulate neurons within the central nervous system (CNS).

Guadeloupe parkinsonism (G-PDC) The form of parkinsonism of the French island of Guadeloupe, which is associated with the consumption of the fruit of the soursop (*Annona muricata*). The features of G-PDC are similar in many respects to those of ALS-PDC and PSP.

Gulf War Syndrome A collection of often overlapping diseases of unknown origin associated with those who served with the Coalition forces in the first Gulf War of 1990–91. Of particular interest, many of the symptoms are neurological, and a subgroup of those with Gulf War Syndrome have ALS.

haecceity The "whatness" of a thing or person. Haecceity considers the things that make any individual person or object unique, even in the context of similar things or persons.

Hill criteria British statistician A. B. Hill set out to aid epidemiological studies in distinguishing simple correlated events from those that might be causal. He described nine criteria by which to do so. The satisfaction of at least a particular four of the nine allows for some confidence that a causal relationship may be present. Note, however, that even satisfying all nine of these rules does not "prove" causality, but merely strengthens the hypothesis that a causal relationship exists.

hippocampus A structure located in the temporal lobe in humans and higher primates that forms part of the limbic system and **is** involved in short-term memory. Damage to cells in various parts of the hippocampus impacts memory formation. The hippocampus is damaged in Alzheimer's disease, and damage to this region was also noted in the domoic acid poisoning cluster.

Holmberg's mistake Allan R. Holmberg was a cultural anthropologist. In the 1940s, he lived with a primitive tribe in South America and concluded from his studies that the level of cultural and material achievements of the tribe reflected their closeness to a natural state of being. What Holmberg did not realize was that the people he studied were the remnant population of a vastly more complex civilization that had been virtually wiped out by invasion and disease.

hormone A molecule formed in one type of cell or organ and carried by the blood as a chemical signal to other cells.

Huntington's disease A genetically-based neurological disease involving the loss of cells in the striatum.

hypothesis An idea or proposal about how some aspect of the natural world works that must be confirmed – or refuted – by experiment. A hypothesis that survives experimental testing, along with similar experimental and theoretical data, can become part of a theory.

immune system The system comprising cells and molecules that provide protection from viral and bacterial pathogens. The immune system is typically considered to consist of "innate" and "adaptive" components.

immunoglobulin *See* **antibody**.

incidence The frequency of some condition, described in terms of the new numbers of people affected (usually per 100 000 persons), in a certain time period. The latter is typically measured over a set period in years. Incidence is used to calculate changing rates of the condition.

inflammasome An intracellular, multiprotein complex that controls the activation of pro-inflammatory caspases, primarily caspase-1. The complex generally has three main components: a cytosolic pattern-recognition receptor known as the nucleotide-binding oligomerization domain receptor (NOD)-like receptor (NLR), the enzyme caspase-1 (part of the apoptosis pathway), and an adaptor protein known as apoptosis-associated speck-like protein (ASC), which facilitates the interaction between the NLR and caspase-1. The NLR subfamilies include NLRP3, the best studied of this group.

Koch's postulates Dr. Robert Heinrich Herman Koch (1843–1910) is considered to be the founder of modern bacteriology. In attempting to satisfy the conditions needed to assign infectious diseases to particular pathogens, he promoted the following postulates: (i) The presumed infectious microorganism has to be found in high levels in those with the disease, but not in those who do not have the disease; (ii) The microorganism has to be isolatable from those who suffer from the disease; (iii) The microorganism, when given to healthy subjects, should induce the disease; (iv) The microorganism isolated from the secondarily infected host should display the same identity as the first.

lathyrism A motor disorder arising from the consumption of legumes containing the neurotoxin and AMPA receptor agonist, BOAA. Lathyrism has a long history, but it came to the attention of neurologists after it was found in those incarcerated in some prisoner-of-war camps following World War II.

Lewy body A protein inclusion in cells of the *substantia nigra* (SN) and elsewhere in Parkinson's disease, some other parkinsonisms, and other neurological diseases. It consists of α-synuclein and ubiquitin.

lytico The ALS form of neurological disease of Guam.

macrophagic myofasciitis (MMF) A neuromuscular disorder that arises following the injection of an aluminum hydroxide vaccine adjuvant. It is characterized as a form of ASIA.

microglia Scavenger cells of the nervous system. Microglia are activated by neuronal injury and are commonly observed as a pathological feature in neurological diseases. There are different types of microglia which serve either to protect neurons from injury or to destroy them.

mild cognitive impairment (MCI) A form of cognitive decline, one of the outcomes of MMF and other neurological disorders. It may also be a precursor to later dementias such as Alzheimer's disease.

model system Any experimental preparation designed to mimic, in whole or in part, the conditions in a living organism. At least at they apply to neurological disease research, models may be computer-based, *in vitro* (cell culture), or *in vivo* (whole animal).

motor neuron A specialized neuron whose axon connects to other motor neurons or to muscle fibers. Motor neurons are the type of neural cells targeted by the neurodegenerative processes of ALS.

multiple-hit model *See* **one-hit model**.

mutant SOD1 (mSOD1) A mutation of the gene coding for the protein superoxide dismutase (SOD), one of the body's key antioxidant molecules, which is linked to fALS. Currently, over 180 variant mutations of this gene are known. m*SOD1* has been used to model ALS *in vivo* in various animal models.

necroptosis A form of programmed cell death that, however, morphologically resembles necrosis. Unlike apoptosis, it is independent of caspase function. Necroptosis relies on the function of the necrosome, made up of the protein kinases RIP1, RIP3, and MLKL. These kinases function to induce cell death by permeablizing the plasma membrane via mechanisms still to be determined.

Necroptosis is thought to be a failsafe mechanism that can induce cell death when apoptosis is inhibited.

necrosis A form of cell death normally occurring following injury.

nerve cell *See* **neuron**.

neural Pertaining to neurons and glia.

neurofibrillary tangle (NFT) An accumulation of twisted protein fragments located inside nerve cells in certain regions of the central nervous system (CNS). The protein in question is a hyperphosphorylated form of tau protein. NFTs are one of the hallmark structural abnormalities found in the post-mortem brains of Alzheimer's disease victims and are used as positive markers of the disease. The second hallmark feature in Alzheimer's is the presence of amyloid plaques. NFTs also occur in FTD associated with cases of ALS, PSP, and other neurological diseases, especially ALS-PDC. On Guam, many Chamorros without signs or symptoms of ALS-PDC show the presence of NFTs.

neuron A specialized cell consisting of a cell body (soma), dendrites, and an axon. The cell-surface membrane is semi-permeable to ions such as sodium, potassium, chloride, and calcium. Most neurons are able to conduct fast electrical signals along their axons.

neurotransmitter A molecule that activates a specific class and subtype of receptor on a neural cell. Neurotransmitters can be amino acids (e.g., glutamate and related amino acids), peptides (opioids and others), amines (acetylcholine), catecholamines (dopamine, serotonin, adrenaline), or a host of other molecules.

nucleotides The building blocks of DNA: adenine, thymine (sometimes replaced by uracil), cytosine, and guanine.

one-hit model The notion that one type of negative impact is sufficient to trigger the death or dysfunction of a particular kind of cell or organ. The multiple-hit model suggests that interactive, multiple events are more likely.

oxidative stress The situation that arises when free-radical production exceeds the ability of the body's or the cell's antioxidant defense mechanisms.

Parkinson's disease A movement disorder caused by the loss of cells in the SN. Patients may also exhibit cognitive function losses and other behaviors.

parkinsonism Any of the various types of neurological disease broadly similar to Parkinson's disease. Examples are ALS-PDC, G-PDC, PSP, and others.

pathology The branch of medicine that studies disease.

plaques Clumps of Aβ protein that surround and engulf cells in regions of the brain in Alzheimer's disease victims.

prevalence The total number of individuals afflicted by some condition at any given time point.

progressive *(in regard to neurological diseases)* Briefly, a disease process that does not abate, but continues to worsen over time. Progressive neurological diseases include Parkinson's disease, ALS, and Alzheimer's disease.

progressive supranuclear palsy (PSP) A type of parkinsonism featuring a strong cognitive decline and many of the pathological features of Alzheimer's disease.

quiddity The essence of a thing or person.

randomized controlled trial The form of clinical trial that is considered the "gold standard" for evaluation of therapeutic efficacy. Other types of epidemiological evaluation (e.g., case–control, cohort, and case studies) are considered to be scientifically inferior.

receptor *(neurotransmitter)* At a molecular level, a receptor is a protein usually contained within the surface membrane of neural cells. Receptors are specifically sensitive to particular neurotransmitters/neuromodulators. For example, the amino acid neurotransmitter glutamate has a number of glutamate receptor classes and, within classes, various subtypes. The first are the "ionotropic" receptors, named for particular glutamate agonists (e.g., AMPA, kainite, NMDA). Ionotropic receptors are themselves ion channels and are responsible for all fast synaptic transmission in the nervous system. When activated by glutamate ionotropic receptors, they allow specific ions to enter the neuron. For example, AMPA receptors flux sodium and calcium; NMDA receptors flux calcium; kainic acid receptors allow both sodium and calcium to enter. Other glutamate receptors are termed "metabotropic." When activated by glutamate, they turn on signaling cascades inside the neuron. They are also called "G-protein receptors." Neurotransmitters may have both ionotropic and G-protein receptor targets, or only one of these types. For each neurotransmitter, there are usually numerous subtypes of receptors of whichever class.

receptor *(sensory)* A specialized cell that transduces environmental energy into an electrical signal. Examples include photoreceptors in the retina (light), pain receptors in the skin (damage), and hair cells in the inner ear (vibration).

reductionism The view that complex natural processes can be studied using simplified model systems in which as many variables as possible are controlled by the experimenter.

resting tremor Shaking of a limb or portion of a limb at rest that tends to decrease with voluntary motion.

signal transduction The process of converting one form of information into another. In the nervous system, this is usually accomplished at a chemical synapse where the electrical signal in the axon causes the release of neurotransmitter molecules. The neurotransmitter then activates receptors on the target neuron, converting the chemical signal back into an electrical one. At the level of sensory receptors, signal transduction refers to a change from environmental to electrical signals (e.g., conversion of light energy into electrical activity in retinal photoreceptors).

sporadic ALS (sALS) ALS of unknown origin. Typically, this is distinguished from fALS, which is often thought to arise as the result of some genetic mutation.

stem cells Undifferentiated cells that can differentiate into specialized cells. There are two kinds of stem cell in mammals: embryonic and adult. Stem-cell therapies have been proposed for various diseases, including those that affect the nervous system. In this case, the goal is to have stem cells from either source differentiate into neurons to replace those lost to the disease.

steryl glucoside A subtype of steroid. A steryl molecule is composed of a tetracyclic structure, with the four carbon rings labeled A through D. An aliphatic side chain is often attached at the C-17 position. The glucoside consists of a glucose moiety (there can be more than one) at the C3 position.

***substantia nigra* (SN)** Part of the basal ganglia, a region in the midbrain, so named because of its black appearance, caused by the molecule neuromelanin. As neurons in the SN die off in Parkinson's disease, a loss of specific motor functions ensues.

synapse The connection between two neurons. Various types of synapse exist, but the most common is between the axon of one neuron and the processes (dendrites) or cell body (soma) of another. Neurotransmitters are released from the axon (pre-synaptic site) and diffuse across to the target neuron (post-synaptic site).

A specialized form of synapse, the end plate, is the junction between motor neuron axons and muscle fibers. Electrical synapses also exist.

synergy The idea that the result of combining two or more elements is a greater response than that produced by the simple addition of the responses of the individual elements.

tangle *See* **neurofibrillary tangle (NFT).**

tardive Late onset. Can involve dyskinesias and dystonias. Parkinson's disease can be considered to have features of tardive dyskinesias. Tardive dyskinesias are characterized by involuntary, repetitive, purposeless movements, including of the facial muscles and limbs.

tau protein The major protein that makes up NFT, found in some degenerating nerve cells. Tau is normally involved in maintaining the structure of neuronal microtubules. In Alzheimer's disease, tau protein is abnormally processed and phosphorylated, forming NFTs, a hallmark feature of the disease.

Th1/Th2 The two types of T (thymus-derived) helper cell, each designed to eliminate different types of pathogen. Th1 cells produce interferon γ and act to stimulate the bactericidal actions of macrophages and to induce B cells to make complement-fixing antibodies. These responses are the basis of cell-mediated immunity. The Th2 response involves the release of interleukin 5 (IL-5), acting to induce eosinophils to clear parasites. It also produces IL-4, which facilitates B-cell isotype switching. In general, Th1 responses are directed against intracellular pathogens (viruses and bacteria), while Th2 responses act against extracellular bacteria, other pathogenic parasites, and toxins.

theory A well-substantiated explanation for some aspect of the natural world, based on evidence and careful reasoning, and encompassed in a large body of knowledge of the subject area.

toxin Strictly speaking, a toxin is any biological molecule that poisons or can harm cells. More general usage includes molecules such as heavy metals, aluminum, etc. Cytotoxins are those that cause harm to cells in general. Neurotoxins are those that are specifically harmful for neural cells. Excitotoxins such as glutamate or related amino acids specifically activate classes of glutamate receptors and lead to cell overstimulation, followed by cell death.

true narrative representation (TNR) Any event in which the general formula S π O applies, where S represents a signal, π the mapping of this signal, and O the object onto which S is mapped. The overall accuracy of a TNR reflects the accuracy of its parts.

vaccine An artificial means of stimulating an immune response against some pathogen that might cause infectious disease. Vaccines can use whole cells or viruses or partial cells or viruses to activate an immune response. When the cells or viruses are intact, they are typically killed or inactivated so that they cannot cause disease. Vaccine formulations that use only part of a cell or virus typically require the assistance of an adjuvant, or helper, to adequately activate the immune response. Various aluminum salts are used for this purpose.

References

Abel, E.L. (2007) Football increases the risk for Lou Gehrig's disease, amyotrophic lateral sclerosis. *Percept Mot Skills*, **104**(3 Pt. 2), 1251–1254.

Agmon-Levin, N., Paz, Z., Israeli, E. and Shoenfeld, Y. (2009) Vaccines and autoimmunity. *Nat Rev Rheumatol*, **5** (11), 648–652.

Ahmed, Z., Mackenzie, I.R., Hutton, M.L. and Dickson, D.W. (2007) Progranulin in frontotemporal lobar degeneration and neuroinflammation. *J Neuroinflammation*, **4** (7), 1–13.

Ahn, S.-W., Kim, J.-E., Sung, J.-J. *et al.* (2011) Asymmetry of motor unit number estimate and its rate of decline in patients with amyotrophic lateral sclerosis. *J Clin Neurophysiol*, **28** (5), 528–532.

Aisen, P.S., Gauthier, S., Ferris, S.H. *et al.* (2011) Tramiprosate in mild-to-moderate Alzheimer's disease – a randomized, double-blind, placebo-controlled, multi-centre study (the ALPHASE Study). *Arch Med Sci*, **7** (1), 102–111.

Akihisa, T., Kokke, W.C.M. and Tamura, T. (1991) Naturally occurring sterols and related compounds from plants, in *Physiology and Biochemistry of Sterols*, (eds G.W. Patterson and W.D. Nes), American Oil Chemist's Soceity, Champaign, IL, pp. 172–228).

Akiyama, H., Barger, S., Barnum, S. *et al.* (2000) Inflammation and Alzheimer's disease. *Neurobiol Aging*, **21** (3), 383–421.

Akushevich, I., Kravchenko, J., Ukraintseva, S. *et al.* (2013) Time trends of incidence of age-associated diseases in the US elderly population: Medicare-based analysis. *Age Ageing*, **42** (4), 494–500.

Al-Chalabi, A., Andersen, P.M., Nilsson, P. *et al.* (1999) Deletions of the heavy neurofilament subunit tail in amyotrophic lateral sclerosis. *Hum Mol Genet*, **8** (2), 157–164.

Al-Chalabi, A., Jones, A., Troakes, C. *et al.* (2012) The genetics and neuropathology of amyotrophic lateral sclerosis. *Acta Neuropathol*, **124** (3), 339–352.

Al-Saif, A., Al-Mohanna, F. and Bohlega, S. (2011) A mutation in sigma-1 receptor causes juvenile amyotrophic lateral sclerosis. *Ann Neurol*, **70** (6), 913–919.

Alfahad, T. and Nath, A. (2013) Retroviruses and amyotrophic lateral sclerosis. *Antiviral Res*, **99** (2), 180–187.

Alonso Vilatela, M.E., López-López, M. and Yescas-Gómez, P. (2012) Genetics of Alzheimer's disease. *Arch Med Res*, **43** (8), 622–631.

ALS Canada. (2013). 2013 annual report: power through collective action. Avaialable from: http://www.als.ca/sites/default/files/files/ALS%20Canada%202013%20Annual %20Report_Layout%201.pdf (last accessed September 23, 2016).

Alzheimer, A. (1906) Uber einen eigenartigen schweren Krankheitsprozess der Hirnrinde. *Zentralblatt fur Nervenkrankheiten*, **25**, 1134.

Alzheimer's Association (2014) 2014 Alzheimer's disease facts and figures. *Alzheimers Dement*, **10** (2), e47–e92.

Alzheimer's Association (2015a) 2015 Alzheimer's disease facts and figures. *Alzheimers Dement*, **11** (3), 332–384.

Alzheimer's Association. (2015b). What is Alzheimer's? Available from: http://www.alz.org/alzheimers_disease_what_is_alzheimers.asp (last accessed September 23, 2016).

Alzheimer's Society of Canada. (2010). *Rising Tide: The Impact of Dementia on Canadian Society.* Available from: http://www.alzheimer.ca/~/media/Files/national/Advocacy/ASC_Rising_Tide_Full_Report_e.pdf (last accessed September 23, 2016).

Alzheimer's Society of Canada. (2012). A new way of looking at the impact of dementia in Canada. Available from: http://www.beingblocked.com/wp/wp-content/uploads/2014/02/A-new-way-of-looking-at-the-impact-of-dementia-in-Canada.pdf (last accessed September 23, 2016).

American Psychiatric Association (2013) *Diagnostic and Statistical Manual of Mental Disorders*, (5 edn.). American Psychiatric Publishing, Arlington, VA.

Amtul, Z. and Rahman, A.-U. (2015) Naturaceuticals neuroprotect naturally, in *Studies in Natural Products Chemistry (Bioactive Natural Product)*, (ed. A.-U. Rahman), Elsevier, Oxford.

Andersen, P.M., Nilsson, P., Keranen, M.-L. *et al.* (1997) Phenotypic heterogeneity in motor neuron disease patients with CuZn-superoxide dismutase mutations in Scandinavia. *Brain*, **120**, 1723–1737.

Anderson, V., Spencer-Smith, M. and Wood, A. (2011) Do children really recover better? Neurobehavioural plasticity after early brain insult. *Brain*, **134** (8), 1297–2221.

Andersson, S., Gustafsson, N., Warner, M. and Gustafsson, J.-Å. (2005) Inactivation of liver X receptor β leads to adult-onset motor neuron degeneration in male mice. *Proc Natl Acad Sci U S A*, **102** (10), 3857–3862.

Andrási, E., Páli, N., Molnár, Z. and Kösel, S. (2005) Brain aluminum, magnesium and phosphorus contents of control and Alzheimer-diseased patients. *J Alzheimers Dis*, **7** (4), 273–284.

Andreose, J.S., Fumagalli, G. and Lømo, T. (1995) Number of junctional acetylcholine receptors: control by neural and muscular influences in the rat. *J Physiol*, **483** (2), 397–406.

Angelidou, A., Asadi, S., Alysandratos, K.-D. *et al.* (2012) Perinatal stress, brain inflammation and risk of autism – review and proposal. *BMC Pediatr*, **12** (1), 89.

Appel, S.H., Smith, R.G., Engelhardt, J.I. and Stefani, E. (1994) Evidence for autoimmunity in amyotrophic lateral sclerosis. *J Neurol Sci*, **124**(Suppl.), 14–19.

Aremu, D.A. and Meshitsuka, S. (2005) Accumulation of aluminum by primary cultured astrocytes from aluminum amino acid complex and its apoptotic effect. *Brain Res*, **1031** (2), 284–296.

Arendt, H. (2006) What is freedom? in *Between Past and Future: Eight Exercises in Political Thought*, (ed. H. Arendt), Penguin, New York.

Arrode-Brusés, G. and Brusés, J.L. (2012) Maternal immune activation by poly (I : C) induces expression of cytokines IL-1beta and IL-13, chemokine MCP-1 and colony stimulating factor VEGF in fetal mouse brain. *J Neuroinflammation*, **9** (8), 1–16.

Arseneault, L., Cannon, M., Fisher, H.L. *et al.* (2011) Childhood trauma and children's emerging psychotic symptoms: a genetically sensitive longitudinal cohort study. *Am J Psychiatry*, **168** (1), 65–72.

Asarnow, R.F. and Forsyth, J.K. (2013) Genetics of childhood-onset schizophrenia. *Child Adolesc Psychiatr Clin N Am*, **22** (4), 675–687.

Asarnow, R.F., Nuechterlein, K.H., Fogelson, D. *et al.* (2001) Schizophrenia and schizophrenia-spectrum personality disorders in the first-degree relatives of children with schizophrenia: the UCLA family study. *Arch Gen Psychiatry*, **58** (6), 581–588.

Ash, P.E.A., Zhang, Y.-J., Roberts, C.M. *et al.* (2010) Neurotoxic effects of TDP-43 overexpression in C. elegans. *Hum Mol Genet*, **19** (16), 3206–3218.

Ash, P.E.A., Bieniek, K.F., Gendron, T.F. *et al.* (2013) Unconventional translation of C9ORF72 GGGGCC expansion generates insoluble polypeptides specific to c9FTD/ALS. *Neuron*, **77** (4), 639.

Ashlock, M.A. and Olson, E.R. (2011) Therapeutics development for cystic fibrosis: a successful model for a multisystem genetic disease. *Annu Rev Med*, **62** (1), 107–125.

Ashwood, P. and van de Water, J. (2004) A review of autism and the immune response. *Clin Dev Immunol*, **11** (2), 165–174.

Ashwood, P., Wills, S. and Van de Water, J. (2006) The immune response in autism: a new frontier for autism research. *J Leukoc Biol*, **80** (1), 1–15.

Ashwood, P., Enstrom, A., Krakowiak, P. *et al.* (2008) Decreased transforming growth factor beta1 in autism: a potential link between immune dysregulation and impairment in clinical behavioral outcomes. *J Neuroimmunol*, **204** (1–2), 149–153.

Ashwood, P., Krakowiak, P., Hertz-Picciotto, I. *et al.* (2011) Altered T cell responses in children with autism. *Brain Behav Immun*, **25** (5), 840–849.

Assous, M., Had-Aissouni, L., Gubellini, P. *et al.* (2014) Progressive parkinsonism by acute dysfunction of excitatory amino acid transporters in the rat substantia nigra. *Neurobiol Dis*, **65**, 69–81.

Atladóttir, H., Thorsen, P., Østergaard, L. *et al.* (2010) Maternal infection requiring hospitalization during pregnancy and autism spectrum disorders. *J Autism Dev Disord*, **40** (12), 1423–1430.

Authier, F.-J., Cherin, P., Creange, A. *et al.* (2001) Central nervous system disease in patients with macrophagic myofasciitis. *Brain*, **124** (5), 974–983.

Azevedo, F.A.C., Carvalho, L.R.B., Grinberg, L.T. *et al.* (2009) Equal numbers of neuronal and nonneuronal cells make the human brain an isometrically scaled-up primate brain. *J Comp Neurol*, **513** (5), 532–541.

Bacchelli, E. and Maestrini, E. (2006) Autism spectrum disorders: molecular genetic advances. *Am J Med Genet C Semin Med Genet*, **142** (1), 13–23.

Bailey, A., Le Couteur, A., Gottesman, I. *et al.* (1995) Autism as a strongly genetic disorder: evidence from a British twin study. *Psychol Med*, **25** (01), 63–77.

Ballaban-Gil, K. and Tuchman, R. (2000) Epilepsy and epileptiform EEG: association with autism and language disorders. *Ment Retard Dev Disabil Res Rev*, **6** (4), 300–308.

Balzola, F., Clauser, D., Gandione, M. *et al.* (2005) Autistic enterocolitis: confirmation of a new inflammatory bowel disease in an Italian cohort of patients. *Gastroenterology*, **128** (4), A303–A303.

Banerjee, R., Starkov, A.A., Beal, M.F. and Thomas, B. (2009) Mitochondrial dysfunction in the limelight of Parkinson's disease pathogenesis. *Biochim Biophys Acta*, **1792** (7), 651–663.

Banjo, O. C. (2009). A Phenotypic and Neuropathological Assessment of the Impact of Fetal and Secondary Adult Re-exposure to Steryl Glucosides in Mice. MSc thesis. Vancouver: University of British Columbia.

Banjo, O. C., Kwok, D., Rosenberg, J. T., Gould, T. M., Grant, S. C., Swinton, P., and Shaw, C. A. (2009a). Fetal and secondary adult treatment with steryl glucosides produces differential behavioral and neuropathological outcomes ain male and female mice. 20th International Symposium on ALS/MND Abstract.

Banjo, O. C., Kwok, D., and Shaw, C. A. (2009b). Developmental and adult re-exposures to cycad steryl glucosides produce different pathological outcomes in male and female mice. Society for Neuroscience Abstract.

Barker, D.J.P. and Osmond, C. (1986) Infant mortality, chidhood nutrition, and ischaemic heart disease in England and Wales. *Lancet*, **327** (8489), 1077–1081.

Barker, R.A., Barrett, J., Mason, S.L. and Björklund, A. (2013) Fetal dopaminergic transplantation trials and the future of neural grafting in Parkinson's disease. *Lancet Neurol*, **12** (1), 84–91.

Barlow, B.K., Richfield, E.K., Cory-Slechta, D.A. and Thiruchelvam, M. (2004) A fetal risk factor for Parkinson's disease. *Dev Neurosci*, **26** (1), 11–23.

Barrientos, R.M., Frank, M.G., Watkins, L.R. and Maier, S.F. (2012) Aging-related changes in neuroimmune-endocrine function: implications for hippocampal-dependent cognition. *Horm Behav*, **62** (3), 219–227.

Bashan, A., Berezin, Y., Buldyrev, S.V. and Havlin, S. (2013) The extreme vulnerability of interdependent spatially embedded networks. *Nat Phys.*, doi: 10.1038/nphys2727

Bateman, A. and Bennett, H.P.J. (2009) The granulin gene family: from cancer to dementia. *BioEssays*, **31** (11), 1245–1254.

Bäumer, D., Hilton, D., Paine, S.M.L. *et al.* (2010) Juvenile ALS with basophilic inclusions is a FUS proteinopathy with FUS mutations. *Neurology*, **75** (7), 611–618.

Baxter . (2013). Baxter announces topline results of Phase III study of immunoglobulin for Alzheimer's disease. News Release, May 7. Available from: http://investor.baxter.com/phoenix.zhtml?c=86121&p=irol-newsArticle&ID=1816190 (last accessed September 23, 2016).

Bayer, T.A. (2015) Proteinopathies, a core concept for understanding and ultimately treating degenerative disorders? *Eur Neuropsychopharmacol*, **25** (5), 713–724.

Beers, D.R., Henkel, J.S., Zhao, W. *et al.* (2011) Endogenous regulatory T lymphocytes ameliorate amyotrophic lateral sclerosis in mice and correlate with disease progression in patients with amyotrophic lateral sclerosis. *Brain*, **134** (5), 1293–1314.

Behari, M. and Shrivastava, M. (2013) Role of platelets in neurodegenerative diseases: a universal pathophysiology. *Int J Neurosci*, **123** (5), 287–299.

Bekris, L.M., Yu, C.-E., Bird, T.D. and Tsuang, D.W. (2010) Review article: genetics of Alzheimer disease. *J Geriatr Psychiatry Neurol*, **23** (4), 213–227.

Bell, E.A. and O'Donovan, J.P. (1966) The isolation of α- and γ-oxalyl derivatives of α,γ-diaminobutyric acid from seeds of *Lathyrus latifolius*, and the detection of the α-oxalyl isomer of the neurotoxin α-amino-β-oxalylaminopropionic acid which occurs together with the neurotoxin in this and other species. *Phytochemistry*, **5** (6), 1211–1219.

Bell, R. and Zlokovic, B. (2009) Neurovascular mechanisms and blood–brain barrier disorder in Alzheimer's disease. *Acta Neuropathol*, **118** (1), 103–113.

Bellingham, M.C. (2011) A review of the neural mechanisms of action and clinical efficiency of riluzole in treating amyotrophic lateral sclerosis: what have we learned in the last decade? *CNS Neurosci Ther*, **17** (1), 4–31.

Belmonte, M.K., Allen, G., Beckel-Mitchener, A. *et al.* (2004) Autism and abnormal development of brain connectivity. *J Neurosci*, **24** (42), 9228–9231.

Belzung, C. and Lemoine, M. (2011) Criteria of validity for animal models of psychiatric disorders: focus on anxiety disorders and depression. *Biol Mood Anxiety Disord*, **1**, 9.

Benabid, A.L., Pollak, P., Louveau, A. *et al.* (1987) Combined (thalamotomy and stimulation) stereotactic surgery of the VIM thalamic nucleus for bilateral Parkinson disease. *Appl Neurophysiol*, **50** (1–6), 344–346.

Benabid, A.L., Chabardes, S., Torres, N. *et al.* (2009) Functional neurosurgery for movement disorders: a historical perspective. *Prog Brain Res*, **175**, 379–391.

Ben-Ari, Y. (2008) Neuro-archaeology: pre-symptomatic architecture and signature of neurological disorders. *Trends Neurosci*, **31** (12), 626–636.

Bennett, C. M., Baird, A. A., Miller, M. B., and Wolford, G. L. (2009). Neural correlates of interspecies perspective taking in the post-mortem Atlantic salmon: an argument for proper multiple comparisons correction. 15th Annual Meeting of the Organization for Human Brain Mapping Abstract.

Bergeron, C. and Steele, J.C. (1990) Guam Parkinson-dementia complex and amyotrophic lateral sclerosis. A clinico-pathological study of seven cases, in *Amyotrophic Lateral Sclerosis. New Advances in Toxicology and Epidemiology*, (eds F.C. Rose and F.H. Norris), Smith-Gordon, London, pp. 89–98.

Besedovsky, H.O. and Rey, A.D. (2007) Physiology of psychoneuroimmunology: a personal view. *Brain Behav Immun*, **21** (1), 34–44.

Besedovsky, H.O. and Rey, A.D. (2008) Brain cytokines as integrators of the immune–neuroendocrine network, in *Handbook of Neurochemistry and Molecular Neurobiology: Neuroimmunology*, (eds A. Lajtha, A. Galoyan and H.O. Besedovsky), Springer, Vienna, pp. 3–17.

Besedovsky, H.O. and Rey, A.D. (2011) Central and peripheral cytokines mediate immune-brain connectivity. *Neurochem Res*, **36** (1), 1–6.

Betarbet, R., Sherer, T.B., MacKenzie, G. *et al.* (2000) Chronic systemic pesticide exposure reproduces features of Parkinson's disease. *Nat Neurosci*, **3** (12), 1301–1306.

Betarbet, R., Sherer, T.B. and Greenamyre, J.T. (2002) Animal models of Parkinson's disease. *BioEssays*, **24** (4), 308–318.

Bhalla, U.S. and Iyengar, R. (1999) Emergent properties of networks of biological signaling pathways. *Science*, **283** (5400), 381–387.

Bharadwaj, P.R., Bates, K.A., Porter, T. *et al.* (2013) Latrepirdine: molecular mechanisms underlying potential therapeutic roles in Alzheimer's and other neurodegenerative diseases. *Transl Psychiatry*, **3**, e332.

Biagi, E., Candela, M., Turroni, S. *et al.* (2013) Ageing and gut microbes: perspectives for health maintenance and longevity. *Pharmacol Res*, **69** (1), 11–20.

Bierut, L.J., Goate, A.M., Breslau, N. *et al.* (2012) ADH1B is associated with alcohol dependence and alcohol consumption in populations of European and African ancestry. *Mol Psychiatry*, **17** (4), 445–450.

Bilbo, S.D., Biedenkapp, J.C., Der-Avakian, A. *et al.* (2005a) Neonatal infection-induced memory impairment after lipopolysaccharide in adulthood is prevented via caspase-1 inhibition. *J Neurosci*, **25** (35), 8000–8009.

Bilbo, S.D., Levkoff, L.H., Mahoney, J.H. *et al.* (2005b) Neonatal infection induces memory impairments following an immune challenge in adulthood. *Behav Neurosci*, **119** (1), 293–301.

Binetti, G., Signorini, S., Squitti, R. *et al.* (2003) Atypical dementia associated with a novel presenilin-2 mutation. *Ann Neurol*, **54** (6), 832–836.

Blaylock, R.L. (2012) Aluminum induced immunoexcitotoxicity in neurodevelopmental and neurodegenerative disorders. *Curr Inorg Chem*, **2** (1), 46–53.

Blaylock, R.L. and Maroon, J. (2011) Immunoexcitotoxicity as a central mechanism in chronic traumatic encephalopathy – A unifying hypothesis. *Surg Neurol Int*, **2**, 107.

Blaylock, R.L. and Strunecka, A. (2009) Immune-glutamatergic dysfunction as a central mechanism of the autism spectrum disorders. *Curr Med Chem*, **16** (2), 157–170.

Blesa, J., Juri, C., Collantes, M. *et al.* (2010) Progression of dopaminergic depletion in a model of MPTP-induced Parkinsonism in non-human primates. An 18F-DOPA and 11C-DTBZ PET study. *Neurobiol Dis*, **38** (3), 456–463.

Blizzard, C.A., Southam, K.A., Dawkins, E. *et al.* (2015) Identifying the primary site of pathogenesis in amyotrophic lateral sclerosis – vulnerability of lower motor neurons to proximal excitotoxicity. *Dis Model Mech*, **8** (3), 215–224.

Blum, D., Torch, S., Lambeng, N. *et al.* (2001) Molecular pathways involved in the neurotoxicity of 6-OHDA, dopamine and MPTP: contribution to the apoptotic theory in Parkinson's disease. *Prog Neurobiol*, **65** (2), 135–172.

Boissé, L., Mouihate, A., Ellis, S. and Pittman, Q.J. (2004) Long-term alterations in neuroimmune responses after neonatal exposure to lipopolysaccharide. *J Neurosci*, **24** (21), 4928–4934.

Bojinov, S. (1971) Encephalitis with acute parkinsonian syndrome and bilateral inflammatory necrosis of the substantia nigra. *J Neurol Sci*, **12** (4), 383–415.

Boll, W., Wagner, P. and Mantei, N. (1991) Structure of the chromosomal gene and cDNAs coding for lactase-phlorizin hydrolase in humans with adult-type hypolactasia or persistence of lactase. *Am J Hum Genet*, **48** (5), 889.

Bolognin, S., Messori, L., Drago, D. *et al.* (2011) Aluminum, copper, iron and zinc differentially alter amyloid-Aβ1–42 aggregation and toxicity. *Int J Biochem Cell Biol*, **43** (6), 877–885.

Bonaparte, J., Grant, I., Benstead, T. *et al.* (2007) ALS incidence in Nova Scotia over a 20-year-period: a prospective study. *Can J Neurol Sci*, **34** (1), 69–73.

Bonifati, V., Rizzu, P., van Baren, M.J. *et al.* (2003) Mutations in the DJ-1 gene associated with autosomal recessive early-onset parkinsonism. *Science*, **299** (5604), 256–259.

Borenstein, A.R., Mortimer, J.A., Schofield, E. *et al.* (2007) Cycad exposure and risk of dementia, MCI, and PDC in the Chamorro population of Guam. *Neurology*, **68** (21), 1764–1771.

Borgohain, R., Szasz, J., Stanzione, P. *et al.* (2014) Randomized trial of safinamide add-on to levodopa in Parkinson's disease with motor fluctuations. *Mov Disord*, **29** (2), 229–237.

Boulanger, L.M. (2009) Immune proteins in brain development and synaptic plasticity. *Neuron*, **64** (1), 93–109.

Bowler, J.V., Munoz, D.G., Merskey, H. and Hachinski, V. (1998) Factors affecting the age of onset and rate of progression of Alzheimer's disease. *J Neurol Neurosurg Psychiatr*, **65** (2), 184–190.

Bozik, M.E., Mitsumoto, H., Brooks, B.R. *et al.* (2014) A post hoc analysis of subgroup outcomes and creatinine in the phase III clinical trial (EMPOWER) of dexpramipexole in ALS. *Amyotroph Lateral Scler Frontotemporal Degener*, **15** (5–6), 406–413.

Braak, H. and Braak, E. (1990) Cognitive impairment in Parkinson's disease: amyloid plaques, neurofibrillary tangles, and neuropil threads in the cerebral cortex. *J Neural Transm Park Dis Dement Sect*, **2** (1), 45–57.

Braak, H. and Braak, E. (1991) Neuropathological stageing of Alzheimer-related changes. *Acta Neuropathol*, **82** (4), 239–259.

Braak, H., Tredici, K.D., Rüb, U. *et al.* (2003) Staging of brain pathology related to sporadic Parkinson's disease. *Neurobiol Aging*, **24** (2), 197–211.

Bradley, W.G., Borenstein, A.R., Nelson, L.M. *et al.* (2013) Is exposure to cyanobacteria an environmental risk factor for amyotrophic lateral sclerosis and other neurodegenerative diseases? *Amyotroph Lateral Scler Frontotemporal Degener*, **14** (5–6), 325–333.

Brent, B.K., Thermenos, H.W., Keshavan, M.S. and Seidman, L.J. (2013) Gray matter alterations in schizophrenia high-risk youth and early-onset schizophrenia: a review of structural MRI findings. *Child Adolesc Psychiatr Clin N Am*, **22** (4), 689–714.

Brice, A. (2005) Genetics of Parkinson's disease: LRRK2 on the rise. *Brain*, **128** (12), 2760–2762.

Brinkmann, J.R., Andres, P., Mendoza, M. and Sanjak, M. (1997) Guidelines for the use and performance of quantitative outcome measures in ALS clinical trials. *J Neurol Sci*, **147** (1), 97–111.

Brites, D. and Vaz, A.R. (2014) Microglia centered pathogenesis in ALS: insights in cell interconnectivity. *Front Cell Neurosci*, **8**, 117.

Broad Institute. (2014). Stanley Center for Psychiatric Research. Available from: https://www.broadinstitute.org/scientific-community/science/programs/psychiatric-disease/stanley-center-psychiatric-research/stanle (last accessed September 23, 2016).

Bronstein, J.M., Tagliati, M., Alterman, R.L. *et al.* (2011) Deep brain stimulation for Parkinson disease: an expert consensus and review of key issues. *Arch Neurol*, **68** (2), 165.

Brooks, B.R. (1994) El escorial World Federation of Neurology criteria for the diagnosis of amyotrophic lateral sclerosis. *J Neurol Sci*, **124**(Suppl.), 96–107.

Brooks, B.R., Miller, R.G., Swash, M. and Munsat, T.L. (2000) El Escorial revisited: revised criteria for the diagnosis of amyotrophic lateral sclerosis. *Amyotroph Lateral Scler*, **1** (5), 293–299.

Brown, A.S. and Derkits, E.J. (2010) Prenatal infection and schizophrenia: a review of epidemiologic and translational studies. *Am J Psychiatry*, **167** (3), 261–280.

Brown, J.R. and Hartwick, E.B. (1988) Influences of temperature, salinity and available food upon suspended culture of the Pacific oyster, *Crassotrea gigas*: I. Absolute and allometric growth. *Aquaculture*, **70** (3), 231–251.

Bruijn, L.I., Becher, M.W., Lee, M.K. *et al.* (1997) ALS-linked SOD1 mutant G85R mediates damage to astrocytes and promotes rapidly progressive disease with SOD1-containing inclusions. *Neuron*, **18** (2), 327–338.

Bruijn, L.I., Miller, T.M. and Cleveland, D.W. (2004) Unraveling the mechanisms involved in motor neuron degeneration in ALS. *Annu Rev Neurosci*, **27** (1), 723–749.

Brunner, R., Jensen-Jarolim, E. and Pali-Schöll, I. (2010) The ABC of clinical and experimental adjuvants – a brief overview. *Immunol Lett*, **128** (1), 29–35.

Buldyrev, S.V., Parshani, R., Paul, G. *et al.* (2010) Catastrophic cascade of failures in interdependent networks. *Nature*, **464** (7291), 1025–1028.

Buller, K.M. and Day, T.A. (2002) Systemic administration of interleukin-1β activates select populations of central amygdala afferents. *J Comp Neurol*, **452** (3), 288–296.

Burd, L. and Kerbeshian, J. (1987) A North Dakota prevalence study of schizophrenia presenting in childhood. *J Am Acad Child Adolesc Psychiatry*, **26** (3), 347–350.

Burnashev, N., Monyer, H., Seeburg, P.H. and Sakmann, B. (1992) Divalent ion permeability of AMPA receptor channels is dominated by the edited form of a single subunit. *Neuron*, **8** (1), 189–198.

Burns, T.C., Li, M.D., Mehta, S. *et al.* (2015) Mouse models rarely mimic the transcriptome of human neurodegenerative diseases: a systematic bioinformatics-based critique of preclinical models. *Eur J Pharmacol*, **759**, 101–117.

Burt, B.A. (1978) Influences for change in the dental health status of populations: an historical perspective. *J Public Health Dent*, **38** (4), 272–288.

Bush, V.J., Moyer, T.P., Batts, K.P. and Parisi, J.E. (1995) Essential and toxic element concentrations in fresh and formalin-fixed human autopsy tissues. *Clin Chem*, **41** (2), 284–294.

Byrne, S., Walsh, C., Lynch, C. *et al.* (2011) Rate of familial amyotrophic lateral sclerosis: a systematic review and meta-analysis. *J Neurol Neurosurg Psychiatr*, **82** (6), 623–627.

Bystron, I., Blakemore, C. and Rakic, P. (2008) Development of the human cerebral cortex: Boulder Committee revisited. *Nat Rev Neurosci*, **9** (2), 110–122.

Caller, T.A., Field, N.C., Chipman, J.W. *et al.* (2012) Spatial clustering of amyotrophic lateral sclerosis and the potential role of BMAA. *Amyotroph Lateral Scler*, **13** (1), 25–32.

Calne, D.B. and Eisen, A. (1989) The relationship between Alzheimer's disease, Parkinson's disease and motor neuron disease. *Can J Neurol Sci*, **16** (Suppl. 4), 547–550.

Campbell, A.K., Waud, J.P. and Matthews, S.B. (2009) The molecular basis of lactose intolerance. *Sci Prog*, **92** (3–4), 241–287.

Campbell, R.J., Steele, J.C., Cox, T.A. *et al.* (1993) Pathologic findings in the retinal pigment epitheliopathy associated with the amyotrophic lateral sclerosis/parkinsonism-dementia complex of Guam. *Ophthalmology*, **100** (1), 37–42.

Campion, D., Dumanchin, C., Hannequin, D. *et al.* (1999) Early-onset autosomal dominant Alzheimer disease: prevalence, genetic heterogeneity, and mutation spectrum. *Am J Hum Genet*, **65** (3), 664–670.

Canadian Institute for Health Information (2007) *The Burden of Neurological Diseases, Disorders and Injuries in Canada*, Canadian Institute for Health Information, Ottawa.

Cannon, J.G., Burton, R.A., Wood, S.G. and Owen, N.L. (2004) Naturally occurring fish poisons from plants. *J Chem Educ*, **81** (10), 1457.

Cannon, W.B. (1939) A law of denervation. *AM J Med Sci*, **198** (6), 737–749.

Cannon, W.B. and Rosenblueth, A. (1949) *The Supersensitivity of Denervated Structures: A Law of Denervation*, Macmillan, London.

Caparros-Lefebvre, D., Sergeant, N., Lees, A. *et al.* (2002) Guadeloupean parkinsonism: a cluster of progressive supranuclear palsy-like tauopathy. *Brain*, **125** (4), 801–811.

Catassi, C., Ratsch, I.-M., Gandolfi, L. *et al.* (1999) Why is coeliac disease endemic in the people of the Sahara? *Lancet*, **354** (9179), 647–648.

Cauwels, A., Vandendriessche, B. and Brouckaert, P. (2013) Of mice, men, and inflammation. *Proc Natl Acad Sci U S A*, **110** (34) E3150.

Cedarbaum, J.M., Stambler, N., Malta, E. *et al.* (1999) The ALSFRS-R: a revised ALS functional rating scale that incorporates assessments of respiratory function. *J Neurol Sci*, **169** (1–2), 13–21.

Centers for Disease Control and Prevention. (2016) Autism specturm disorder (ASD): data & statistics. Available from: http://www.cdc.gov/ncbddd/autism/data.html (last accessed September 23, 2016).

Charcot, J.M. (1865) Sclérose du cordons lateraux del la moelle épiniere chez une femme hysterique atteinte de contracture permaneste des quatres membres. *L' Union Med*, 451–457.

Charcot, J.M. (1880) Lecon sur les maladies du systeme nerveux faites a la Salpetriere. *Delahaye et Lecrosnier II*, **237**.

Chartier-Harlin, M.C., Dachsel, J.C., Vilariño-Güell, C. *et al.* (2011) Translation initiator EIF4G1 mutations in familial Parkinson disease. *Am J Hum Genet*, **89** (3), 398–406.

Chen, B., Girgis, S. and El-Matary, W. (2010) Childhood autism and eosinophilic colitis. *Digestion*, **81** (2), 127–129.

Chen, Y.-Z., Bennett, C.L., Huynh, H.M. *et al.* (2004) DNA/RNA helicase gene mutations in a form of juvenile amyotrophic lateral sclerosis (ALS4). *Am J Hum Genet*, **74** (6), 1128–1135.

Chen, Y., Yang, M., Deng, J. *et al.* (2011) Expression of human FUS protein in Drosophila leads to progressive neurodegeneration. *Protein Cell*, **2** (6), 477–486.

Cherry, J.D., Olschowka, J.A. and O'Banion, M.K. (2014) Are "resting" microglia more "M2"? *Front Immunol*, **5**, 594.

Chevalier-Larsen, E. and Holzbaur, E.L.F. (2006) Axonal transport and neurodegenerative disease. *Biochim Biophys Acta*, **1762** (11–12), 1094–1108.

The Children's Hospital of Philadelphia. (2013). Vaccine Education Center. Available from: http://vec.chop.edu/service/vaccine-education-center (last accessed September 23, 2016).

Chiò, A., Benzi, G., Dossena, M. *et al.* (2005) Severely increased risk of amyotrophic lateral sclerosis among Italian professional football players. *Brain*, **128** (3), 472–476.

Chiò, A., Calvo, A., Dossena, M. *et al.* (2009) ALS in Italian professional soccer players: the risk is still present and could be soccer-specific. *Amyotroph Lateral Scler*, **10** (4), 205–209.

Chiò, A., Calvo, A., Moglia, C., Mazzini, L., Mora, G., and PARALS Study Group (2011) Phenotypic heterogeneity of amyotrophic lateral sclerosis: a population based study. *J Neurol Neurosurg Psychiatr*, **82** (7), 740–746.

Chiò, A., Logroscino, G., Traynor, B.J. *et al.* (2013) Global epidemiology of amyotrophic lateral sclerosis: a systematic review of the published literature. *Neuroepidemiology*, **41** (2), 118–130.

Cho, I. and Blaser, M.J. (2012) The human microbiome: at the interface of health and disease. *Nat Rev Genet*, **13** (4), 260–270.

Chow, C.Y., Landers, J.E., Bergren, S.K. *et al.* (2009) Deleterious variants of FIG4, a phosphoinositide phosphatase, in patients with ALS. *Am J Hum Genet*, **84** (1), 85–88.

Chu, J., Thomas, L.M., Watkins, S.C. *et al.* (2009) Cholesterol-dependent cytolysins induce rapid release of mature IL-1β from murine macrophages in a NLRP3 inflammasome and cathepsin B-dependent manner. *J Leukoc Biol*, **86** (5), 1227–1238.

Chu, Y., Jin, X., Parada, I. *et al.* (2010) Enhanced synaptic connectivity and epilepsy in C1q knockout mice. *Proc Natl Acad Sci U S A*, **107** (17), 7975–7980.

Cifra, A., Mazzone, G.L. and Nistri, A. (2013) Riluzole: what it does to spinal and brainstem neurons and how it does it. *Neuroscientist*, **19** (2), 137–144.

Cirulli, E.T., Lasseigne, B.N., Petrovski, S. *et al.* (2015) Exome sequencing in amyotrophic lateral sclerosis identifies risk genes and pathways. *Science*, **347** (6229), 1436–1441.

Ciura, S., Lattante, S., Le Ber, I. *et al.* (2013) Loss of function of C9orf72 causes motor deficits in a zebrafish model of amyotrophic lateral sclerosis. *Ann Neurol*, **74** (2), 180–187.

Clancy, B., Finlay, B.L., Darlington, R.B. and Anand, K.J.S. (2007) Extrapolating brain development from experimental species to humans. *NeuroToxicology*, **28** (5), 931–937.

Clarke, G., Lumsden, C.J. and McInnes, R.R. (2001) Inherited neurodegenerative diseases: the one-hit model of neurodegeneration. *Hum Mol Genet*, **10** (20), 2269–2275.

Clement, A.M., Nguyen, M.D., Roberts, E.A. *et al.* (2003) Wild-type nonneuronal cells extend survival of SOD1 mutant motor neurons in ALS mice. *Science*, **302** (5642), 113–117.

Clowry, G.J., Moss, J.A. and Clough, R.L. (2005) An immunohistochemical study of the development of sensorimotor components of the early fetal human spinal cord. *J Anat*, **207** (4), 313–324.

Codolo, G., Plotegher, N., Pozzobon, T. *et al.* (2013) Triggering of inflammasome by aggregated α–synuclein, an inflammatory response in synucleinopathies. *PLoS ONE*, **8** (1) e55375.

Cohen, A.D. and Shoenfeld, Y. (1996) Vaccine-induced autoimmunity. *J Autoimmun*, **9** (6), 699–703.

Colton, C., Mott, R., Sharpe, H. *et al.* (2006) Expression profiles for macrophage alternative activation genes in AD and in mouse models of AD. *J Neuroinflammation*, **3** (1), 27.

Contag, C.H., Harty, J.T. and Plagemann, P.G. (1989) Dual virus etiology of age-dependent poliomyelitis of mice. A potential model for human motor neuron diseases. *Microb Pathog*, **6** (6), 391–401.

Conti, B., Tabarean, I., Andrei, C. and Bartfai, T. (2004) Cytokines and fever. *Front Biosci*, **9**, 1433–1449.

Cook, E.H., Lindgren, V., Leventhal, B.L. *et al.* (1997) Autism or atypical autism in maternally but not paternally derived proximal 15q duplication. *Am J Hum Genet*, **60** (4), 928–934.

Corcia, P., Mayeux-Portas, V., Khoris, J. *et al.* (2002) Abnormal SMN1 gene copy number is a susceptibility factor for amyotrophic lateral sclerosis. *Ann Neurol*, **51** (2), 243–246.

Corder, E., Saunders, A., Strittmatter, W. *et al.* (1993) Gene dose of apolipoprotein E type 4 allele and the risk of Alzheimer's disease in late onset families. *Science*, **261** (5123), 921–923.

Costa, J., Resende, C. and De Carvalho, M. (2003) Motor-axonal polyneuropathy associated with hepatitis C virus. *Eur J Neurol*, **10** (2), 183–185.

Costa, J., Swash, M. and de Carvalho, M. (2012) Awaji criteria for the diagnosis of amyotrophic lateral sclerosis: a systematic review. *Arch Neurol*, **69** (11), 1410–1416.

Costa, L.G. and Furlong, C.E. (2002) *Paraoxonase (PON1) in Health and Disease: Basic and Clinical Aspects*, Springer Science and Business Media, Medford, MA.

Cotzias, G.C., Papavasiliou, P., Ginos, J. *et al.* (1971) Metabolic modification of Parkinson's disease and of chronic manganese poisoning. *Annu Rev Med*, **22** (1), 305–326.

Cotzias, G.C., Papavasiliou, P.S., Mena, I. *et al.* (1974) Manganese and catecholamines. *Adv Neurol*, **5**, 235–243.

Couette, M., Boisse, M.-F., Maison, P. *et al.* (2009) Long-term persistence of vaccine-derived aluminum hydroxide is associated with chronic cognitive dysfunction. *J Inorg Biochem*, **103** (11), 1571–1578.

Cowley, M. and Oakey, R.J. (2013) Transposable elements re-wire and fine-tune the transcriptome. *PLoS Genet*, **9** (1) e1003234.

Cox, G. (2011). Are mice a good model for human ALS? 22nd International Symposium on ALS/MND Abstract.

Cox, P.A. and Sacks, O.W. (2002) Cycad neurotoxins, consumption of flying foxes, and ALS-PDC disease in Guam. *Neurology*, **58** (6), 956–959.

Cox, P.A., Davis, D.A., Mash, D.C. *et al.* (2016) Dietary exposure to an environmental toxin triggers neurofibrillary tangles and amyloid deposits in the brain. *Proc R Soc B*, **283** (1823).

Cox, T.A., McDarby, J.V., Lavine, L. *et al.* (1989) A retinopathy on Guam with high prevalence in Lytico-Bodig. *Ophthalmology*, **96** (12), 1731–1735.

Craft, S., Cholerton, B. and Baker, L.D. (2013) Insulin and Alzheimer's disease: untangling the web. *J Alzheimers Dis*, **33**, S263–S275.

Crépeaux, G., Eidi, H., David, M.-O. *et al.* (2015) Highly delayed systemic translocation of aluminum-based adjuvant in CD1 mice following intramuscular injections. *J Inorg Biochem*, **152**, 199–205.

Crépeaux, G., Eidi, H., David, M.-O., Baba-Amer, Y., Tzavara, E., Giros, B., et al. (in press, 2016). Non-linear dose-response of aluminium hydroxide adjuvant particles: selective low dose neurotoxicity. *Toxicology*.

Crick, F. and Koch, C. (2003) A framework for consciousness. *Nat Neurosci*, **6** (2), 119–126.

Cronin, S., Berger, S., Ding, J. *et al.* (2008) A genome-wide association study of sporadic ALS in a homogenous Irish population. *Hum Mol Genet*, **17** (5), 768–774.

Cruchaga, C., Karch, C.M., Jin, S.C. *et al.* (2014) Rare coding variants in the phospholipase D3 gene confer risk for Alzheimer's disease. *Nature*, **505** (7484), 550–554.

Cruts, M. and Van Broeckhoven, C. (2008) Loss of progranulin function in frontotemporal lobar degeneration. *Trend Genet*, **24** (4), 186–194.

Cruts, M., Theuns, J. and Van Broeckhoven, C. (2012) Locus-specific mutation databases for neurodegenerative brain diseases. *Hum Mutat*, **33** (9), 1340–1344.

Cruz-Aguado, R., Winkler, D. and Shaw, C.A. (2006) Lack of behavioral and neuropathological effects of dietary β-methylamino-l-alanine (BMAA) in mice. *Pharmacol Biochem Behav*, **84** (2), 294–299.

CTV News. (2015). Whole genome sequencing reveals, "each child with autism is like a snowflake." *CTV News*. Available from: http://www.ctvnews.ca/health/whole-genome-sequencing-reveals-each-child-with-autism-is-like-a-snowflake-1.2206000 (last accessed September 23, 2016).

Cudkowicz, M.E., Shefner, J.M., Schoenfeld, D.A. *et al.* (2006) Trial of celecoxib in amyotrophic lateral sclerosis. *Ann Neurol*, **60** (1), 22–31.

Cudkowicz, M.E., van den Berg, L.H., Shefner, J.M. *et al.* (2013) Dexpramipexole versus placebo for patients with amyotrophic lateral sclerosis (EMPOWER): a randomised, double-blind, phase 3 trial. *Lancet Neurol*, **12** (11), 1059–1067.

Cudkowicz, M.E., Titus, S., Kearney, M. *et al.* (2014) Safety and efficacy of ceftriaxone for amyotrophic lateral sclerosis: a multi-stage, randomised, double-blind, placebo-controlled trial. *Lancet Neurol*, **13** (11), 1083–1091.

Cummins, A.G. and Roberts-Thomson, I.C. (2009) Prevalence of celiac disease in the Asia–Pacific region. *J Gastroenterol Hepatol*, **24** (8), 1347–1351.

Curtis, B., Liberato, N., Rulien, M. *et al.* (2015) Examination of the safety of pediatric vaccine schedules in a non-human primate model: assessments of neurodevelopment, learning, and social behavior. *Environ Health Perspect*, **123**, 579–589.

The Cycad Pages. (1998–2012). Welcome to the intriguing world of cycads: survivors from before the dinosaurs! Royal Botanic Gardens Sydney. Available from: http://plantnet.rbgsyd.nsw.gov.au/PlantNet/cycad/ (last accessed September 23, 2016).

Czaplinski, A., Yen, A.A. and Appel, S.H. (2006) Forced vital capacity (FVC) as an indicator of survival and disease progression in an ALS clinic population. *J Neurol Neurosurg Psychiatr*, **77** (3), 390–392.

D'Andrea, M.R. (2005) Evidence that immunoglobulin-positive neurons in Alzheimer's disease are dying via the classical antibody-dependent complement pathway. *Am J Alzheimers Dis Other Demen*, **20** (3), 144–150.

D'Arcy, R.C.N., Lindsay, D.S., Song, X. *et al.* (2016) Long-term motor recovery after severe traumatic brain injury: beyond established limits. *J Head Trauma Rehabil*, **31** (5), E50–E58.

Dahlström, A., Wigander, A., Lundmark, K. *et al.* (1990) Investigations on auto-antibodies in Alzheimer's and Parkinson's diseases, using defined neuronal cultures, in *Neurotransmitter Actions and Interactions*, vol. **29**, (eds M.H. Youdim and K. Tipton), Springer, Vienna, pp. 195–206.

Dantzer, R. and Kelley, K.W. (2007) Twenty years of research on cytokine-induced sickness behavior. *Brain Behav Immun*, **21** (2), 153–160.

Dastur, D.K. (1964) Cycad toxicity in monkeys: clinical, pathological and biochemical aspects. *Fed Proc*, **23**, 1368–1369.

Dastur, D.K., Palekar, R. and Manghani, D. (1990) Toxicity of various forms of Cycas circinalis in rhesus monkeys – pathology of brain, spinal cord and liver, in *ALS. New Advances in Toxicology and Epidemiology*, (eds F.C. Rose and F.H. Norris), Smith Gordon, New York.

Dauer, W. and Przedborski, S. (2003) Parkinson's disease: mechanisms and models. *Neuron*, **39** (6), 889–909.

Davenward, S., Bentham, P., Wright, J. *et al.* (2013) Silicon-rich mineral water as a non-invasive test of the "aluminum hypothesis" in Alzheimer's disease. *J Alzheimers Dis*, **33**, 423–430.

David, S. and Kroner, A. (2011) Repertoire of microglial and macrophage responses after spinal cord injury. *Nat Rev Neurosci*, **12** (7), 388–399.

Davies, M.J., Spencer, A.J. and Slade, G.D. (1997) Trends in dental caries experience of school children in Australia – 1977 to 1993. *Aust Dent J*, **42** (6), 389–394.

Davis, E.P. and Granger, D.A. (2009) Developmental differences in infant salivary alpha-amylase and cortisol responses to stress. *Psychoneuroendocrinology*, **34** (6), 795–804.

Dawber, T.R., Meadors, G.F. and Moore, F.E. (1951) Epidemiological approaches to heart disease: the Framingham Study. *Am J Public Health Nations Health*, **41** (3), 279–286.

Dawber, T.R., Kannel, W.B., Revotskie, N. *et al.* (1959) Some factors associated with the development of coronary heart disease – six years' follow-up experience in the Framingham Study. *Am J Public Health Nations Health*, **49** (10), 1349–1356.

Dawber, T.R. (1980) *The Framingham Study: The Epidemiology of Atherosclerotic Disease*, Harvard University Press, Cambridge, MA.

de Carvalho, M., Dengler, R., Eisen, A. *et al.* (2008) Electrodiagnostic criteria for diagnosis of ALS. *Clin Neurophysiol*, **119** (3), 497–503.

de Jong, S.W., Huisman, M.H.B., Sutedja, N.A. *et al.* (2012) Smoking, alcohol consumption, and the risk of amyotrophic lateral sclerosis: a population-based study. *Am J Epidemiol*, **176** (3), 233–239.

de Munck, E., Muñoz-Sáez, E., Miguel, B.G. *et al.* (2013) β-N-methylamino-l-alanine causes neurological and pathological phenotypes mimicking Amyotrophic Lateral Sclerosis (ALS): the first step towards an experimental model for sporadic ALS. *Environ Toxicol Pharmacol*, **36** (2), 243–255.

De Muynck, L. and Van Damme, P. (2011) Cellular effects of progranulin in health and disease. *J Mol Neurosci*, **45** (3), 549–560.

De Strooper, B., Saftig, P., Craessaerts, K. *et al.* (1998) Deficiency of presenilin-1 inhibits the normal cleavage of amyloid precursor protein. *Nature*, **391** (6665), 387–390.

DeJesus-Hernandez, M., Mackenzie, I.R., Boeve, B.F. *et al.* (2011) Expanded GGGGCC hexanucleotide repeat in noncoding region of C9ORF72 causes chromosome 9p-linked FTD and ALS. *Neuron*, **72** (2), 245–256.

Del Tredici, K., Hawkes, C., Ghebremedhin, E. and Braak, H. (2010) Lewy pathology in the submandibular gland of individuals with incidental Lewy body disease and sporadic Parkinson's disease. *Acta Neuropathol*, **119** (6), 703–713.

Deng, H.-X., Chen, W., Hong, S.-T. *et al.* (2011) Mutations in UBQLN2 cause dominant X-linked juvenile and adult-onset ALS and ALS/dementia. *Nature*, **477** (7363), 211–215.

Denys, D. and Mantione, M. (2009) Deep brain stimulation in obsessive–compulsive disorder. *Prog Brain Res*, **175**, 419–427.

Deployment Health Working Group Research Subcommittee. (2001). Annual Report to Congress: Federally Sponsored Research on Gulf War Veterans' Illnesses for 1999. Available from: http://www.research.va.gov/pubs/docs/1999_gulf_war_illnesses.doc (last accessed September 23, 2016).

Derflinger, S., Sorg, C., Gaser, C. *et al.* (2011) Grey-matter atrophy in Alzheimer's disease is asymmetric but not lateralized. *J Alzheimers Dis*, **25** (2), 347–357.

DeStefano, A.L., Golbe, L.I., Mark, M.H. *et al.* (2001) Genome-wide scan for Parkinson's disease: the GenePD Study. *Neurology*, **57** (6), 1124–1126.

Deuschl, G., Schade-Brittinger, C., Krack, P. *et al.* (2006) A randomized trial of deep-brain stimulation for Parkinson's disease. *N Engl J Med*, **355** (9), 896–908.

Devine, M.S., Kiernan, M.C., Heggie, S. *et al.* (2014) Study of motor asymmetry in ALS indicates an effect of limb dominance on onset and spread of weakness, and an important role for upper motor neurons. *Amyotroph Lateral Scler Frontotemporal Degener*, **15** (7–8), 481–487.

Dewey, C.M., Cenik, B., Sephton, C.F. *et al.* (2012) TDP-43 aggregation in neurodegeneration: are stress granules the key? *Brain Res*, **1462**, 16–25.

Di Fede, G., Catania, M., Morbin, M. *et al.* (2009) A recessive mutation in the APP gene with dominant-negative effect on amyloidogenesis. *Science*, **323** (5920), 1473–1477.

Di Fonzo, A., Rohé, C.F., Ferreira, J. *et al.* (2005) A frequent LRRK2 gene mutation associated with autosomal dominant Parkinson's disease. *Lancet*, **365** (9457), 412–415.

Di Fonzo, A., Dekker, M.C.J., Montagna, P. *et al.* (2009) FBXO7 mutations cause autosomal recessive, early-onset parkinsonian-pyramidal syndrome. *Neurology*, **72** (3), 240–245.

Dietert, R.R. and Dietert, J.M. (2008) Potential for early-life immune insult including developmental immunotoxicity in autism and autism spectrum disorders: focus on critical windows of immune vulnerability. *J Toxicol Environ Health B*, **11** (8), 660–680.

Dinarello, C.A. (1999) Cytokines as endogenous pyrogens. *J Infect Dis*, **179** (Suppl. 2), S294–S304.

Do, C.B., Tung, J.Y., Dorfman, E. *et al.* (2011) Web-based genome-wide association study identifies two novel loci and a substantial genetic component for Parkinson's disease. *PLoS Genet*, **7** (6e1002141).

Döllken, V. (1897) Über die Wirkung des Aluminiums mit besonderer Berucksichtigung der durch das Aluminium verursachten Lasionen im Centralnervensystem. *Arch Exp Pathol Pharmacol*, 98–120.

Dominov, J.A., Uyan, Ö., Sapp, P.C. *et al.* (2014) A novel dysferlin mutant pseudoexon bypassed with antisense oligonucleotides. *Ann Clin Transl Neurol*, **1** (9), 703–720.

Doody, R.S., Raman, R., Farlow, M. *et al.* (2013) A phase 3 trial of semagacestat for treatment of Alzheimer's disease. *N Engl J Med*, **369** (4), 341–350.

Doody, R.S., Thomas, R.G., Farlow, M. *et al.* (2014) Phase 3 trials of solanezumab for mild-to-moderate Alzheimer's disease. *N Engl J Med*, **370** (4), 311–321.

Doty, R.L. (2012) Olfactory dysfunction in Parkinson disease. *Nat Rev Neurol*, **8** (6), 329–339.

Douglass, C.P., Kandler, R.H., Shaw, P.J. and McDermott, C.J. (2010) An evaluation of neurophysiological criteria used in the diagnosis of motor neuron disease. *J Neurol Neurosurg Psychiatr*, **81** (6), 646–649.

Douillet, P. and Orgogozo, J.M. (2009) What we have learned from the xaliproden Sanofi-aventis trials. *J Nutr Health Aging*, **13** (4), 365–366.

Dranoff, G. (2004) Cytokines in cancer pathogenesis and cancer therapy. *Nat Rev Cancer*, **4** (1), 11–22.

Droppelmann, C.A., Wang, J., Campos-Melo, D. *et al.* (2013) Detection of a novel frameshift mutation and regions with homozygosis within ARHGEF28 gene in familial amyotrophic lateral sclerosis. *Amyotroph Lateral Scler Frontotemporal Degener*, **14** (5–6), 444–451.

Du, X., Fleiss, B., Li, H. *et al.* (2011) Systemic stimulation of TLR2 impairs neonatal mouse brain development. *PLoS ONE*, **6** (5e19583).

Dubois, P.C., Trynka, G., Franke, L. *et al.* (2010) Multiple common variants for celiac disease influencing immune gene expression. *Nat Genet*, **42** (4), 295–302.

Dubový, P., Brázda, V., Klusáková, I. and Hradilová-Svíženská, I. (2013) Bilateral elevation of interleukin-6 protein and mRNA in both lumbar and cervical dorsal root ganglia following unilateral chronic compression injury of the sciatic nerve. *J Neuroinflammation*, **10** (55), 22.

Duesberg, P., Mandrioli, D., McCormack, A. and Nicholson, J.M. (2011) Is carcinogenesis a form of speciation? *Cell Cycle*, **10** (13), 2100–2114.

Duncan, J.A., Gao, X., Huang, M.T.-H. *et al.* (2009) Neisseria gonorrhoeae activates the proteinase cathepsin B to mediate the signaling activities of the NLRP3 and ASC-containing inflammasome. *J Immunol*, **182** (10), 6460–6469.

Duncan, M. (1991) Role of the cycad neurotoxin BMAA in the amyotrophic lateral sclerosi-parkisonism dementia complex of the western Pacific. *Adv Neurol*, **56**, 301–310.

Duncan, M., Marini, A., Watters, R. *et al.* (1992) Zinc, a neurotoxin to cultured neurons, contaminates cycad flour prepared by traditional guamanian methods. *J Neurosci*, **12** (4), 1523–1537.

Dunlop, R.A., Cox, P.A., Banack, S.A. and Rodgers, K.J. (2013) The non-protein amino acid BMAA is misincorporated into human proteins in place of l-serine causing protein misfolding and aggregation. *PLoS ONE*, **8** (9), e75376.

Dunn, A.J. (1995) Interactions between the nervous system and the immune system: implications for psychopharmacology, in *Psychopharmacology: The Fourth Generation of Progress*, 4 edn (eds F.E. Bloom and D.J. Kupfer), Lippincott Williams & Wilkins, Philadelphia, PA, pp. 719–733.

Dunn, A.J. (2006) Effects of cytokines and infections on brain neurochemistry. *Clin Neurosci Res*, **6** (1–2), 52–68.

Edenberg, H.J. (2007) The genetics of alcohol metabolism: role of alcohol dehydrogenase and aldehyde dehydrogenase variants. *Alcohol Res Health*, **30**, 5–13.

Edenberg, H.J. and Bosron, W.F. (2010) Alcohol dehydrogenases, in *Comprehensive Toxiclogy*, 2 edn (ed. C.A. McQueen), Elsevier, Oxford, pp. 111–130.

Edenberg, H.J. and Foroud, T. (2013) Genetics and alcoholism. *Nature Rev Gastroenterol Hepatol*, **10** (8), 487–494.

Edvardson, S., Cinnamon, Y., Ta-Shma, A. *et al.* (2012) A deleterious mutation in *DNAJC6* encoding the neuronal-specific clathrin-uncoating co-chaperone auxilin, is associated with juvenile parkinsonism. *PLoS ONE*, **7** (5) e36458.

Eftychiadis, A.C. and Chen, T.S.N. (2001) Saint Vitus and his dance. *J Neurol Neurosurg Psychiatr*, **70** (1), 14.

Ehlers, C.L., Spence, J.P., Wall, T.L. *et al.* (2004) Association of ALDH1 promoter polymorphisms with alcohol-related phenotypes in Southwest California Indians. *Alcohol Clin Exp Res*, **28** (10), 1481–1486.

Eisen, A. (2010). Prenatal origin of ALS. 2010 ALS Canada Research Forum Abstract.

Eisenbarth, S.C., Colegio, O.R., O'Connor, W. *et al.* (2008) Crucial role for the Nalp3 inflammasome in the immunostimulatory properties of aluminium adjuvants. *Nature*, **453** (7198), 1122–1126.

Elden, A.C., Kim, H.-J., Hart, M.P. *et al.* (2010) Ataxin-2 intermediate-length polyglutamine expansions are associated with increased risk for ALS. *Nature*, **466** (7310), 1069–1075.

Elenkov, I.J. and Chrousos, G.P. (1999) Stress hormones, Th1/Th2 patterns, pro/anti-inflammatory cytokines and susceptibility to disease. *Trends Endocrinol Metab*, **10** (9), 359–368.

Elenkov, I.J., Wilder, R.L., Chrousos, G.P. and Vizi, E.S. (2000) The sympathetic nerve – an integrative interface between two supersystems: the brain and the immune system. *Pharmacol Rev*, **52** (4), 595–638.

Elinder, C.G., Ahrengart, L., Lidums, V. *et al.* (1991) Evidence of aluminium accumulation in aluminium welders. *Br J Ind Med*, **48** (11), 735–738.

Elizan, T.S., Chen, K.-M., Mathai, K. *et al.* (1966) Amyotrophic lateral sclerosis and parkinsonism-dementia complex: a study in non-Chamorros of the Mariana and Caroline Islands. *Arch Neurol*, **14** (4), 347.

Eloe-Fadrosh, E.A. and Rasko, D.A. (2013) The human microbiome: from symbiosis to pathogenesis. *Annu Rev Med*, **64**, 145.

Enattah, N.S., Sahi, T., Savilahti, E. *et al.* (2002) Identification of a variant associated with adult-type hypolactasia. *Nat Genet*, **30** (2), 233–237.

Enattah, N.S., Jensen, T.G.K., Nielsen, M. *et al.* (2008) Independent introduction of two lactase-persistence alleles into human populations reflects different history of adaptation to milk culture. *Am J Hum Genet*, **82** (1), 57–72.

The ENCODE Project Consortium (2012) An integrated encyclopedia of DNA elements in the human genome. *Nature*, **489** (7414), 57–74.

Ertelt, D., Hemmelmann, C., Dettmers, C. *et al.* (2012) Observation and execution of upper-limb movements as a tool for rehabilitation of motor deficits in paretic stroke patients: protocol of a randomized clinical trial. *BMC Neurol*, **12**, 42.

Escott-Price, V.; International Parkinson's Disease Genomics Consortium, Nalls, M. A., Morris, H. R., Lubbe, S., Brice, A., et al (2015) Polygenic risk of Parkinson disease is correlated with disease age at onset. *Ann Neurol*, **77** (4), 582–591.

Eskandari, F., Webster, J.I. and Sternberg, E.M. (2003) Neural immune pathways and their connection to inflammatory diseases. *Arthritis Res Ther*, **5** (6), 251–265.

Exley, C. (2003) A biogeochemical cycle for aluminium? *J Inorg Biochem*, **97** (1), 1–7.

Exley, C. (2004) The pro-oxidant activity of aluminum. *Free Radic Biol Med*, **36** (3), 380–387.

Exley, C. (2009) Darwin, natural selection and the biological essentiality of aluminium and silicon. *Trends Biochem Sci*, **34** (12), 589–593.

Exley, C. (2012) The coordination chemistry of aluminium in neurodegenerative disease. *Coord Chem Rev*, **256** (19), 2142–2146.

Exley, C. and Esiri, M.M. (2006) Severe cerebral congophilic angiopathy coincident with increased brain aluminium in a resident of Camelford, Cornwall, UK. *J Neurol Neurosurg Psychiatr*, **77** (7), 877–879.

Exley, C., Burgess, E., Day, J.P. *et al.* (1996) Aluminum toxicokinetics. *J Toxicol Environ Health*, **48** (6), 569–584.

Exley, C., Siesjö, P. and Eriksson, H. (2010) The immunobiology of aluminium adjuvants: how do they really work? *Trend Immunol*, **31** (3), 103–109.

Fahn, S., Elton, R.L. and UPDRS program members (1987) Unified Parkinson's disease rating scale, in *Recent Developments in Parkinson's Disease*, vol. **2** (eds S. Fahn, C.D. Marsden, M. Goldstein and D.B. Calne), Macmillan Healthcare Information, Florham Park, NJ, pp. 153–163 293–304.

Fallat, R.J., Norris, F.H., Holden, D. *et al.* (1987) Respiratory monitoring and treatment: objective treatments using non-invasive measurements, in *Amyotrophic Lateral Sclerosis*, vol. **209**, (eds V. Cosi, A. Kato, W. Parlette *et al.*), Springer, New York, pp. 191–200.

Fecto, F., Yan, J., Vemula, S. *et al.* (2011) SQSTM1 mutations in familial and sporadic amyotrophic lateral sclerosis. *Arch Neurol*, **68** (11), 1440–1446.

Feldman, H.H., Doody, R.S., Kivipelto, M. *et al.* (2010) Randomized controlled trial of atorvastatin in mild to moderate Alzheimer disease: LEADe. *Neurology*, **74** (12), 956–964.

Fenn, A.M., Hall, J.C.E., Gensel, J.C. *et al.* (2014) IL-4 signaling drives a unique arginase+/IL-1β+ microglia phenotype and recruits macrophages to the inflammatory CNS: consequences of age-related deficits in IL-4Rα after traumatic spinal cord injury. *J Neurosci*, **34** (26), 8904–8917.

Ferraiuolo, L., Kirby, J., Grierson, A.J. *et al.* (2011) Molecular pathways of motor neuron injury in amyotrophic lateral sclerosis. *Nat Rev Neurol*, **7** (11), 616–630.

Ferrarese, C., Zoia, C., Pecora, N. *et al.* (1999) Reduced platelet glutamate uptake in Parkinson's disease. *J Neural Transm*, **106** (7–8), 685–692.

Figlewicz, D., Krizus, A., Martinoli, M.G. *et al.* (1994) Variants of the heavy neurofilament subunit are associated with the development of amyotrophic lateral sclerosis. *Hum Mol Genet*, **3** (10), 1757–1761.

Finkelstein, Y., Markowitz, M.E. and Rosen, J.F. (1998) Low-level lead-induced neurotoxicity in children: an update on central nervous system effects. *Brain Res Rev*, **27** (2), 168–176.

Fischer, J.A.B.A.J. and McCray, P.B. (2008) Innate immune functions of the airway epithelium. *Trends Innate Immun*, **15**, 147–163.

Fischer, L.R., Culver, D.G., Tennant, P. *et al.* (2004) Amyotrophic lateral sclerosis is a distal axonopathy: evidence in mice and man. *Exp Neurol*, **185** (2), 232–240.

Folstein, S. and Rutter, M. (1977) Infantile autism: a genetic study of 21 twin pairs. *J Child Psychol Psychiatry*, **18** (4), 297–321.

Fombonne, E. (1999) The epidemiology of autism: a review. *Psychol Med*, **29** (04), 769–786.

Fombonne, E. (2003) Epidemiological surveys of autism and other pervasive developmental disorders: an update. *J Autism Dev Disord*, **33** (4), 365–382.

Fox, S.H., Chuang, R. and Brotchie, J.M. (2008) Parkinson's disease – opportunities for novel therapeutics to reduce the problems of levodopa therapy, in *Progress in Brain*

Research, vol. **172**, (eds G. Di Giovanni, V. Di Matteo and E. Ennio), Elsevier, Oxford, pp. 479–494.

Franco, R., Li, S., Rodriguez-Rocha, H. *et al.* (2010) Molecular mechanisms of pesticide-induced neurotoxicity: relevance to Parkinson's disease. *Chem Biol Interact*, **188** (2), 289–300.

Frank, M.G., Miguel, Z.D., Watkins, L.R. and Maier, S.F. (2009) Prior exposure to glucocorticoids sensitizes the neuroinflammatory and peripheral inflammatory responses to E. coli lipopolysaccharide. *Brain Behav Immun*, **24** (1), 19–30.

Freischmidt, A., Wieland, T., Richter, B. *et al.* (2015) Haploinsufficiency of TBK1 causes familial ALS and fronto-temporal dementia. *Nat Neurosci*, **18** (5), 631–636.

Freitag, C., Staal, W., Klauck, S. *et al.* (2010) Genetics of autistic disorders: review and clinical implications. *Eur Child Adolesc Psychiatry*, **19** (3), 169–178.

Fujita, M., Ichise, M., Zoghbi, S.S. *et al.* (2006) Widespread decrease of nicotinic acetylcholine receptors in Parkinson's disease. *Ann Neurol*, **59** (1), 174–177.

Fukunishi, R. (1973) Acute hepatic lesions induced by cycasin. *Pathol Int*, **23** (3), 639–646.

Fullmer, H.M., Siedler, H.D., Krooth, R.S. and Kurland, L.T. (1960) A cutaneous disorder of connective tissue in amyotrophic lateral sclerosis: a histochemical study. *Neurology*, **10** (8), 717.

Fumimura, Y., Ikemura, M., Saito, Y. *et al.* (2007) Analysis of the adrenal gland is useful for evaluating pathology of the peripheral autonomic nervous system in Lewy body disease. *J Neuropathol Exp Neurol*, **66** (5), 354–362.

Funayama, M., Ohe, K., Amo, T. *et al.* (2015) CHCHD2 mutations in autosomal dominant late-onset Parkinson's disease: a genome-wide linkage and sequencing study. *Lancet Neurol*, **14** (3), 274–282.

Gajdusek, D.C. and Salazar, A.M. (1982) Amyotrophic lateral sclerosis and parkinsonian syndromes in high incidence among the Auyu and Jakai people of West New Guinea. *Neurology*, **32** (2), 107.

Galasko, D., Salmon, D.P., Craig, U.-K. *et al.* (2002) Clinical features and changing patterns of neurodegenerative disorders on Guam, 1997–2000. *Neurology*, **58** (1), 90–97.

Galic, M.A., Riazi, K., Heida, J.G. *et al.* (2008) Postnatal inflammation increases seizure susceptibility in adult rats. *J Neurosci*, **28** (27), 6904–6913.

Galic, M.A., Spencer, S.J., Mouihate, A. and Pittman, Q.J. (2009) Postnatal programming of the innate immune response. *Integr Comp Biol*, **49** (3), 237–245.

Garay, P.A. and McAllister, A.K. (2010) Novel roles for immune molecules in neural development: implications for neurodevelopmental disorders. *Front Synaptic Neurosci*, **2**, 136.

Garay, P.A., Hsiao, E.Y., Patterson, P.H. and McAllister, A.K. (2012) Maternal immune activation causes age- and region-specific changes in brain cytokines in offspring throughout development. *Brain Behav Immun*, **31** (0), 54–68.

Garcia, R.I. and Sohn, W. (2012) The paradigm shift to prevention and its relationship to dental education. *J Dent Educ*, **76** (1), 36–45.

Gardner, M.B. (1985) Retroviral spongiform polioencephalomyelopathy. *Rev Infect Dis*, 7 (1), 99–110.

Garruto, R.M. (1996) Early environment, long latency and slow progression of late onset neuro-degenerative disorders, in *Long-Term Consequences of Early Environment: Growth, Development, and the Lifespan Developmental Perspective*, (eds C.J.K. Henry and S.J. Ulijaszek), Cambridge University Press, Melbourne, p. 219.

Garruto, R.M., Shankar, S.K., Yanagihara, R. *et al.* (1989) Low-calcium, high-aluminum diet-induced motor neuron pathology in cynomolgus monkeys. *Acta Neuropathol*, **78** (2), 210–219.

Gendron, T. and Petrucelli, L. (2011) Rodent models of TDP-43 proteinopathy: investigating the mechanisms of TDP-43-mediated neurodegeneration. *J Mol Neurosci*, **45** (3), 486–499.

Gherardi, R. and Authier, F. (2012) Macrophagic myofasciitis: characterization and pathophysiology. *Lupus*, **21** (2), 184–189.

Gherardi, R., Coquet, M., Cherin, P. *et al.* (2001) Macrophagic myofasciitis lesions assess long-term persistence of vaccine-derived aluminium hydroxide in muscle. *Brain*, **124** (9), 1821–1831.

Giaccone, G., Morbin, M., Moda, F. *et al.* (2010) Neuropathology of the recessive A673V APP mutation: Alzheimer disease with distinctive features. *Acta Neuropathol*, **120** (6), 803–812.

Giasson, B.I., Duda, J.E., Quinn, S.M. *et al.* (2002) Neuronal α-synucleinopathy with severe movement disorder in mice expressing A53T human α-synuclein. *Neuron*, **34** (4), 521–533.

Gies, W.J. (1911) Some objections to the use of alum baking-powder. *JAMA*, **LVII** (10), 816–821.

Gigerenzer, G. and Goldstein, D.G. (1996) Mind as computer: birth of a metaphor. *Creat Res J*, **9** (2–3), 131–144.

Gijselinck, I., Van Langenhove, T., van der Zee, J. *et al.* (2012) A C9orf72 promoter repeat expansion in a Flanders-Belgian cohort with disorders of the frontotemporal lobar degeneration-amyotrophic lateral sclerosis spectrum: a gene identification study. *Lancet Neurol*, **11** (1), 54–65.

Gilli, M. and Rossier, E. (1981) Understanding complex systems. *Automatica*, **17** (4), 647–652.

Gillies, G.E., Pienaar, I.S., Vohra, S. and Qamhawi, Z. (2014) Sex differences in Parkinson's disease. *Front Neuroendocrinol*, **35** (3), 370–384.

Gitcho, M.A., Baloh, R.H., Chakraverty, S. *et al.* (2008) TDP-43 A315T mutation in familial motor neuron disease. *Ann Neurol*, **63** (4), 535–538.

Gitelman, H.J., Alderman, F.R., Kurs-Lasky, M. and Rockette, H.E. (1995) Serum and urinary aluminum levels of workers in the aluminum industry. *Ann Occup Hyg*, **39** (2), 181–191.

Gladman, M., Dharamshi, C. and Zinman, L. (2014) Economic burden of amyotrophic lateral sclerosis: a Canadian study of out-of-pocket expenses. *Amyotroph Lateral Scler Frontotemporal Degener*, **15** (5–6), 426–432.

Glasson, E.J., Bower, C., Petterson, B. *et al.* (2004) Perinatal factors and the development of autism: a population study. *Arch Gen Psychiatry*, **61** (6), 618–627.

Glover, J.C. (2008) Can we use human embryonic stem cells to treat brain and spinal cord injury and disease? in *Stem Cells, Human Embryos and Ethics*, (ed. L. Østnor), Springer, Vienna, pp. 55–70.

Glover, D. and Rhoads, D. (eds) (2006) *Environmental Guide for Congregations, Their Buildings, and Grounds*, Web of Creation. Available from: http://www.webofcreation .org/Environmental%20Guide.pdf (last accessed September 23, 2016).

Goate, A., Chartier-Harlin, M.-C., Mullan, M. *et al.* (1991) Segregation of a missense mutation in the amyloid precursor protein gene with familial Alzheimer's disease. *Nature*, **349** (6311), 704–706.

Goedert, M., Spillantini, M.G., Del Tredici, K. and Braak, H. (2013) 100 years of Lewy pathology. *Nat Rev Neurol*, **9** (1), 13–24.

Goetz, C.G., Poewe, W., Rascol, O. *et al.* (2004) Movement Disorder Society Task Force report on the Hoehn and Yahr staging scale: status and recommendations. *Mov Disord*, **19** (9), 1020–1028.

Goetz, C.G., Damier, P., Hicking, C. *et al.* (2007a) Sarizotan as a treatment for dyskinesias in Parkinson's disease: a double-blind placebo-controlled trial. *Mov Disord*, **22** (2), 179–186.

Goetz, C.G., Fahn, S., Martinez-Martin, P. *et al.* (2007b) Movement Disorder Society-sponsored revision of the Unified Parkinson's Disease Rating Scale (MDS-UPDRS): process, format, and clinimetric testing plan. *Mov Disord*, **22** (1), 41–47.

Goines, P.E. and Ashwood, P. (2012) Cytokine dysregulation in autism spectrum disorders (ASD): possible role of the environment. *Neurotoxicol Teratol*, **36**, 67–81.

Gold, M., Alderton, C., Zvartau-Hind, M. *et al.* (2009) Effects of rosiglitazone as monotherapy in APOE4-stratified subjects with mild-to-moderate Alzheimer's disease. *Alzheimers Dement*, **5** (Suppl. 4), 86.

Goldman, S.M. (2013) Environmental toxins and Parkinson's disease. *Pharmacol Toxicol*, **54**, 141–164.

Goldstein, R. A. (2015). Newron announces phase 2 clinical trial of sNN0029 (VEGF). January 27. Available from: http://blogs.als.net/post/Newron-Announces-Phase-2-Clinical-Trial-of-sNN0029-(VEGF).aspx?utm_source=contactologyandutm_medium=emailandutm_campaign=Feb2015MonthlyUpdate (last accessed September 23, 2016).

Gómez-Isla, T., Growdon, W.B., McNamara, M.J. *et al.* (1999) The impact of different presenilin 1 andpresenilin 2 mutations on amyloid deposition, neurofibrillary changes and neuronal loss in the familial Alzheimer's disease brain: evidence for other phenotype-modifying factors. *Brain*, **122** (9), 1709–1719.

Goodson, A., Robin, H., Summerfield, W. and Cooper, I. (2004) Migration of bisphenol A from can coatings – effects of damage, storage conditions and heating. *Food Addit Contam*, **21** (10), 1015–1026.

Gordon, P.H., Moore, D.H., Miller, R.G. *et al.* (2007) Efficacy of minocycline in patients with amyotrophic lateral sclerosis: a phase III randomised trial. *Lancet Neurol*, **6** (12), 1045–1053.

Gorrie, G.H., Fecto, F., Radzicki, D. *et al.* (2014) Dendritic spinopathy in transgenic mice expressing ALS/dementia-linked mutant UBQLN2. *Proc Natl Acad Sci U S A*, **111** (40), 14524–14529.

Gould, S.J. and Lewontin, R.C. (1979) The spandrels of San Marco and the Panglossian paradigm: a critique of the adaptationist programme. *Proc R Soc Lond B Biol Sci*, **205** (1161), 581–598.

Grad, L.I. and Cashman, N.R. (2014) Prion-like activity of Cu/Zn superoxide dismutase. *Prion*, **8** (1), 33–41.

Grad, L.I., Fernando, S.M. and Cashman, N.R. (2015) From molecule to molecule and cell to cell: prion-like mechanisms in amyotrophic lateral sclerosis. *Neurobiol Dis*, **77**, 257–265.

Graf, M., Ecker, D., Horowski, R. *et al.* (2005) High dose vitamin E therapy in amyotrophic lateral sclerosis as add-on therapy to riluzole: results of a placebo-controlled double-blind study. *J Neural Transm*, **112** (5), 649–660.

Gray, M.T. and Woulfe, J.M. (2015) Striatal blood-brain barrier permeability in Parkinson's disease. *J Cereb Blood Flow Metab*, **35** (5), 747–750.

Greco, L., Romino, R., Coto, I. *et al.* (2002) The first large population based twin study of coeliac disease. *Gut*, **50** (5), 624–628.

Green, R.C., Schneider, L.S., Amato, D.A. *et al.* (2009) Effect of tarenflurbil on cognitive decline and activities of daily living in patients with mild Alzheimer disease: a randomized controlled trial. *JAMA*, **302** (23), 2557–2564.

Greenway, M.J., Alexander, M.D., Ennis, S. *et al.* (2004) A novel candidate region for ALS on chromosome 14q11.2. *Neurology*, **63** (10), 1936–1938.

Greenway, M.J., Andersen, P.M., Russ, C. *et al.* (2006) ANG mutations segregate with familial and "sporadic" amyotrophic lateral sclerosis. *Nat Genet*, **38** (4), 411–413.

Griesenbach, U., McLachlan, G., Owaki, T. *et al.* (2011) Validation of recombinant Sendai virus in a non-natural host model. *Gene Ther*, **18** (2), 182–188.

Griesmaier, E. and Keller, M. (2012) Glutamate receptors – prenatal insults, long-term consequences. *Pharmacol Biochem Behav*, **100** (4), 835–840.

Gros-Louis, F., Larivière, R., Gowing, G. *et al.* (2004) A frameshift deletion in peripherin gene associated with amyotrophic lateral sclerosis. *J Biol Chem*, **279** (44), 45951–45956.

Gross, R.E., Watts, R.L., Hauser, R.A. *et al.* (2011) Intrastriatal transplantation of microcarrier-bound human retinal pigment epithelial cells versus sham surgery in patients with advanced Parkinson's disease: a double-blind, randomised, controlled trial. *Lancet Neurol*, **10** (6), 509–519.

Grünblatt, E., Mandel, S., Jacob-Hirsch, J. *et al.* (2004) Gene expression profiling of parkinsonian substantia nigra pars compacta; alterations in ubiquitin-proteasome, heat shock protein, iron and oxidative stress regulated proteins, cell adhesion/cellular matrix and vesicle trafficking genes. *J Neural Transm*, **111** (12), 1543–1573.

Gryder, B., Nelson, C. and Shepard, S. (2013) Biosemiotic entropy of the genome: mutations and epigenetic imbalances resulting in cancer. *Entropy*, **15** (1), 234–261.

Guerreiro, R., Wojtas, A., Bras, J. *et al.* (2013) TREM2 variants in Alzheimer's disease. *N Engl J Med*, **368** (2), 117–127.

Guillette, E.A., Meza, M.M., Aquilar, M.G. *et al.* (1998) An anthropological approach to the evaluation of preschool children exposed to pesticides in Mexico. *Environ Health Perspect*, **106** (6), 347–353.

Gunnar, M.R. (1992) Reactivity of the hypothalamic-pituitary-adrenocortical system to stressors in normal infants and children. *Pediatrics*, **90** (3), 491–497.

Gunnar, M.R., Talge, N.M. and Herrera, A. (2009) Stressor paradigms in developmental studies: what does and does not work to produce mean increases in salivary cortisol. *Psychoneuroendocrinology*, **34** (7), 953–967.

Gurney, M., Pu, H., Chiu, A. *et al.* (1994) Motor neuron degeneration in mice that express a human Cu, Zn superoxide dismutase mutation. *Science*, **264** (5166), 1772–1775.

Hadano, S., Hand, C.K., Osuga, H. *et al.* (2001) A gene encoding a putative GTPase regulator is mutated in familial amyotrophic lateral sclerosis 2. *Nat Genet*, **29** (2), 166–173.

Hadlock, K.G., Miller, R.G., Jin, X. *et al.* (2004) Elevated rates of antibody reactivity to HML-2/Herv-K but not other endogenous retroviruses in ALS. *Neurology*, **62** (7), A37–A38.

Hales, C.N., Barker, D.J., Clark, P.M. *et al.* (1991) Fetal and infant growth and impaired glucose tolerance at age 64. *BMJ*, **303** (6809), 1019–1022.

Haley, R.W. (2003) Excess incidence of ALS in young Gulf War veterans. *Neurology*, **61** (6), 750–756.

Haley, R.W., Hom, J., Roland, P.S. *et al.* (1997) Evaluation of neurologic function in Gulf War veterans: a blinded case-control study. *JAMA*, **277** (3), 223–230.

Halle, A., Hornung, V., Petzold, G.C. *et al.* (2008) The NALP3 inflammasome is involved in the innate immune response to amyloid-[beta]. *Nat Immunol*, **9** (8), 857–865.

Hallett, P.J., Deleidi, M., Astradsson, A. *et al.* (2015) Successful function of autologous iPSC-derived dopamine neurons following transplantation in a non-human primate model of Parkinson's disease. *Cell Stem Cell*, **16** (3), 269–274.

Hallmayer, J., Cleveland, S., Torres, A. *et al.* (2011) Genetic heritability and shared environmental factors among twin pairs with autism. *Arch Gen Psychiatry*, **68** (11), 1095–1102.

Hamza, R.T., Hewedi, D.H. and Ismail, M.A. (2010a) Basal and adrenocorticotropic hormone stimulated plasma cortisol levels among Egyptian autistic children: relation to disease severity. *Ital J Pediatr*, **36**, 71.

Hamza, T.H., Zabetian, C.P., Tenesa, A. *et al.* (2010b) Common genetic variation in the HLA region is associated with late-onset sporadic Parkinson's disease. *Nat Genet*, **42** (9), 781–785.

Hansen, S.N., Schendel, D.E. and Parner, E.T. (2015) Explaining the increase in the prevalence of autism spectrum disorders: the proportion attributable to changes in reporting practices. *JAMA Pediatr*, **169** (1), 56–62.

Hardiman, O., van den Berg, L.H. and Kiernan, M.C. (2011) Clinical diagnosis and management of amyotrophic lateral sclerosis. *Nat Rev Neurol*, **7** (11), 639–649.

Harms, M.B. and Baloh, R.H. (2013) Clinical neurogenetics: amyotrophic lateral sclerosis. *Neurol Clin*, **31** (4), 929–950.

Harold, D., Abraham, R., Hollingworth, P. *et al.* (2009) Genome-wide association study identifies variants at CLU and PICALM associated with Alzheimer's disease. *Nat Genet*, **41** (10), 1088–1093.

Hauser, R.A., Hsu, A., Kell, S. *et al.* (2013) Extended-release carbidopa-levodopa (IPX066) compared with immediate-release carbidopa-levodopa in patients with Parkinson's disease and motor fluctuations: a phase 3 randomised, double-blind trial. *Lancet Neurol*, **12** (4), 346–356.

Hawkes, C. (2003) Olfaction in neurodegenerative disorder. *Mov Disord*, **18** (4), 364–372.

Hawkes, D., Benhamu, J., Sidwell, T. *et al.* (2015) Revisiting adverse reactions to vaccines: a critical appraisal of Autoimmune Syndrome Induced by Adjuvants (ASIA). *J Autoimmun*, **59**, 77–84.

He, B.P. and Strong, M.J. (2000) Motor neuronal death in sporadic amyotrophic lateral sclerosis (ALS) is not apoptotic. A comparative study of ALS and chronic aluminium chloride neurotoxicity in New Zealand white rabbits. *Neuropathol Appl Neurobiol*, **26** (2), 150–160.

He, Z. and Bateman, A. (2003) Progranulin (granulin-epithelin precursor, PC-cell-derived growth factor, acrogranin) mediates tissue repair and tumorigenesis. *J Mol Med*, **81** (10), 600–612.

Hebert, L.E., Weuve, J., Scherr, P.A. and Evans, D.A. (2013) Alzheimer disease in the United States (2010–2050) estimated using the 2010 census. *Neurology*, **80** (19), 1778–1783.

Hemmer, B., Glocker, F., Kaiser, R. *et al.* (1997) Generalised motor neuron disease as an unusual manifestation of Borrelia burgdorferi infection. *J Neurol Neurosurg Psychiatr*, **63** (2), 257–258.

Heneka, M.T., Kummer, M.P., Stutz, A. *et al.* (2013) NLRP3 is activated in Alzheimer's disease and contributes to pathology in APP/PS1 mice. *Nature*, **493** (7434), 674–678.

Heneka, M.T., Carson, M.J., Khoury, J.E. *et al.* (2015) Neuroinflammation in Alzheimer's disease. *Lancet Neurol*, **14** (4), 388–405.

Herbert, M.R., Ziegler, D.A., Deutsch, C.K. *et al.* (2003) Dissociations of cerebral cortex, subcortical and cerebral white matter volumes in autistic boys. *Brain*, **126** (5), 1182–1192.

Hertz-Picciotto, I., Park, H.-Y., Dostal, M. *et al.* (2008) Prenatal exposures to persistent and non-persistent organic compounds and effects on immune system development. *Basic Clin Pharmacol Toxicol*, **102** (2), 146–154.

Hewitson, L., Lopresti, B.J., Stott, C. *et al.* (2010) Influence of pediatric vaccines on amygdala growth and opioid ligand binding in rhesus macaque infants: a pilot study. *Acta Neurobiol Exp (Wars)*, **70** (2), 147–164.

Hill, A.B. (1965) The environment and disease: association or causation? *Proc R Soc Med*, **58** (5), 295–300.

Hirano, A., Kurland, L.T., Krooth, R.S. and Lessell, S. (1961) Parkinsonism-dementia complex, an endemic disease on the island of Guam. I. Clinical features. *Brain*, **84** (4), 642–661.

Hjalgrim, L.L., Westergaard, T., Rostgaard, K. *et al.* (2003) Birth weight as a risk factor for childhood leukemia: a meta-analysis of 18 epidemiologic studies. *Am J Epidemiol*, **158** (8), 724–735.

Hobert, O., Johnston, R.J. and Chang, S. (2002) Left-right asymmetry in the nervous system: the Caenorhabditis elegans model. *Nat Rev Neurosci*, **3** (8), 629–640.

Hoegen, T., Tremel, N., Klein, M. *et al.* (2011) The NLRP3 inflammasome contributes to brain injury in pneumococcal meningitis and is activated through ATP-dependent lysosomal cathepsin B release. *J Immunol*, **187** (10), 5440–5451.

Hoehn, M.M. and Yahr, M.D. (1967) Parkinsonism: onset, progression, and mortality. *Neurology*, **17**, 427–442.

Hoeppner, M.P., White, S., Jeffares, D.C. and Poole, A.M. (2009) Evolutionarily stable association of intronic snoRNAs and microRNAs with their host genes. *Genome Biol Evol*, **1**, 420–428.

Hollingworth, P., Harold, D., Sims, R. *et al.* (2011) Common variants at ABCA7, MS4A6A/MS4A4E, EPHA1, CD33 and CD2AP are associated with Alzheimer's disease. *Nat Genet*, **43** (5), 429–435.

Holmes, G. (1909) The pathology of amyotrophic lateral sclerosis. *Rev Neurol Psychiatry*, **7**, 693–725.

Holzbaur, E.L.F., Howland, D.S., Weber, N. *et al.* (2006) Myostatin inhibition slows muscle atrophy in rodent models of amyotrophic lateral sclerosis. *Neurobiol Dis*, **23** (3), 697–707.

Hooli, B.V., Mohapatra, G., Mattheisen, M. *et al.* (2012) Role of common and rare APP DNA sequence variants in Alzheimer disease. *Neurology*, **78** (16), 1250–1257.

Hooten, K., Beers, D., Zhao, W. and Appel, S. (2015) Protective and toxic neuroinflammation in amyotrophic lateral sclerosis. *Neurotherapeutics*, **12** (2), 364–375.

Hornung, V., Bauernfeind, F., Halle, A. *et al.* (2008) Silica crystals and aluminum salts activate the NALP3 inflammasome through phagosomal destabilization. *Nat Immunol*, **9** (8), 847–856.

Hornykiewicz, O. and Kish, S.J. (1987) Biochemical pathophysiology of Parkinson's disease. *Adv Neurol*, **45**, 19–34.

Hosler, B.A., Siddique, T., Sapp, P.C. *et al.* (2000) Linkage of familial amyotrophic lateral sclerosis with frontotemporal dementia to chromosome 9q21-q22. *JAMA*, **284** (13), 1664–1669.

Hotopf, M., David, A., Hull, L. *et al.* (2000) Role of vaccinations as risk factors for ill health in veterans of the Gulf war: cross sectional study. *BMJ*, **320** (7246), 1363–1367.

Hsiao, E.Y., McBride, S.W., Chow, J. *et al.* (2012) Modeling an autism risk factor in mice leads to permanent immune dysregulation. *Proc Natl Acad Sci U S A*, **109** (31), 12776–12781.

Hsiao, E.Y., McBride, S.W., Hsien, S. *et al.* (2013) Microbiota modulate behavioral and physiological abnormalities associated with neurodevelopmental disorders. *Cell*, **155** (7), 1451–1463.

Hu, X., Li, P., Guo, Y. *et al.* (2012) Microglia/macrophage polarization dynamics reveal novel mechanism of injury expansion after focal cerebral ischemia. *Stroke*, **43** (11), 3063–3070.

Huang, C., Zhou, H., Tong, J. *et al.* (2011) FUS transgenic rats develop the phenotypes of amyotrophic lateral sclerosis and frontotemporal lobar degeneration. *PLoS Genet*, **7** (3) e1002011.

Huang, E., Strober, J., and Lomen-Hoerth, C. (2009). Demyelination and severe loss of spinal motor neurons following HPV vaccination. American Neurological Association 134th Annual Meeting Abstract.

Hubel, D.H. and Wiesel, T.N. (1962) Receptive fields, binocular interaction and functional architecture in the cat's visual cortex. *J Physiol*, **160** (1), 106–154.

Hüe, S., Mention, J.-J., Monteiro, R.C. *et al.* (2004) A direct role for NKG2D/MICA interaction in villous atrophy during celiac disease. *Immunity*, **21** (3), 367–377.

Hughes, A., Mann, D. and Pickering-Brown, S. (2003) Tau haplotype frequency in frontotemporal lobar degeneration and amyotrophic lateral sclerosis. *Exp Neurol*, **181** (1), 12–16.

Hughes, C.P., Berg, L., Danziger, W.L. *et al.* (1982) A new clinical scale for the staging of dementia. *Br J Psychiatry*, **140** (6), 566–572.

Hughes, J.T. (1982) Pathology of amyotrophic lateral sclerosis. *Adv Neurol*, **36**, 61–74.

Huh, G.S., Boulanger, L.M., Du, H. *et al.* (2000) Functional requirement for class I MHC in CNS development and plasticity. *Science*, **290** (5499), 2155–2159.

Hui, J., Hung, L.-H., Heiner, M. *et al.* (2005) Intronic CA-repeat and CA-rich elements: a new class of regulators of mammalian alternative splicing. *EMBO J*, **24** (11), 1988–1998.

Hunter, J.W., Mullen, G.P., McManus, J.R. *et al.* (2010) Neuroligin-deficient mutants of C. elegans have sensory processing deficits and are hypersensitive to oxidative stress and mercury toxicity. *Dis Model Mech*, **3** (5–6), 366–376.

Huntington, G. (1872) On chorea. *The Medical and Surgical Reporter: A Weekly Journal*, **26** (15), 317–321.

Hurd, M.D., Martorell, P., Delavande, A. *et al.* (2013) Monetary costs of dementia in the United States. *N Engl J Med*, **368** (14), 1326–1334.

Hurley, T.D. and Edenberg, H.J. (2012) Genes encoding enzymes involved in ethanol metabolism. *Alcohol Res*, **34** (3), 339–344.

Hyman, B.T. and Yuan, J. (2012) Apoptotic and non-apoptotic roles of caspases in neuronal physiology and pathophysiology. *Nat Rev Neurosci*, **13** (6), 395–406.

Hyman, S.E. (2012) *The Changing Global Neuroscience Ecosystem: Why it Matters to our Future*, Paper presented at the Society for Neuroscience, New Orleans.

Hyun, C.H., Yoon, C.Y., Lee, H.-J. and Lee, S.-J. (2013) LRRK2 as a potential genetic modifier of synucleinopathies: interlacing the two major genetic factors of Parkinson's disease. *Exp Neurobiol*, **22** (4), 249–257.

Ibi, D., Nagai, T., Kitahara, Y. *et al.* (2009) Neonatal polyI:C treatment in mice results in schizophrenia-like behavioral and neurochemical abnormalities in adulthood. *Neurosci Res*, **64** (3), 297–305.

Ichinohe, T., Lee, H.K., Ogura, Y. *et al.* (2009) Inflammasome recognition of influenza virus is essential for adaptive immune responses. *J Exp Med*, **206** (1), 79–87.

Iheozor-Ejiofor, Z., Worthington, H.V., Walsh, T. *et al.* (2015) Water fluoridation for the prevention of dental caries. *Cochrane Database Syst Rev*, **6**, CD010856.

Ikemura, M., Saito, Y., Sengoku, R. *et al.* (2008) Lewy body pathology involves cutaneous nerves. *J Neuropathol Exp Neurol*, **67** (10), 945–953.

Ingram, C.J., Elamin, M.F., Mulcare, C.A. *et al.* (2007) A novel polymorphism associated with lactose tolerance in Africa: multiple causes for lactase persistence? *Hum Genet*, **120** (6), 779–788.

Instituto Grifols. (2015). A study to evaluate albumin and immunoglobulin in Alzheimer's disease (AMBAR). Available from: https://clinicaltrials.gov/ct2/show/record/ NCT01561053?term=nct01561053andrank=1 (last accessed September 23, 2016).

International Parkinson Disease Genomics Consortium, Nalls, M. A., Plagnol, V., Hernandez, D. G., Sharma, M., Sheerin, U. M., et al (2011) Imputation of sequence variants for identification of genetic risks for Parkinson's disease: a meta-analysis of genome-wide association studies. *Lancet*, **377** (9766), 641–649.

International Parkinson Disease Genomics Consortium and Wellcome Trust Case Control Consortium 2 (2011) A two-stage meta-analysis identifies several new loci for Parkinson's disease. *PLoS Genet*, **7** (6) e1002142.

Ioannidis, J.P. (2005) Why most published research findings are false. *PLoS Med*, **2** (8e124).

Irwin, D., Lippa, C.F. and Swearer, J.M. (2007) Cognition and amyotrophic lateral sclerosis (ALS). *Am J Alzheimers Dis Other Demen*, **22** (4), 300–312.

Irwin, D., Lippa, C.F. and Rosso, A. (2009) Progranulin (PGRN) expression in ALS: an immunohistochemical study. *J Neurol Sci*, **276** (1–2), 9–13.

Israeli, E., Agmon-Levin, N., Blank, M. and Shoenfeld, Y. (2009) Adjuvants and autoimmunity. *Lupus*, **18** (13), 1217–1225.

Iwanaga, K., Wakabayashi, K., Yoshimoto, M. *et al.* (1999) Lewy body-type degeneration in cardiac plexus in Parkinson's and incidental Lewy body diseases. *Neurology*, **52** (6), 1269.

Jacobsen, L.K., Giedd, J.N., Vaituzis, A.C. *et al.* (1996) Temporal lobe morphology in childhood-onset schizophrenia. *Am J Psychiatry*, **153** (3), 355–361.

James, J. and Nordberg, A. (1995) Genetic and environmental aspects of the role of nicotinic receptors in neurodegenerative disorders: emphasis on Alzheimer's disease and Parkinson's disease. *Behav Genet*, **25** (2), 149–159.

Janeway, C.A., Travers, P., Walport, M. and Capra, J.D. (1999) *Immunobiology: The Immune System in Health and Disease*, vol. **157**, Current Biology Publications, New York.

Jansen, L.M., Gispen-de Wied, C.C., Van der Gaag, R.J. *et al.* (2000) Unresponsiveness to psychosocial stress in a subgroup of autistic-like children, multiple complex developmental disorder. *Psychoneuroendocrinology*, **25** (8), 753–764.

Jass, J.R. (2005) The intestinal lesion of autistic spectrum disorder. *Eur J Gastroenterol Hepatol*, **17** (8), 821–822.

Jenner, P. and Marsden, C.D. (1986) The actions of 1-methyl-4-phenyl-1,2,3,6-tetrahydropyridine in animals as a model of Parkinson's disease. *J Neural Transm Suppl*, **20**, 11–39.

Jia, J., Zhu, F., Ma, X. *et al.* (2009) Mechanisms of drug combinations: interaction and network perspectives. *Nat Rev Drug Discov*, **8** (2), 111–128.

Johnson, J.O., Mandrioli, J., Benatar, M. *et al.* (2010) Exome sequencing reveals VCP mutations as a cause of familial ALS. *Neuron*, **68** (5), 857–864.

Johnson, R. and Brooks, B. (1984) Possible viral etiology of amyotrophic lateral sclerosis. *Neuromuscul Dis*, 353–359.

Johnston, M.V. (1995) Neurotransmitters and vulnerability of the developing brain. *Brain and Development*, **17** (5), 301–306.

Jolicoeur, P., Nicolaiew, N., DesGroseillers, L. and Rassart, E. (1983) Molecular cloning of infectious viral DNA from ecotropic neurotropic wild mouse retrovirus. *J Virol*, **45** (3), 1159–1163.

Jones, S., Burt, B.A., Petersen, P.E. and Lennon, M.A. (2005) The effective use of fluorides in public health. *Bull World Health Organ*, **83**, 670–676.

Jonsson, P.A., Graffmo, K.S., Brännström, T. *et al.* (2006) Motor neuron disease in mice expressing the wild type-like D90A mutant superoxide dismutase-1. *J Neuropathol Exp Neurol*, **65** (12), 1126–1136.

Jonsson, T., Stefansson, H., Steinberg, S. *et al.* (2013) Variant of TREM2 associated with the risk of Alzheimer's disease. *N Engl J Med*, **368** (2), 107–116.

Joyce, P., Fratta, P., Fisher, E.C. and Acevedo-Arozena, A. (2011) SOD1 and TDP-43 animal models of amyotrophic lateral sclerosis: recent advances in understanding disease toward the development of clinical treatments. *Mamm Genome*, **22** (7–8), 420–448.

Just, M.A., Cherkassky, V.L., Keller, T.A. and Minshew, N.J. (2004) Cortical activation and synchronization during sentence comprehension in high-functioning autism: evidence of underconnectivity. *Brain*, **127** (8), 1811–1821.

Kabashi, E., Valdmanis, P.N., Dion, P. and Rouleau, G.A. (2007) Oxidized/misfolded superoxide dismutase-1: the cause of all amyotrophic lateral sclerosis? *Ann Neurol*, **62** (6), 553–559.

Kabashi, E., Valdmanis, P.N., Dion, P. *et al.* (2008) TARDBP mutations in individuals with sporadic and familial amyotrophic lateral sclerosis. *Nat Genet*, **40** (5), 572–574.

Kabashi, E., Lin, L., Tradewell, M.L. *et al.* (2010) Gain and loss of function of ALS-related mutations of TARDBP (TDP-43) cause motor deficits in vivo. *Hum Mol Genet*, **19** (4), 671–683.

Kannel, W.B. (2011) Sixty years of preventive cardiology: a Framingham perspective. *Clin Cardiol*, **34** (6), 342–343.

Karlik, S.J., Eichhorn, G.L., Lewis, P.N. and Crapper, D.R. (1980) Interaction of aluminum species with deoxyribonucleic acid. *Biochemistry*, **19** (26), 5991–5998.

Kato, S. (2008) Amyotrophic lateral sclerosis models and human neuropathology: similarities and differences. *Acta Neuropathol*, **115** (1), 97–114.

Keele University. (2015). Keele Meetings. Available from: http://www.keele.ac.uk/ aluminium/keelemeetings/ (last accessed September 23, 2016).

Keshavan, M.S. and Hogarty, G.E. (1999) Brain maturational processes and delayed onset in schizophrenia. *Dev Psychopathol*, **11** (03), 525–543.

Kett, L.R., Stiller, B., Bernath, M.M. *et al.* (2015) α-synuclein-independent histopathological and motor deficits in mice lacking the endolysosomal parkinsonism protein Atp13a2. *J Neurosci*, **35** (14), 5724–5742.

Khabazian, I., Bains, J.S., Williams, D.E. *et al.* (2002) Isolation of various forms of sterol β-D-glucoside from the seed of Cycas circinalis: neurotoxicity and implications for ALS-parkinsonism dementia complex. *J Neurochem*, **82** (3), 516–528.

Khan, Z., Combadiere, C., Authier, F.-J. *et al.* (2013) Slow CCL2-dependent translocation of biopersistent particles from muscle to brain. *BMC Med*, **11** (1), 99.

Kihira, T., Yoshida, S., Mitani, K. *et al.* (1993) ALS in the Kii Peninsula of Japan, with special reference to neurofibrillary tangles and aluminum. *Neuropathology*, **13** (2), 125–136.

Kim, C.-Y., Quarsten, H., Bergseng, E. *et al.* (2004) Structural basis for HLA-DQ2-mediated presentation of gluten epitopes in celiac disease. *Proc Natl Acad Sci U S A*, **101** (12), 4175–4179.

Kim, H.-J., Fan, X., Gabbi, C. *et al.* (2008) Liver X receptor β (LXRβ): a link between β-sitosterol and amyotrophic lateral sclerosis–Parkinson's dementia. *Proc Natl Acad Sci U S A*, **105** (6), 2094–2099.

Kim, H.J., Kim, N.C., Wang, Y.-D. *et al.* (2013) Mutations in prion-like domains in hnRNPA2B1 and hnRNPA1 cause multisystem proteinopathy and ALS. *Nature*, **495** (7442), 467–473.

Kim, Y.I., Lømo, T., Lupa, M.T. and Thesleff, S. (1984) Miniature end-plate potentials in rat skeletal muscle poisoned with botulinum toxin. *J Physiol*, **356** (1), 587–599.

Kimberly, W.T., LaVoie, M.J., Ostaszewski, B.L. *et al.* (2003) γ-Secretase is a membrane protein complex comprised of presenilin, nicastrin, aph-1, and pen-2. *Proc Natl Acad Sci U S A*, **100** (11), 6382–6387.

Kimura, F., Fujimura, C., Ishida, S. *et al.* (2006) Progression rate of ALSFRS-R at time of diagnosis predicts survival time in ALS. *Neurology*, **66** (2), 265–267.

Kinch, C.D., Ibhazehiebo, K., Jeong, J.-H. *et al.* (2015) Low-dose exposure to bisphenol A and replacement bisphenol S induces precocious hypothalamic neurogenesis in embryonic zebrafish. *Proc Natl Acad Sci U S A*, **112** (5), 1475–1480.

Kisby, G. (2000) β-N-methylamino-L-alanine, in *Experimental and Clinical Neurotoxicology*, 2 edn (eds P.S. Spencer, H.H. Schaumburg and A.C. Ludolph), Oxford University Press, Oxford.

Kisby, G., Kabel, H., Hugon, J. and Spencer, P.S. (1999) Damage and repair of nerve cell DNA in toxic stress. *Drug Metab Rev*, **31** (3), 589–618.

Kish, S.J., Shannak, K. and Hornykiewicz, O. (1988) Uneven pattern of dopamine loss in the striatum of patients with idiopathic Parkinson's disease. *N Engl J Med*, **318** (14), 876–880.

Kitada, T., Asakawa, S., Hattori, N. *et al.* (1998) Mutations in the parkin gene cause autosomal recessive juvenile parkinsonism. *Nature*, **392** (6676), 605–608.

Klauck, S.M. (2006) Genetics of autism spectrum disorder. *Eur J Hum Genet*, **14** (6), 714–720.

Kleinschnitz, C., Brinkhoff, J., Sommer, C. and Stoll, G. (2005) Contralateral cytokine gene induction after peripheral nerve lesions: dependence on the mode of injury and NMDA receptor signaling. *Mol Brain Res*, **136** (1–2), 23–28.

Kobayashi, A. (1972) Cycasin in cycad materials used in Japan. *Paper presented at the Federation proceedings.*

Koçer, A., Yaman, A., Niftaliyev, E. *et al.* (2013) Assessment of platelet indices in patients with neurodegenerative diseases: mean platelet volume was increased in patients with Parkinson's disease. *Curr Gerontol Geriatr Res*, **2013**, 986254.

Koch, A.L. (2003) Cell wall-deficient (CWD) bacterial pathogens: could amylotrophic lateral sclerosis (ALS) be due to one? *Crit Rev Microbiol*, **29** (3), 215–221.

Koch, C. (2012) *Consciousness: Confessions of a Romantic Reductionist*, MIT Press, Cambridge, MA.

Konat, G.W., Lally, B.E., Toth, A.A. and Salm, A.K. (2011) Peripheral immune challenge with viral mimic during early postnatal period robustly enhances anxiety-like behavior in young adult rats. *Metab Brain Dis*, **26** (3), 237–240.

Kovacs, D.M., Fausett, H.J., Page, K.J. *et al.* (1996) Alzheimer-associated presenilins 1 and 2: neuronal expression in brain and localization to intracellular membranes in mammalian cells. *Nat Med*, **2** (2), 224–229.

Koval, E.D., Shaner, C., Zhang, P. *et al.* (2013) Method for widespread microRNA-155 inhibition prolongs survival in ALS-model mice. *Hum Mol Genet*, **22** (20), 4127–4135.

Kowal, S.L., Dall, T.M., Chakrabarti, R. *et al.* (2013) The current and projected economic burden of Parkinson's disease in the United States. *Mov Disord*, **28** (3), 311–318.

Krebs, C.E., Karkheiran, S., Powell, J.C. *et al.* (2013) The Sac1 domain of SYNJ1 identified mutated in a family with early-onset progressive parkinsonism with generalized seizures. *Hum Mutat*, **34** (9), 1200–1207.

Krewski, D. (2014a) Systemic review of factors influencing the onset of neurological conditions, in *Neurological Health Charities Canada and Public Health Agency of Canada,* Mapping Connections: An Understanding of Neurological Conditions in Canada, The National Population Health Study of Neurological Conditions, Ottawa.

Krewski, D. (2014b) Systemic review of factors influencing the progression of neurological conditions, in *Neurological Health Charities Canada and Public Health Agency of Canada,* Mapping Connections: An Understanding of Neurological Conditions in Canada, The National Population Health Study of Neurological Conditions, Ottawa.

Krewski, D., Yokel, R.A., Nieboer, E. *et al.* (2007) Human health risk assessment for aluminium, aluminium oxide, and aluminium hydroxide. *J Toxicol Environ Health B*, **10** (Suppl. 1), 1–269.

Krieger, C., Hu, J.H. and Pelech, S. (2003) Aberrant protein kinases and phosphoproteins in amyotrophic lateral sclerosis. *Trends Pharmacol Sci*, **24** (10), 535–541.

Krooth, R.S., Macklin, M.T. and Hilbish, T.F. (1961) Diaphysial aclasis (multiple exotoses) on Guam. *Am J Hum Genet*, **13** (3), 340–347.

Kumar, R.A., KaraMohamed, S., Sudi, J. *et al.* (2008) Recurrent 16p11.2 microdeletions in autism. *Hum Mol Genet*, **17** (4), 628–638.

Kumra, S., Ashtari, M., Cervellione, K.L. *et al.* (2005) White matter abnormalities in early-onset schizophrenia: a voxel-based diffusion tensor imaging study. *J Am Acad Child Adolesc Psychiatry*, **44** (9), 934–941.

Kurakin, A. (2005) Self-organization vs. watchmaker: stochastic gene expression and cell differentiation. *Dev Genes Evol*, **215** (1), 46–52.

Kurland, L.T. (1972) An appraisal of the neurotoxicity of cycad and the etiology of amyotrophic lateral sclerosis on Guam. *Fed Proc*, **31** (5), 1540–1542.

Kurland, L.T. (1988) Amyotrophic lateral sclerosis and parkinson's disease complex on Guam linked to an environmental neurotoxin. *Trends Neurosci*, **11** (2), 51–54.

Kurland, L.T. and Mulder, D.W. (1954) Epidemiologic investigations of amyotrophic lateral sclerosis: 1. Preliminary report on geographic distribution, with special reference to the Mariana islands, including clinical and pathologic observations. *Neurology*, **4** (5), 355–355.

Kurosinski, P., Guggisberg, M. and Götz, J. (2002) Alzheimer's and Parkinson's disease – overlapping or synergistic pathologies? *Trends Mol Med*, **8** (1), 3–5.

Kwiatkowski, T.J., Bosco, D.A., LeClerc, A.L. *et al.* (2009) Mutations in the FUS/TLS gene on chromosome 16 cause familial amyotrophic lateral sclerosis. *Science*, **323** (5918), 1205–1208.

Labra, J., Menon, P., Byth, K. *et al.* (2016) Rate of disease progression: a prognostic biomarker in ALS. *J Neurol Neurosurg Psychiatr*, **87** (6), 628–632.

Ladd, A.N. and Cooper, T.A. (2002) Finding signals that regulate alternative splicing in the post-genomic era. *Genome Biol*, **3** (11), 1–16.

Lagier-Tourenne, C., Baughn, M., Rigo, F. *et al.* (2013) Targeted degradation of sense and antisense C9orf72 RNA foci as therapy for ALS and frontotemporal degeneration. *Proc Natl Acad Sci U S A*, **110** (47), E4530–E4539.

Lain, E., Carnejac, S., Escher, P. *et al.* (2009) A novel role for embigin to promote sprouting of motor nerve terminals at the neuromuscular junction. *J Biol Chem*, **284** (13), 8930–8939.

Lambert, J.-C., Ibrahim-Verbaas, C.A., Harold, D. *et al.* (2013) Meta-analysis of 74,046 individuals identifies 11 new susceptibility loci for Alzheimer's disease. *Nat Genet*, **45** (12), 1452–1458.

Lambrechts, D., Storkebaum, E., Morimoto, M. *et al.* (2003) VEGF is a modifier of amyotrophic lateral sclerosis in mice and humans and protects motoneurons against ischemic death. *Nat Genet*, **34** (4), 383–394.

Landers, J.E., Melki, J., Meininger, V. *et al.* (2009) Reduced expression of the Kinesin-Associated Protein 3 (KIFAP3) gene increases survival in sporadic amyotrophic lateral sclerosis. *Proc Natl Acad Sci U S A*, **106** (22), 9004–9009.

Landfield, P., Baskin, R. and Pitler, T. (1981) Brain aging correlates: retardation by hormonal-pharmacological treatments. *Science*, **214** (4520), 581–584.

Langston, J., Ballard, P., Tetrud, J. and Irwin, I. (1983) Chronic parkinsonism in humans due to a product of meperidine-analog synthesis. *Science*, **219** (4587), 979–980.

Lanson, N.A. and Pandey, U.B. (2012) FUS-related proteinopathies: lessons from animal models. *Brain Res*, **1462**, 44–60.

Larkindale, J., Yang, W., Hogan, P.F. *et al.* (2014) Cost of illness for neuromuscular diseases in the United States. *Muscle Nerve*, **49** (3), 431–438.

Lau, C., Rogers, J.M., Desai, M. and Ross, M.G. (2011) Fetal programming of adult disease: implications for prenatal care. *Obstet Gynecol*, **117** (4), 978–985.

Lauria, G., Dalla Bella, E., Antonini, G. *et al.* (2015) Erythropoietin in amyotrophic lateral sclerosis: a multicentre, randomised, double blind, placebo controlled, phase III study. *J Neurol Neurosurg Psychiatr*, **86** (8), 879–886.

Lauritsen, M.B., Als, T.D., Dahl, H.A. *et al.* (2005) A genome-wide search for alleles and haplotypes associated with autism and related pervasive developmental disorders on the Faroe Islands. *Mol Psychiatry*, **11** (1), 37–46.

Leblond, C.S., Kaneb, H.M., Dion, P.A. and Rouleau, G.A. (2014) Dissection of genetic factors associated with amyotrophic lateral sclerosis. *Exp Neurol*, **262** (B), 91–101.

Lederer, C.W., Torrisi, A., Pantelidou, M. *et al.* (2007) Pathways and genes differentially expressed in the motor cortex of patients with sporadic amyotrophic lateral sclerosis. *BMC Genomics*, **8**, 26.

Ledford, H. (2015). End of cancer-genome project prompts rethink. *Nature*. January 5. Available from: http://www.nature.com/news/end-of-cancer-genome-project-prompts-rethink-1.16662 (last accessed September 23, 2016).

Lee, A.L., Ogle, W.O. and Sapolsky, R.M. (2002) Stress and depression: possible links to neuron death in the hippocampus. *Bipolar disorders*, **4** (2), 117–128.

Lee, G. and Shaw, C.A. (2012) Early exposure to environmental toxin contributes to neuronal vulnerability and axonal pathology in familial ALS. *Neurosci Med*, **3** (4), 404–417.

Lee, G., Chu, T. and Shaw, C.A. (2009) The primary locus of motor neuron death in an ALS-PDC mouse model. *Neuroreport*, **20** (14), 1284.

Lee, Y.-B., Chen, H.-J., Peres, J.N. *et al.* (2013) Hexanucleotide repeats in ALS/FTD form length-dependent RNA foci, sequester RNA binding proteins, and are neurotoxic. *Cell Rep*, **5** (5), 1178–1186.

Lees, A., Fahn, S., Eggert, K.M. *et al.* (2012) Perampanel, an AMPA antagonist, found to have no benefit in reducing "off" time in Parkinson's disease. *Mov Disord*, **27** (2), 284–288.

Lehrer, J. (2010) The truth wears off. *New Yorker, December*, **13**, 52.

Lehrich, J.R., Oger, J. and Arnason, B.G. (1974) Neutralizing antibodies to poliovirus and mumps virus in amyotrophic lateral sclerosis. *J Neurol Sci*, **23** (4), 537–540.

Leinenga, G. and Götz, J. (2015) Scanning ultrasound removes amyloid-β and restores memory in an Alzheimer's disease mouse model. *Sci Transl Med*, **7** (278), 278ra233.

Leis, A.A., Stokic, D.S., Webb, R.M. *et al.* (2003) Clinical spectrum of muscle weakness in human West Nile virus infection. *Muscle Nerve*, **28** (3), 302–308.

Leiser, D. (2001) Scattered naive theories: why the human mind is isomorphic to the internet web. *New Ideas Psychol*, **19** (3), 175–202.

Lenglet, T., Lacomblez, L., Abitbol, J.L. *et al.* (2014) A phase II–III trial of olesoxime in subjects with amyotrophic lateral sclerosis. *Eur J Neurol*, **21** (3), 529–536.

Lévesque, L., Mizzen, C.A., McLachlan, D.R. and Fraser, P.E. (2000) Ligand specific effects on aluminum incorporation and toxicity in neurons and astrocytes. *Brain Res*, **877** (2), 191–202.

Levin, H.L. and Moran, J.V. (2011) Dynamic interactions between transposable elements and their hosts. *Nat Rev Genet*, **12** (9), 615–627.

Levin, M.C., Lee, S.M., Kalume, F. *et al.* (2002) Autoimmunity due to molecular mimicry as a cause of neurological disease. *Nat Med*, **8** (5), 509–513.

Levy, R., Shohat, L. and Solomon, B. (1998) Specificity of an anti-aluminium monoclonal antibody toward free and protein-bound aluminium. *J Inorg Biochem*, **69** (3), 159–163.

Levy-Lahad, E., Wijsman, E.M., Nemens, E. *et al.* (1995) A familial Alzheimer's disease locus on chromosome 1. *Science*, **269** (5226), 970–973.

Li, C. and Naren, A.P. (2005) Macromolecular complexes of cystic fibrosis transmembrane conductance regulator and its interacting partners. *Pharmacol Ther*, **108** (2), 208–223.

Li, D., Zhao, H. and Gelernter, J. (2011) Strong association of the alcohol dehydrogenase 1B gene (ADH1B) with alcohol dependence and alcohol-induced medical diseases. *Biol Psychiatry*, **70** (6), 504–512.

Li, D., Zhao, H. and Gelernter, J. (2012) Strong protective effect of the aldehyde dehydrogenase gene (ALDH2) 504lys (*2) allele against alcoholism and alcohol-induced medical diseases in Asians. *Hum Genet*, **131** (5), 725–737.

Li, D., Li, Y., and Shaw, C. A. (2015). Gene-toxin synergy in the brain of autistic mouse model. 11th Keele Meeting on Aluminum Abstract.

Li, D., Tomljenovic, L., Li, Y., and Shaw, C.A. (2017, in press) Activation of innate immune genes by aluminum injection in mouse brain. *J Inorg Biochem*.

Li, H., Nookala, S. and Re, F. (2007) Aluminum hydroxide adjuvants activate caspase-1 and induce IL-1β and IL-18 release. *J Immunol*, **178** (8), 5271–5276.

Li, H., Willingham, S.B., Ting, J.P.-Y. and Re, F. (2008) Cutting edge: inflammasome activation by alum and alum's adjuvant effect are mediated by NLRP3. *J Immunol*, **181** (1), 17–21.

Li, X.-B., Zheng, H., Zhang, Z.-R. *et al.* (2009) Glia activation induced by peripheral administration of aluminum oxide nanoparticles in rat brains. *Nanomedicine*, **5** (4), 473–479.

Li, Y., Ray, P., Rao, E.J. *et al.* (2010) A Drosophila model for TDP-43 proteinopathy. *Proc Natl Acad Sci U S A*, **107** (7), 3169–3174.

Lidsky, T.I. (2014) Is the aluminum hypothesis dead? *J Occup Environ Med*, **56** (Suppl. 5), S73–S79.

Lidsky, T.I. and Schneider, J.S. (2003) Lead neurotoxicity in children: basic mechanisms and clinical correlates. *Brain*, **126** (Pt. 1), 5–19.

Liu, H.-N., Sanelli, T., Horne, P. *et al.* (2009) Lack of evidence of monomer/misfolded superoxide dismutase-1 in sporadic amyotrophic lateral sclerosis. *Ann Neurol*, **66** (1), 75–80.

Liu, H.-N., Tjostheim, S., DaSilva, K. *et al.* (2012) Targeting of monomer/misfolded SOD1 as a therapeutic strategy for amyotrophic lateral sclerosis. *J Neurosci*, **32** (26), 8791–8799.

Lix, L.M., Hobson, D.E., Azimaee, M. *et al.* (2010) Socioeconomic variations in the prevalence and incidence of Parkinson's disease: a population-based analysis. *J Epidemiol Community Health*, **64** (4), 335–340.

Ljunggren, K.G., Lidums, V. and Sjögren, B. (1991) Blood and urine concentrations of aluminium among workers exposed to aluminium flake powders. *Br J Ind Med*, **48** (2), 106–109.

Louveau, A., Smirnov, I., Keyes, T.J. *et al.* (2015) Structural and functional features of central nervous system lymphatic vessels. *Nature*, **523** (7560), 337–341.

Lowe, J. (1994) New pathological findings in amyotrophic lateral sclerosis. *J Neurol Sci*, **124** (Suppl.), 38–51.

Ludvigsson, J.F., Montgomery, S.M., Ekbom, A. *et al.* (2009) Small-intestinal histopathology and mortality risk in celiac disease. *JAMA*, **302** (11), 1171–1178.

Luján, L., Pérez, M., Salazar, E. *et al.* (2013) Autoimmune/autoinflammatory syndrome induced by adjuvants (ASIA syndrome) in commercial sheep. *Immunol Res*, **56** (2–3), 317–324.

Lukiw, W. and Bazan, N. (2000) Neuroinflammatory signaling upregulation in Alzheimer's disease. *Neurochem Res*, **25** (9–10), 1173–1184.

Lukiw, W.J., Alexandrov, P.N., Zhao, Y. *et al.* (2012) Spreading of Alzheimer's disease inflammatory signaling through soluble micro-RNA. *NeuroReport*, **23** (10), 621–626.

Lundin, K.E.A., Scott, H., Hansen, T. *et al.* (1993) Gliadin-specific, HLA-DQ restricted T cells isolated from the small intestinal mucosa of coeliac disease patients. *J Exp Med*, **178**, 187–196.

Lundin, K.E.A., Scott, H., Fausa, O. *et al.* (1994) T cells from the small intestinal Mucosa of a DR4, DQ7/DR4. DQ8 celiac disease patient preferentially recognize gliadin when presented by DQ8. *Hum Immunol*, **41** (4), 285–291.

Luo, Y., Kuang, S.Y. and Hoffer, B. (2009) How useful are stem cells in PD therapy? *Parkinsonism Relat Disord*, **15**, S171–S175.

Mackenzie, I.R.A., Bigio, E.H., Ince, P.G. *et al.* (2007) Pathological TDP-43 distinguishes sporadic amyotrophic lateral sclerosis from amyotrophic lateral sclerosis with SOD1 mutations. *Ann Neurol*, **61** (5), 427–434.

Macmillan, M. and Lena, M.L. (2010) Rehabilitating Phineas Gage. *Neuropsychol Rehabil*, **20** (5), 641–658.

Majoor-Krakauer, D., Ottman, R., Johnson, W.G. and Rowland, L.P. (1994) Familial aggregation of amyotrophic lateral sclerosis, dementia, and Parkinson's disease: evidence of shared genetic susceptibility. *Neurology*, **44** (10), 1872.

Majounie, E., Renton, A.E., Mok, K. *et al.* (2012) Frequency of the C9orf72 hexanucleotide repeat expansion in patients with amyotrophic lateral sclerosis and frontotemporal dementia: a cross-sectional study. *Lancet Neurol*, **11** (4), 323–330.

Malekzadeh, R., Sachdev, A. and Fahid Ali, A. (2005) Coeliac disease in developing countries: Middle East, India and North Africa. *Best Pract Res Clin Gastroenterol*, **19** (3), 351–358.

Malkova, N.V., Yu, C.Z., Hsiao, E.Y. *et al.* (2012) Maternal immune activation yields offspring displaying mouse versions of the three core symptoms of autism. *Brain Behav Immun*, **26** (4), 607–616.

Mann, C.C. (2005) *1491: New Revelations of the Americas before Columbus*, Alfred A. Knopf, New York.

Marangi, G. and Traynor, B.J. (2015) Genetic causes of amyotrophic lateral sclerosis: new genetic analysis methodologies entailing new opportunities and challenges. *Brain Res*, **1607**, 75–93.

Mariathasan, S., Weiss, D.S., Newton, K. *et al.* (2006) Cryopyrin activates the inflammasome in response to toxins and ATP. *Nature*, **440** (7081), 228–232.

Marler, T.E., Lee, V., Chung, J. and Shaw, C.A. (2006) Steryl glucoside concentration declines with Cycas micronesica seed age. *Funct Plant Biol*, **33** (9), 857–862.

Marler, T.E., Snyder, L.R. and Shaw, C.A. (2010) Cycas micronesica (Cycadales) plants devoid of endophytic cyanobacteria increase in β-methylamino-l-alanine. *Toxicon*, **56** (4), 563–568.

Marsden, C.D. (1994) Problems with long-term levodopa therapy for Parkinson's disease. *Clin Neuropharmacol*, **17** (Suppl. 2), S32–44.

Martin, L.J., Pan, Y., Price, A.C. *et al.* (2006) Parkinson's disease α-synuclein transgenic mice develop neuronal mitochondrial degeneration and cell death. *J Neurosci*, **26** (1), 41–50.

Martinez, F.O. and Gordon, S. (2014) The M1 and M2 paradigm of macrophage activation: time for reassessment. *F1000Prime Rep*, **6**, 13.

Martinon, F., Petrilli, V., Mayor, A. *et al.* (2006) Gout-associated uric acid crystals activate the NALP3 inflammasome. *Nature*, **440** (7081), 237–241.

Maruyama, H., Morino, H., Ito, H. *et al.* (2010) Mutations of optineurin in amyotrophic lateral sclerosis. *Nature*, **465** (7295), 223–226.

Masliah, E., Rockenstein, E., Veinbergs, I. *et al.* (2000) Dopaminergic loss and inclusion body formation in α-synuclein mice: implications for neurodegenerative disorders. *Science*, **287** (5456), 1265–1269.

Maslowski, K.M. and Mackay, C.R. (2011) Diet, gut microbiota and immune responses. *Nat Immunol*, **12** (1), 5–9.

Matsumoto, H. and Strong, F.M. (1963) The occurrence of methylazoxymethanol in Cycas circinalis L. *Arch Biochem Biophys*, **101** (2), 299–310.

Matsuoka, Y., Vila, M., Lincoln, S. *et al.* (2001) Lack of nigral pathology in transgenic mice expressing human α-synuclein driven by the tyrosine hydroxylase promoter. *Neurobiol Dis*, **8** (3), 535–539.

Mattman, L.H. (2000) *Cell Wall Deficient Forms: Stealth Pathogens*, CRC Press, Boca Raton, FL.

Mattson, M.P. (2000) Apoptosis in neurodegenerative disorders. *Nat Rev Mol Cell Biol*, **1** (2), 120–130.

Matzilevich, D.A., Rall, J.M., Moore, A.N. *et al.* (2002) High-density microarray analysis of hippocampal gene expression following experimental brain injury. *J Neurosci Res*, **67** (5), 646–663.

Maynard, T.M., Sikich, L., Lieberman, J.A. and LaMantia, A.-S. (2001) Neural development, cell-cell signaling, and the "two-hit" hypothesis of schizophrenia. *Schizophr Bull*, **27** (3), 457–476.

McManus, R., Wilson, A.G., Mansfield, J. *et al.* (1996) TNF2, a polymorphism of the tumour necrosis-α gene promoter, is a component of the celiac disease major histocompatibility complex haplotype. *Eur J Immunol*, **26** (9), 2113–2118.

McDowell, I., Hill, G., Nilsson, T.H. and Kozma, A. (2000) The incidence of dementia in Canada. *Neurology*, **55**, 66.

McLachlan, D.R., Kruck, T.P., Lukiw, W.J. and Krishnan, S.S. (1991) Would decreased aluminum ingestion reduce the incidence of Alzheimer's disease? *CMAJ*, **145** (7), 793–804.

McNaught, K.S.P., Belizaire, R., Isacson, O. *et al.* (2003) Altered proteasomal function in sporadic Parkinson's disease. *Exp Neurol*, **179** (1), 38–46.

Movement Disorder Society. (2014). MDS-UPDRS. Available from: http://www .movementdisorders.org/MDS-Files1/PDFs/Rating-Scales/MDS-UPDRSfinal_Update .pdf (last accessed September 23, 2016).

Mega, M.S., Cummings, J.L., Fiorello, T. and Gornbein, J. (1996) The spectrum of behavioral changes in Alzheimer's disease. *Neurology*, **46** (1), 130–135.

Mehal, J.M., Holman, R.C., Schonberger, L.B. and Sejvar, J.J. (2013) Amyotrophic lateral sclerosis/motor neuron disease deaths in the United States, 1999–2009. *Amyotroph Lateral Scler Frontotemporal Degener*, **14** (5–6), 346–352.

Mehta, P., Antao, V., Kaye, W. *et al.* (2014) Prevalence of amyotrophic lateral sclerosis – United States, 2010–2011. *MMWR Surveill Summ*, **63** (Suppl. 7), 1–14.

Meininger, V., Bensimon, G., Bradley, W.R. *et al.* (2004) Efficacy and safety of xaliproden in amyotrophic lateral sclerosis: results of two phase III trials. *Amyotroph Lateral Scler Other Motor Neuron Disord*, **5** (2), 107–117.

Meininger, V., Asselain, B., Guillet, P. *et al.* (2006) Pentoxifylline in ALS: a double-blind, randomized, multicenter, placebo-controlled trial. *Neurology*, **66** (1), 88–92.

Meininger, V., Drory, V.E., Leigh, P.N. *et al.* (2009) Glatiramer acetate has no impact on disease progression in ALS at 40 mg/day: a double- blind, randomized, multicentre, placebo-controlled trial. *Amyotroph Lateral Scler*, **10** (5–6), 378–383.

Meissner, F., Molawi, K. and Zychlinsky, A. (2010) Mutant superoxide dismutase 1-induced IL-1β accelerates ALS pathogenesis. *Proc Natl Acad Sci U S A*, **107** (29), 13046–13050.

Meister, G. and Tuschl, T. (2004) Mechanisms of gene silencing by double-stranded RNA. *Nature*, **431** (7006), 343–349.

Mendes Soares, L.M. and Valcárcel, J. (2006) The expanding transcriptome: the genome as the "Book of Sand.". *EMBO J*, **25** (5), 923–931.

Merolla, P.A., Arthur, J.V., Alvarez-Icaza, R. *et al.* (2014) A million spiking-neuron integrated circuit with a scalable communication network and interface. *Science*, **345** (6197), 668–673.

Meroni, P.L. (2011) Autoimmune or auto-inflammatory syndrome induced by adjuvants (ASIA): old truths and a new syndrome? *J Autoimmun*, **36** (1), 1–3.

Mettler, F.A. and Stern, G.M. (1963) Observations on the toxic effects of yellow star thistle. *J Neuropathol Exp Neurol*, **22** (1), 164–169.

The Michael Stern Parkinson's Research Foundation. (2013). The economic impact of Parkinson's disease. Available from: https://web.archive.org/web/20130409115707/ http://www.parkinsoninfo.org/about-parkinsons-disease/economic-impact/ [archived] (last accessed September 23, 2016).

Michels, K.B., Trichopoulos, D., Robins, J.M. *et al.* (1996) Birthweight as a risk factor for breast cancer. *Lancet*, **348** (9041), 1542–1546.

Milane, A., Tortolano, L., Fernandez, C. *et al.* (2009) Brain and plasma riluzole pharmacokinetics: effect of minocycline combination. *J Pharm Pharm Sci*, **12** (2), 209–217.

Miles, J., Takahashi, T., Bagby, S. *et al.* (2005) Essential versus complex autism: definition of fundamental prognostic subtypes. *Am J Med Genet A*, **135** (2), 171–180.

Miller, R., Bradley, W., Cudkowicz, M. *et al.* (2007) Phase II/III randomized trial of TCH346 in patients with ALS. *Neurology*, **69** (8), 776–784.

Minami, S.S., Min, S.-W., Krabbe, G. *et al.* (2014) Progranulin protects against amyloid-beta deposition and toxicity in Alzheimer's disease mouse models. *Nat Med*, **20** (10), 1157–1164.

Minshall, C., Nadal, J. and Exley, C. (2014) Aluminium in human sweat. *J Trace Elem Med Biol*, **28** (1), 87–88.

Miocinovic, S., Somayajula, S., Chitnis, S. and Vitek, J.L. (2013) History, applications, and mechanisms of deep brain stimulation. *JAMA Neurol*, **70** (2), 163–171.

Miossec, L., Le Deuff, R., and Goulletquer, P. (2009). ICES Cooperative Research Report No. 299: Alien species alert: *Crassostrea gigas* (Pacific oyster). Available from: http://docs.lib.noaa.gov/noaa_documents/NOAA_related_docs/ICES_Report/CRR-299.pdf (last accessed September 23, 2016).

Mitchell, J., Paul, P., Chen, H.-J. *et al.* (2010) Familial amyotrophic lateral sclerosis is associated with a mutation in D-amino acid oxidase. *Proc Natl Acad Sci U S A*, **107** (16), 7556–7561.

Mitsumoto, H., Brooks, B.R. and Silani, V. (2014) Clinical trials in amyotrophic lateral sclerosis: why so many negative trials and how can trials be improved? *Lancet Neurol*, **13** (11), 1127–1138.

Mizielinska, S., Grönke, S., Niccoli, T. *et al.* (2014) C9orf72 repeat expansions cause neurodegeneration in Drosophila through arginine-rich proteins. *Science*, **345** (6201), 1192–1194.

Mizuno, Y., Kondo, T., and the Japanese Istradefylline Study, G (2013) Adenosine A2A receptor antagonist istradefylline reduces daily OFF time in Parkinson's disease. *Mov Disord*, **28** (8), 1138–1141.

Moisse, K., Volkening, K., Leystra-Lantz, C. *et al.* (2009) Divergent patterns of cytosolic TDP-43 and neuronal progranulin expression following axotomy: implications for TDP-43 in the physiological response to neuronal injury. *Brain Res*, **1249**, 202–211.

Molloy, C.A., Morrow, A.L., Meinzen-Derr, J. *et al.* (2006) Elevated cytokine levels in children with autism spectrum disorder. *J Neuroimmunol*, **172** (1–2), 198–205.

Monahan, A.J., Warren, M. and Carvey, P.M. (2008) Neuroinflammation and peripheral immune infiltration in Parkinson's disease: an autoimmune hypothesis. *Cell Transplant*, **17** (4), 363–372.

Mondal, T., Rasmussen, M., Pandey, G.K. *et al.* (2010) Characterization of the RNA content of chromatin. *Genome Res*, **20** (7), 899–907.

Monteys, A.M., Spengler, R.M., Wan, J. *et al.* (2010) Structure and activity of putative intronic miRNA promoters. *RNA*, **16** (3), 495–505.

Morrice J. R., Tomljenovic L., White R., Shaw C. A. (Scheduled 2017) A retrospective analysis of specific vaccines in relation to infectious disease incidence. In Shaw C.A. Editor, Lujan L. Editor, Dwoskin C. Editor, Tomljenovic L. Editor (Eds), *Controversies in Vaccine Safety: A critical review*, Elsevier, scheduled for publication in 2017.

Morris, H.R., Steele, J.C., Crook, R. *et al.* (2004) Genome-wide analysis of the parkinsonism-dementia complex of guam. *Arch Neurol*, **61** (12), 1889–1897.

Moser, H., Moser, A., Hollandsworth, K. *et al.* (2007) "Lorenzo's oil" therapy for X-linked adrenoleukodystrophy: rationale and current assessment of efficacy. *J Mol Neurosci*, **33** (1), 105–113.

Mosser, D.M. and Edwards, J.P. (2008) Exploring the full spectrum of macrophage activation. *Nat Rev Immunol*, **8** (12), 958–969.

Mueller, S., Saunier, K., Hanisch, C. *et al.* (2006) Differences in fecal microbiota in different european study populations in relation to age, gender, and country: a cross-sectional study. *Appl Environ Microbiol*, **72** (2), 1027–1033.

Mulcare, C.A., Weale, M.E., Jones, A.L. *et al.* (2004) The T allele of a single-nucleotide polymorphism 13.9 kb upstream of the lactase gene (LCT) (C−13.9kbT) does not predict or cause the lactase-persistence phenotype in Africans. *Am J Hum Genet*, **74** (6), 1102–1110.

Müller, W. and Schaltenbrand, G. (1979) Attempts to reproduce amyotrophic lateral sclerosis in laboratory animals by inoculation of Schu virus isolated from a patient with apparent amyotrophic lateral sclerosis. *J Neurol*, **220** (1), 1–19.

Münch, C., Sedlmeier, R., Meyer, T. *et al.* (2004) Point mutations of the p150 subunit of dynactin (DCTN1) gene in ALS. *Neurology*, **63** (4), 724–726.

Munson, J., Dawson, G., Abbott, R. *et al.* (2006) Amygdalar volume and behavioral development in autism. *Arch Gen Psychiatry*, **63** (6), 686–693.

Murata, M., Hasegawa, K. and Kanazawa, I. (2007) Zonisamide improves motor function in Parkinson disease: a randomized, double-blind study. *Neurology*, **68** (1), 45–50.

Murre, J.M.J. and Sturdy, D.P.F. (1995) The connectivity of the brain: multi-level quantitative analysis. *Biol. Cybern.*, **73** (6), 529–545.

Muslimovic, D., Post, B., Speelman, J.D. *et al.* (2009) Cognitive decline in Parkinson's disease: a prospective longitudinal study. *J Int Neuropsychol Soc*, **15** (3), 426–437.

Myrexis. (2008). Open-label treatment with MPC-7869 for patients with Alzheimer's who previously participated in an MPC-7869 Protocol. Available from: https://clinicaltrials.gov/ct2/show/NCT00380276?term=NCT00380276andrank=1 (last accessed September 23, 2016).

Nadeau, S. and Rivest, S. (2003) Glucocorticoids play a fundamental role in protecting the brain during innate immune response. *J Neurosci*, **23** (13), 5536–5544.

Naj, A.C., Jun, G., Beecham, G.W. *et al.* (2011) Common variants at MS4A4/MS4A6E, CD2AP, CD33 and EPHA1 are associated with late-onset Alzheimer's disease. *Nat Genet*, **43** (5), 436–441.

Nalls, M.A., Plagnol, V., Hernandez, D. *et al.* (2011) Imputation of sequence variants for identification of genetic risks for Parkinson's disease: a meta-analysis of genome-wide association studies. *Lancet*, **377** (9766), 641–649.

Nalls, M.A., Pankratz, N., Lill, C.M. *et al.* (2014) Large-scale meta-analysis of genome-wide association data identifies six new risk loci for Parkinson's disease. *Nat Genet*, **46** (9), 989–993.

The National Institute on Aging and Reagan Institute Working Group on Diagnostic Criteria for the Neuropathological Assessment of Alzheimer's Disease (1997) Consensus recommendations for the postmortem diagnosis of Alzheimer's disease. *Neurobiol Aging*, **18** (4 Suppl. 1), S1–S2.

Nature Neuroscience Editorial (2000) Mysterianism lite. *Nat Neurosci*, **3** (3), 199–199.

Nebert, D.W., Mckinnon, R.A. and Puga, A. (1996) Human drug-metabolizing enzyme polymorphisms: effects on risk of toxicity and cancer. *DNA and Cell Biol*, **15** (4), 273–280.

Neill, D. (2001) Maladaptive and dysfunctional synaptoplasticity in relation to Alzheimer's disease and schizophrenia, in *Toward a Theory of Neuroplasticity*, (eds C.A. Shaw and J. McEachern), Taylor and Francis, Philadelphia, PA.

Neumann, M., Sampathu, D.M., Kwong, L.K. *et al.* (2006) Ubiquitinated TDP-43 in frontotemporal lobar degeneration and amyotrophic lateral sclerosis. *Science*, **314** (5796), 130–133.

Neurological Health Charities Canada and Public Health Agency of Canada (2014) *Mapping Connections: An Understanding of Neurological Conditions in Canada*, The National Population Health Study of Neurological Conditions, Ottawa.

Nevison, C.D. (2014) A comparison of temporal trends in United States autism prevalence to treds in suspected environmental factors. *Environ Health*, **13** (1), 73.

Newschaffer, C.J., Croen, L.A., Daniels, J. *et al.* (2007) The epidemiology of autism spectrum disorders. *Annu Rev Public Health*, **28** (1), 235–258.

Nicholls, J.G., Martin, A.R., Fuchs, P.A. *et al.* (2012) *From Neuron to Brain*, 5 edn, Sinauer Associates, Sunderland, MA.

Nicolescu, R., Petcu, C., Cordeanu, A. *et al.* (2010) Environmental exposure to lead, but not other neurotoxic metals, relates to core elements of ADHD in Romanian children: performance and questionnaire data. *Environ Res*, **110** (5), 476–483.

Nishimura, A.L., Mitne-Neto, M., Silva, H.C.A. *et al.* (2004) A mutation in the vesicle-trafficking protein VAPB causes late-onset spinal muscular atrophy and amyotrophic lateral sclerosis. *Am J Hum Genet*, **75** (5), 822–831.

Nonneman, A., Robberecht, W. and Den Bosch, L.V. (2014) The role of oligodendroglial dysfunction in amyotrophic lateral sclerosis. *Neurodegenr Dis Manag*, **4** (3), 223–239.

Nunomura, A., Tamaoki, T., Motohashi, N. *et al.* (2012) The earliest stage of cognitive impairment in transition from normal aging to Alzheimer disease is marked by prominent RNA oxidation in vulnerable neurons. *J Neuropathol Exp Neurol*, **71** (3), 233–241.

Nurchi, V., Crisponi, G., Bertolasi, V. *et al.* (2012) Aluminium-dependent human diseases and chelating properties of aluminium chelators for biomedical applications, in *Metal Ions in Neurological Systems*, (eds W. Linert and H. Kozlowski), Springer, Vienna, pp. 103–123.

O'Brien, R. (2015). Amyloid-beta and Alzheimer's disease. Science of Aging: *The Buck Institute's Blog*. Available from: http://sage.buckinstitute.org/amyloid-beta-and-alzheimers-disease/ (last accessed September 23, 2016).

O'Donnell, C.J. and Elosua, R. (2008) Cardiovascular risk factors. Insights from Framingham Heart Study. *Revista Española de Cardiología (English Version)*, **61** (3), 299–310.

Ogata, A., Tashiro, K., Nukuzuma, S. *et al.* (1997) A rat model of Parkinson's disease induced by Japanese encephalitis virus. *J Neuroviol*, **3** (2), 141–147.

Ohno, S. (1972) So much "junk" DNA in our genome. *Brookhaven Symp Biol*, **23**, 366–370.

Oizumi, M., Albantakis, L. and Tononi, G. (2014) From the phenomenology to the mechanisms of consciousness: integrated information theory 3.0. *PLoS Comput Biol*, **10** (5) e1003588.

Okun, M.S., Fernandez, H.H., Wu, S.S. *et al.* (2009) Cognition and mood in Parkinson's disease in subthalamic nucleus versus globus pallidus interna deep brain stimulation: the COMPARE Trial. *Ann Neurol*, **65** (5), 586–595.

Olds, L.C. and Sibley, E. (2003) Lactase persistence DNA variant enhances lactase promoter activity in vitro: functional role as a cis regulatory element. *Hum Mol Genet*, **12** (18), 2333–2340.

Oller, J.W. (2013) Pragmatic information, in *Biological Information: New Perspectives*, (eds R. Marks, M. Behe, W. Dembski *et al.*), World Scientific, Singapore.

Oller, J.W. (2014) Biosemiotic entropy: concluding the series. *Entropy*, **16** (7), 4060–4087.

Olney, J.W. (1969) Brain lesions, obesity, and other disturbances in mice treated with monosodium glutamate. *Science*, **164** (3880), 719–721.

Olney, J.W., Zorumski, C., Price, M. and Labruyere, J. (1990) L-cysteine, a bicarbonate-sensitive endogenous excitotoxin. *Science*, **248** (4955), 596–599.

Ono, S., Imai, T., Takahashi, K. *et al.* (1999) Increased type III procollagen in serum and skin of patients with amyotrophic lateral sclerosis. *Acta Neurol Scand*, **100** (6), 377–384.

Orfila, M.J.B. (1814) *Traité des Poisons: tirés des regnes minéral, végétal et animal, ou Toxicologie générale, considerée sous les rapports de la physiologie, de la pathologie et de la médicine légale*, Chez Crochard, libraire, Paris.

Orlacchio, A., Babalini, C., Borreca, A. *et al.* (2010) SPATACSIN mutations cause autosomal recessive juvenile amyotrophic lateral sclerosis. *Brain*, **133** (2), 591–598.

Orton, S.-M., Herrera, B.M., Yee, I.M. *et al.* (2006) Sex ratio of multiple sclerosis in Canada: a longitudinal study. *Lancet Neurol*, **5** (11), 932–936.

Osier, M.V., Pakstis, A.J., Soodyall, H. *et al.* (2002) A global perspective on genetic variation at the ADH genes reveals unusual patterns of linkage disequilibrium and diversity. *Am J Hum Genet*, **71** (1), 84–99.

Oyinbo, C.A. (2011) Secondary injury mechanisms in traumatic spinal cord injury: a nugget of this multiply cascade. *Acta Neurobiol Exp*, **71** (2), 281–299.

Pagliusi, S.R., Gerrard, P., Abdallah, M. *et al.* (1994) Age-related changes in expression of ampa-selective glutamate receptor subunits: is calcium-permeability altered in hippocampal neurons? *Neuroscience*, **61** (3), 429–433.

Paisan-Ruiz, C., Bhatia, K.P., Li, A. *et al.* (2009) Characterization of PLA2G6 as a locus for dystonia-parkinsonism. *Ann Neurol*, **65** (1), 19–23.

Palazzo, A.F. and Gregory, T.R. (2014) The case for junk DNA. *PLoS Genet*, **10** (5) e1004351.

Palmer, C., Bik, E.M., DiGiulio, D.B. *et al.* (2007) Development of the human infant intestinal microbiota. *PLoS Biol*, **5** (7) e177.

Pankratz, N., Wilk, J., Latourelle, J. *et al.* (2009) Genomewide association study for susceptibility genes contributing to familial Parkinson disease. *Hum Genet*, **124** (6), 593–605.

Pankratz, N., Beecham, G.W., DeStefano, A.L. *et al.* (2012) Meta-analysis of Parkinson's Disease: identification of a novel locus, RIT2. *Ann Neurol*, **71** (3), 370–384.

Paolicelli, R.C., Bolasco, G., Pagani, F. *et al.* (2011) Synaptic pruning by microglia is necessary for normal brain development. *Science*, **333** (6048), 1456–1458.

Pardo, C.A., Vargas, D.L. and Zimmerman, A.W. (2005) Immunity, neuroglia and neuroinflammation in autism. *Int Rev Psychiatry*, **17** (6), 485–495.

Paré, B., Touzel-Deschênes, L., Lamontagne, R. *et al.* (2015) Early detection of structural abnormalities and cytoplasmic accumulation of TDP-43 in tissue-engineered skins derived from ALS patients. *Acta Neuropathol Commun*, **3** (1), 1–12.

Parkinson, J. (1817) *An Essay on the Shaking Palsy*, Sherwood, Neely, and Jones, London.

Parkinson, N., Ince, P.G., Smith, M.O. *et al.* (2006) ALS phenotypes with mutations in CHMP2B (charged multivesicular body protein 2B). *Neurology*, **67** (6), 1074–1077.

Parkinson's Disease Foundation. (2010). Understanding Parkinson's: Parkinson's FAQ. Available from: http://www.pdf.org/pdf/fs_frequently_asked_questions_10.pdf (last accessed September 23, 2016).

Parkinson's Disease Foundation. (2015). Understanding Parkinson's. Available from: http://www.pdf.org/en/understanding_pd (last accessed September 23, 2016).

Parkinson Society Canada and Health Canada. (2003). Parkinson's disease: social and economic impact. Available from: http://www.parkinson.ca/atf/cf/%7B9ebd08a9-7886-4b2d-a1c4-a131e7096bf8%7D/PARKINSONSDISEASE_EN.PDF (last accessed September 23, 2016).

Pascuzzi, R.M., Shefner, J., Chappell, A.S. *et al.* (2010) A phase II trial of talampanel in subjects with amyotrophic lateral sclerosis. *Amyotroph Lateral Scler*, **11** (3), 266–271.

Passeri, E., Villa, C., Couette, M. *et al.* (2011) Long-term follow-up of cognitive dysfunction in patients with aluminum hydroxide-induced macrophagic myofasciitis (MMF). *J Inorg Biochem*, **105** (11), 1457–1463.

Pastor, P., Ezquerra, M., Muñoz, E. *et al.* (2000) Significant association between the tau gene A0/A0 genotype and Parkinson's disease. *Ann Neurol*, **47** (2), 242–245.

Patterson, P.H. (2011) Maternal infection and immune involvement in autism. *Trends Mol Med*, **17** (7), 389–394.

Pei, B., Sisu, C., Frankish, A. *et al.* (2012) The GENCODE pseudogene resource. *Genome Biol*, **13** (9), R51.

Pellionisz, A.J., Graham, R., Pellionisz, P.A. and Perez, J.C. (2013) Recursive genome function of the cerebellum: geometric unification of neuroscience and genomics, in *Handbook of the Cerebellum and Cerebellar Disorders*, (eds E. Manto, D. Gruol, J. Schmahmann *et al.*), Springer, Vienna, pp. 1381–1422.

Perego, C., Fumagalli, S. and De Simoni, M.-G. (2011) Temporal pattern of expression and colocalization of microglia/macrophage phenotype markers following brain ischemic injury in mice. *J Neuroinflammation*, **8** (1), 174.

Perl, D.P. (1985) Relationship of aluminum to Alzheimer's disease. *Environ Health Perspect*, **63**, 149–153.

Perl, D.P. and Brody, A. (1980) Alzheimer's disease: X-ray spectrometric evidence of aluminum accumulation in neurofibrillary tangle-bearing neurons. *Science*, **208** (4441), 297–299.

Perl, D.P. and Good, P.F. (1991) Aluminum, Alzheimer's disease, and the olfactory system. *Ann N Y Acad Sci*, **640**, 8–13.

Perl, D.P., Gajdusek, D.C., Garruto, R.M. *et al.* (1982) Intraneuronal aluminum accumulation in amyotrophic lateral sclerosis and parkinsonism dementia of Guam. *Science*, **217** (4564), 1053–1055.

Perl, T.M., Bédard, L., Kosatsky, T. *et al.* (1990) An outbreak of toxic encephalopathy caused by eating mussels contaminated with domoic acid. *N Engl J Med*, **322** (25), 1775–1780.

Perl, D.P., Warren, C.O. and Calne, D. (1998) Alzheimer's disease and Parkinson's disease: distinct entities or extremes of a spectrum of neurodegeneration? *Ann Neurol*, **44** (Suppl. 1), S19–S31.

Perry, T.L., Bergeron, C., Biro, A.J. and Hansen, S. (1989) β-N-methylamino-l-alanine: chronic oral administration is not neurotoxic to mice. *J Neurol Sci*, **94** (1–3), 173–180.

Petkau, T.L. and Leavitt, B.R. (2014) Progranulin in neurodegenerative disease. *Trends Neurosci*, **37** (7), 388–398.

Petrik, M.S., Wilson, J.M.B., Grant, S.C. *et al.* (2007a) Magnetic resonance microscopy and immunohistochemistry of the CNS of the mutant SOD murine model of ALS reveals widespread neural deficits. *Neuromolecular Med*, **9** (3), 216–229.

Petrik, M.S., Wong, M.C., Tabata, R.C. *et al.* (2007b) Aluminum adjuvant linked to Gulf war illness induces motor neuron death in mice. *Neuromolecular Med*, **9** (1), 83–100.

Petrilli, V., Papin, S., Dostert, C. *et al.* (2007) Activation of the NALP3 inflammasome is triggered by low intracellular potassium concentration. *Cell Death Differ*, **14** (9), 1583–1589.

Pettem, K.L., Yokomaku, D., Luo, L. *et al.* (2013) The specific α-neurexin interactor calsyntenin-3 promotes excitatory and inhibitory synapse development. *Neuron*, **80** (1), 113–128.

Philips, T., De Muynck, L., Thu, H.N.T. *et al.* (2010) Microglial upregulation of progranulin as a marker of motor neuron degeneration. *J Neuropathol Exp Neurol*, **69** (12), 1191–1200.

Piccini, P., Pavese, N., Hagell, P. *et al.* (2005) Factors affecting the clinical outcome after neural transplantation in Parkinson's disease. *Brain*, **128** (12), 2977–2986.

Pickard, L., Noël, J., Henley, J.M. *et al.* (2000) Developmental changes in synaptic AMPA and NMDA receptor distribution and AMPA receptor subunit composition in living hippocampal neurons. *J Neurosci*, **20** (21), 7922–7931.

Pickles, A., Bolton, P., Macdonald, H. *et al.* (1995) Latent-class analysis of recurrence risks for complex phenotypes with selection and measurement error: a twin and family history study of autism. *Am J Hum Genet*, **57** (3), 717–726.

Plato, C.C., Garruto, R.M., Galasko, D. *et al.* (2003) Amyotrophic lateral sclerosis and parkinsonism-dementia complex of Guam: changing incidence rates during the past 60 years. *Am J Epidemiol*, **157** (2), 149–157.

Pokrishevsky, E., Grad, L.I., Yousefi, M. *et al.* (2012) Aberrant localization of FUS and TDP43 is associated with misfolding of SOD1 in amyotrophic lateral sclerosis. *PLoS ONE*, **7** (4), e35050.

Polanco, I., Biemond, I., van Leeuwen, A. *et al.* (1981) Gluten sensitive enteropathy in Spain: genetic and environmental factors, in *The Genetics of Coeliac Disease*, (ed. R.B. McConnell), Springer, Dordrecht, pp. 211–234.

Polymeropoulos, M.H., Lavedan, C., Leroy, E. *et al.* (1997) Mutation in the α-synuclein gene identified in families with Parkinson's disease. *Science*, **276** (5321), 2045–2047.

Poot-Poot, W. and Hernandez-Sotomayor, S.M. (2011) Aluminum stress and its role in the phospholipid signaling pathway in plants and possible biotechnological applications. *IUBMB Life*, **63** (10), 864–872.

Porges, S.W. (2005) The vagus: a mediator of behavioral and physiologic features associated with autism, in *The Neurobiology of Autism*, 2 edn (eds M.L. Bauman and T.L. Kemper), Johns Hopkins University Press, Baltimore, MD, pp. 65–78.

Price, K.S., Farley, I.J. and Hornykiewicz, O. (1978) Neurochemistry of Parkinson's disease: relation between striatal and limbic dopamine. *Adv Biochem Psychopharmacol*, **19**, 293–300.

Prickett, M. and Jain, M. (2013) Gene therapy in cystic fibrosis. *Transl Res*, **161** (4), 255–264.

Pritchard, C. and Rosenorm-Lanng, E. (2015) Neurological deaths of American adults (55–74) and the over 75's by sex compared with 20 Western countries 1989–2010: cause for concern. *Surg Neurol Int*, **6** (1), 123.

Pritchard, C., Baldwin, D. and Mayers, A. (2004) Changing patterns of adult (45–74 years) neurological deaths in the major Western world countries 1979–1997. *Public Health*, **118** (4), 268–283.

Prusiner, S.B. (2001) Neurodegenerative diseases and prions. *N Engl J Med*, **344** (20), 1516–1526.

Public Health Agency of Canada. (2015). Canadian Best Practices Portal: Neurological Conditions. Available from: http://cbpp-pcpe.phac-aspc.gc.ca/chronic-diseases/neurological-conditions/ (last accessed September 23, 2016).

Pupillo, E., Messina, P., Logroscino, G. *et al.* (2014) Long-term survival in amyotrophic lateral sclerosis: a population-based study. *Ann Neurol*, **75** (2), 287–297.

Purcell, A.E., Jeon, O.H., Zimmerman, A.W. *et al.* (2001) Postmortem brain abnormalities of the glutamate neurotransmitter system in autism. *Neurology*, **57** (9), 1618–1628.

Quertemont, E. (2004) Genetic polymorphism in ethanol metabolism: acetaldehyde contribution to alcohol abuse and alcoholism. *Mol Psychiatry*, **9** (6), 570–581.

Quick, D.T. and Greer, M. (1967) Pancreatic dysfunction in patients with amyotrophic lateral sclerosis. *Neurology*, **17** (2), 112–112.

Quinn, J.F., Raman, R., Thomas, R.G. *et al.* (2010) Docosahexaenoic acid supplementation and cognitive decline in alzheimer disease: a randomized trial. *JAMA*, **304** (17), 1903–1911.

Raber, J., Wong, D., Yu, G.-Q. *et al.* (2000) Alzheimer's disease: apolipoprotein E and cognitive performance. *Nature*, **404** (6776), 352–354.

Raber, J., Huang, Y. and Ashford, J.W. (2004) ApoE genotype accounts for the vast majority of AD risk and AD pathology. *Neurobiol Aging*, **25** (5), 641–650.

Rademakers, R., Cruts, M. and van Broeckhoven, C. (2004) The role of tau (MAPT) in frontotemporal dementia and related tauopathies. *Hum Mutat*, **24** (4), 277–295.

Rajput, A.H., Sitte, H.H., Rajput, A. *et al.* (2008) Globus pallidus dopamine and Parkinson motor subtypes: clinical and brain biochemical correlation. *Neurology*, **70** 16 Pt. 2, 1403–1410.

Rakhit, R., Cunningham, P., Furtos-Matei, A. *et al.* (2002) Oxidation-induced misfolding and aggregation of superoxide dismutase and its implications for amyotrophic lateral sclerosis. *J Biol Chem*, **277** (49), 47551–47556.

Ramanan, V.K. and Saykin, A.J. (2013) Pathways to neurodegeneration: mechanistic insights from GWAS in Alzheimer's disease, Parkinson's disease, and related disorders. *Am J Neurodegener Dis*, **2** (3), 145–175.

Ramirez, A., Heimbach, A., Grundemann, J. *et al.* (2006) Hereditary parkinsonism with dementia is caused by mutations in ATP13A2, encoding a lysosomal type 5 P-type ATPase. *Nat Genet*, **38** (10), 1184–1191.

Ramlow, J., Alexander, M., LaPorte, R. *et al.* (1992) Epidemiology of the post-polio syndrome. *Am J Epidemiol*, **136** (7), 769–786.

Rankin, C.H. (2004) Invertebrate learning: what can't a worm learn? *Curr Biol*, **14** (15), R617–R618.

Rapin, I. (1997) Autism. *N Engl J Med*, **337** (21), 1556–1557.

Rapoport, J.L., Giedd, J.N., Blumenthal, J. *et al.* (1999) Progressive cortical change during adolescence in childhood-onset schizophrenia: a longitudinal magnetic resonance imaging study. *Arch Gen Psychiatry*, **56** (7), 649–654.

Ravits, J. (2005) Sporadic amyotrophic lateral sclerosis: a hypothesis of persistent (non-lytic) enteroviral infection. *Amyotroph Lateral Scler*, **6** (2), 77–87.

Ravits, J., Appel, S., Baloh, R.H. *et al.* (2013) Deciphering amyotrophic lateral sclerosis: what phenotype, neuropathology and genetics are telling us about pathogenesis. *Amyotroph Lateral Scler Frontotemporal Degener*, **14** (Suppl. 1), 5–18.

Re, D.B., Le Verche, V., Yu, C. *et al.* (2014) Necroptosis drives motor neuron death in models of both sporadic and familial ALS. *Neuron*, **81** (5), 1001–1008.

Recchia, A., Rota, D., Debetto, P. *et al.* (2008) Generation of a α-synuclein-based rat model of Parkinson's disease. *Neurobiol Dis*, **30** (1), 8–18.

Reekum, R.V., Streiner, D.L. and Conn, D.K. (2001) Applying Bradford Hill's criteria for causation to neuropsychiatry. *J Neuropsychiatry Clin Neurosci*, **13** (3), 318–325.

Reisberg, B., Ferris, S.H., de Leon, M.J. and Crook, T. (1982) The Global Deterioration Scale for assessment of primary degenerative dementia. *Am J Psychiatry*, **139** (9), 1136–1139.

Renton, A.E., Majounie, E., Waite, A. *et al.* (2011) A hexanucleotide repeat expansion in C9ORF72 is the cause of chromosome 9p21-linked ALS-FTD. *Neuron*, **72** (2), 257–268.

Renton, A.E., Chio, A. and Traynor, B.J. (2014) State of play in amyotrophic lateral sclerosis genetics. *Nat Neurosci*, **17** (1), 17–23.

Reusche, E., Koch, V., Friedrich, H.J. *et al.* (1996) Correlation of drug-related aluminum intake and dialysis treatment with deposition of argyrophilic aluminum-containing inclusions in CNS and in organ systems of patients with dialysis-associated encephalopathy. *Clin Neuropathol*, **15** (6), 342–347.

Rigolet, M., Aouizerate, J., Couette, M. *et al.* (2014) Clinical features in patients with long-lasting macrophagic myofasciitis. *Front Neurol*, **5**, 230.

Riihimäki, V. and Aitio, A. (2012) Occupational exposure to aluminum and its biomonitoring in perspective. *Crit Rev Toxicol*, **42** (10), 827–853.

Rioux, J.D., Karinen, H., Kocher, K. *et al.* (2004) Genomewide search and association studies in a Finnish celiac disease population: identification of a novel locus and replication of the HLA and CTLA4 loci. *Am J Med Genet A*, **130** (4), 345–350.

Risch, N., Spiker, D., Lotspeich, L. *et al.* (1999) A genomic screen of autism: evidence for a multilocus etiology. *Am J Hum Genet*, **65** (2), 493–507.

Risher, J.F., Murray, H.E. and Prince, G.R. (2002) Organic mercury compounds: human exposure and its relevance to public health. *Toxicol Ind Health*, **18** (3), 109–160.

Robberecht, W. and Philips, T. (2013) The changing scene of amyotrophic lateral sclerosis. *Nat Rev Neurosci*, **14** (4), 248–264.

Rocca, W.A., Bower, J., McDonnell, S. *et al.* (2001) Time trends in the incidence of parkinsonism in Olmsted County, Minnesota. *Neurology*, **57** (3), 462–467.

Rocca, W.A., Petersen, R.C., Knopman, D.S. *et al.* (2011) Trends in the incidence and prevalence of Alzheimer's disease, dementia, and cognitive impairment in the United States. *Alzheimers Dement*, **7** (1), 80–93.

Rogaev, E.I., Sherrington, R., Rogaeva, E.A. *et al.* (1995) Familial Alzheimer's disease in kindreds with missense mutations in a gene on chromosome 1 related to the Alzheimer's disease type 3 gene. *Nature*, **376** (6543), 775–778.

Rojanathammanee, L., Murphy, E.J. and Combs, C.K. (2011) Expression of mutant alpha-synuclein modulates microglial phenotype in vitro. *J Neuroinflammation*, **8** (44), 1742–2094.

Rosen, D.R., Siddique, T., Patterson, D. *et al.* (1993) Mutations in Cu/Zn superoxide dismutase gene are associated with familial amyotrophic lateral sclerosis. *Nature*, **362** (6415), 59–62.

Ross, G.W. and Abbott, R.D. (2014) Living and dying with Parkinson's disease. *Mov Disord*, **29** (13), 1571–1573.

Rosso, I.M., Cannon, T.D., Huttunen, T. *et al.* (2000) Obstetric risk factors for early-onset schizophrenia in a Finnish birth cohort. *Am J Psychiatry*, **157** (5), 801–807.

Rothstein, J.D. (1995) Excitotoxicity and neurodegeneration in amyotrophic lateral sclerosis. *Clin Neurosci*, **3** (6), 348–359.

Rotunno, M.S. and Bosco, D.A. (2013) An emerging role for misfolded wild-type SOD1 in sporadic ALS pathogenesis. *Front Cell Neurosci*, **7**, 253.

Rouse, M. (2006). Definition: tipping point. Available from: http://whatis.techtarget.com/definition/tipping-point (last accessed September 23, 2006).

Ruiz, A., Heilmann, S., Becker, T. *et al.* (2014) Follow-up of loci from the International Genomics of Alzheimer's Disease Project identifies TRIP4 as a novel susceptibility gene. *Transl Psychiatry*, **4**, e358.

Ryan, C., Baranowski, D., Chitramuthu, B. *et al.* (2009) Progranulin is expressed within motor neurons and promotes neuronal cell survival. *BMC Neurosci*, **10** (1), 130.

Sabel, C.E. (2014) Disease clusters, in The Wiley Blackwell Encyclopedia of Health, Illness, Behavior, and Society, (eds W. Cockerham, R. Dingwall and S.R. Quah), Hoboken, NJ, Wiley-Blackwell.

Saccon, R.A., Bunton-Stasyshyn, R.K.A., Fisher, E.M.C. and Fratta, P. (2013) Is SOD1 loss of function involved in amyotrophic lateral sclerosis? *Brain*, **136** (B), 2342–2358.

Sacks, O. (1999) *Awakenings*, Vintage, New York.

Saeed, M., Siddique, N., Hung, W.Y. *et al.* (2006) Paraoxonase cluster polymorphisms are associated with sporadic ALS. *Neurology*, **67** (5), 771–776.

Safford, W.E. (1903) The Chamorro language of Guam: a grammar of the idiom spoken by the inhabitants of the Marianne or Ladrones, Islands. *Am Anthropol*, **5** (2), 289–311.

Sahi, T. (1994) Genetics and epidemiology of adult-type hypolactasia. *Scand J Gastroenterol*, **202**, 7–20.

Saing, T., Dick, M., Nelson, P.T. *et al.* (2012) Frontal cortex neuropathology in dementia pugilistica. *J Neurotrauma*, **29** (6), 1054–1070.

Saiyed, S.M. and Yokel, R.A. (2005) Aluminium content of some foods and food products in the USA, with aluminium food additives. *Food Addit Contam*, **22** (3), 234–244.

Sakamoto, T., Ogasawara, Y., Ishii, K. *et al.* (2004) Accumulation of aluminum in ferritin isolated from rat brain. *Neurosci Lett*, **366** (3), 264–267.

Sakki, T.K., Knuuttila, M.L.E., Vimpari, S.S. and Kivelä, S.-L. (1994) Lifestyle, dental caries and number of teeth. *Community Dent Oral Epidemiol*, **22** 5 Pt. 1, 298–302.

Salazar-Grueso, E. and Roos, R. (1994) Amyotrophic lateral sclerosis and viruses. *Clin Neurosci*, **3** (6), 360–367.

Salloway, S., Sperling, R., Fox, N.C. *et al.* (2014) Two phase 3 trials of bapineuzumab in mild-to-moderate Alzheimer's disease. *N Engl J Med*, **370** (4), 322–333.

Salzberg, Y., Díaz-Balzac, C.A., Ramirez-Suarez, N.J. *et al.* (2013) Skin-derived cues control arborization of sensory dendrites in Caenorhabditis elegans. *Cell*, **155** (2), 308–320.

Sampaio, C., Bronzova, J., Hauser, R.A. *et al.* (2011) Pardoprunox in early Parkinson's disease: results from 2 large, randomized double-blind trials. *Mov Disord*, **26** (8), 1464–1476.

Sandyk, R., Iacono, R.P. and Bamford, C.R. (1987) The hypothalamus in Parkinson disease. *Ital J Neuro Sci*, **8** (3), 227–234.

Sano, M., Bell, K.L., Galasko, D. *et al.* (2011) A randomized, double-blind, placebo-controlled trial of simvastatin to treat Alzheimer disease. *Neurology*, 77 (6), 556–563.

Sapolsky, R.M. (1993) Potential behavioral modification of glucocorticoid damage to the hippocampus. *Behav Brain Res*, **57** (2), 175–182.

Sapone, A., Bai, J.C., Ciacci, C. *et al.* (2012) Spectrum of gluten-related disorders: consensus on new nomenclature and classification. *BMC Med*, **10** (1), 13.

Sapp, P.C., Hosler, B.A., McKenna-Yasek, D. *et al.* (2003) Identification of two novel loci for dominantly inherited familial amyotrophic lateral sclerosis. *Am J Hum Genet*, **73** (2), 397–403.

Sasakura, H. and Mori, I. (2013) Behavioral plasticity, learning, and memory in C. elegans. *Curr Opin Neurobiol*, **23** (1), 92–99.

Satake, W., Nakabayashi, Y., Mizuta, I. *et al.* (2009) Genome-wide association study identifies common variants at four loci as genetic risk factors for Parkinson's disease. *Nat Genet*, **41** (12), 1303–1307.

Schellenberg, G., Bird, T., Wijsman, E. *et al.* (1992) Genetic linkage evidence for a familial Alzheimer's disease locus on chromosome 14. *Science*, **258** (5082), 668–671.

Scheperjans, F., Aho, V., Pereira, P.A.B. *et al.* (2014) Gut microbiota are related to Parkinson's disease and clinical phenotype. *Mov Disord*, **30** (3), 350–358.

Schlenker, E., Jones, Q., Rowland, R. *et al.* (2001) Age-dependent poliomyelitis in mice is associated with respiratory failure and viral replication in the central nervous system and lung. *J Neuroviol*, **7** (3), 265–271.

Schonberger, L.B., Bregman, D.J., Sullivan-Bolyai, J.Z. *et al.* (1979) Guillain-Barre syndrome following vaccination in the national influenza immunization program, United States, 1976–1977. *Am J Epidemiol*, **110** (2), 105–123.

Schooler, J. (2011) Unpublished results hide the decline effect. *Nature*, **470**, 437.

Schulte, J. and Littleton, J.T. (2011) The biological function of the Huntingtin protein and its relevance to Huntington's Disease pathology. *Curr Trends Neurol*, **5**, 65.

Schwab, R.S. and England, A.C. (1969) Projection technique for evaluating surgery in Parkinson's disease, in *Third Symposium on Parkinson's Disease, Royal College of Surgeons in Edinburgh, May 20–22 [1968]*, Livingstone, Edinburgh, pp. 152–157.

Schymick, J.C., Yang, Y., Andersen, P.M. *et al.* (2007) Progranulin mutations and amyotrophic lateral sclerosis or amyotrophic lateral sclerosis-frontotemporal dementia phenotypes. *J Neurol Neurosurg Psychiatr*, **78** (7), 754–756.

Scott, S., Kranz, J.E., Cole, J. *et al.* (2008) Design, power, and interpretation of studies in the standard murine model of ALS. *Amyotroph Lateral Scler*, **9** (1), 4–15.

Sejvar, J.J., Holman, R.C., Bresee, J.S. *et al.* (2005) Amyotrophic lateral sclerosis mortality in the United States, 1979–2001. *Neuroepidemiology*, **25** (3), 144–152.

Sekar, A., Bialas, A.R., de Rivera, H. *et al.* (2016) Schizophrenia risk from complex variation of complement component 4. *Nature*, **530** (7589), 177–183.

Selemon, L.D., Rajkowska, G. and Goldman-Rakic, P.S. (2004) Evidence for progression in frontal cortical pathology in late-stage Huntington's disease. *J Comp Neurol*, **468** (2), 190–204.

Seneff, S., Davidson, R. and Liu, J. (2012) Empirical data confirm autism symptoms related to aluminum and acetaminophen exposure. *Entropy*, **14** (11), 2227–2253.

Seneff, S., Swanson, N. and Li, C. (2015) Aluminum and glyphosate can synergistically induce pineal gland pathology: connection to gut dysbiosis and neurological disease. *Agr Sci*, **6** (01), 42.

Seok, J., Warren, H.S., Cuenca, A.G. *et al.* (2013) Genomic responses in mouse models poorly mimic human inflammatory diseases. *Proc Natl Acad Sci U S A*, **110** (9), 3507–3512.

Service, R. F (2014) The brain chip. *Science*, **345** (6197), 614–616.

Seshadri, S., Fitzpatrick, A.L., Ikram, M.A. *et al.* (2010) Genome-wide analysis of genetic loci associated with Alzheimer disease. *JAMA*, **303** (18), 1832–1840.

Sessa, R., Di Pietro, M., Filardo, S. and Turriziani, O. (2014) Infectious burden and atherosclerosis: a clinical issue. *World J Clin Cases*, **2** (7), 240.

Shatunov, A., Mok, K., Newhouse, S. *et al.* (2010) Chromosome 9p21 in sporadic amyotrophic lateral sclerosis in the UK and seven other countries: a genome-wide association study. *Lancet Neurol*, **9** (10), 986–994.

Shaw, C. and Cynader, M. (1984) Disruption of cortical activity prevents ocular dominance changes in monocularly deprived kittens. *Nature*, **308** (5961), 731–734.

Shaw, C.A. and Höglinger, G. (2008) Neurodegenerative diseases: neurotoxins as sufficient etiologic agents? *Neuromolecular Med*, **10** (1), 1–9.

Shaw, C.A. and McEachern, J.C. (2001) *Toward a Theory of Neuroplasticity*, Taylor and Francis, Philadelphia, PA.

Shaw, C.A. and Petrik, M.S. (2009) Aluminum hydroxide injections lead to motor deficits and motor neuron degeneration. *J Inorg Biochem*, **103** (11), 1555–1562.

Shaw, C.A. and Tomljenovic, L. (2013) Aluminum in the central nervous system (CNS): toxicity in humans and animals, vaccine adjuvants, and autoimmunity. *Immunol Res*, **56** (2–3), 304–316.

Shaw, C.A., Wilkinson, M., Cynader, M. *et al.* (1986) The laminar distributions and postnatal development of neurotransmitter and neuromodulator receptors in cat visual cortex. *Brain Res Bull*, **16** (5), 661–671.

Shaw, C.A., Bains, J.S., Pasqualotto, B.A. and Curry, K. (1999) Methionine sulfoximine shows excitotoxic actions in rat cortical slices. *Can J Physiol Pharmacol*, **77** (11), 871–877.

Shaw, C.A., Kette, S., Davidson, R. and Seneff, S. (2013) Aluminum's role in CNS-immune system interactions leading to neurological disorders. *Immunome Res*, **9** (069), 2.

Shaw, C.A., Li, D. and Tomlijenovic, L. (2014a) Are there negative CNS impacts of aluminum adjuvants in vaccines and immunotherapy? *Immunotherapy*, **6** (10), 1055–1071.

Shaw, C.A., Seneff, S., Kette, S.D. *et al.* (2014b) Aluminum-induced entropy in biological systems: implications for neurological disease. *J Toxicol*, **2014**, 491316.

Shaw, C.A., Sheth, S., Li, D. and Tomlijenovic, L. (2014c) Etiology of autism spectrum disorders: genes, environment, or both? *OA Autism*, **2** (2), 11.

Shaw, L.M., Korecka, M., Clark, C.M. *et al.* (2007) Biomarkers of neurodegeneration for diagnosis and monitoring therapeutics. *Nat Rev Drug Discov*, **6** (4), 295–303.

Sheiham, A. (2005) Oral health, general health and quality of life. *Bull World Health Organ*, **83** (9).

Shen, W.-B., McDowell, K.A., Siebert, A.A. *et al.* (2010) Environmental neurotoxin-induced progressive model of parkinsonism in rats. *Ann Neurol*, **68** (1), 70–80.

Shenton, M.E., Dickey, C.C., Frumin, M. and McCarley, R.W. (2001) A review of MRI findings in schizophrenia. *Schizophr Res*, **49** (1–2), 1–52.

Sherer, T.B. and Mari, Z. (2014) Is Parkinson's one disease or many? *The Michael J. Fox Foundation's Third Thursdays Webinars on Parkinson's Research* [Webinar].

Sherrington, R., Froelich, S., Sorbi, S. *et al.* (1996) Alzheimer's disease associated with mutations in presenilin 2 is rare and variably penetrant. *Hum Mol Genet*, **5** (7), 985–988.

Sheth, S., Li, Y., and Shaw, C. A. (2015). Effects of aluminum adjuvants on social behavior in mice. 11th Keele Meeting on Aluminum Abstract.

Shimmura, C., Suda, S., Tsuchiya, K.J. *et al.* (2011) Alteration of plasma glutamate and glutamine levels in children with high-functioning autism. *PLoS ONE*, **6** (10), e25340.

Shinohe, A., Hashimoto, K., Nakamura, K. *et al.* (2006) Increased serum levels of glutamate in adult patients with autism. *Prog Neuropsychopharmacol Biol Psychiatry*, **30** (8), 1472–1477.

Shoenfeld, Y. and Agmon-Levin, N. (2011) "ASIA" – autoimmune/inflammatory syndrome induced by adjuvants. *J Autoimmun*, **36** (1), 4–8.

Sidransky, E., Nalls, M.A., Aasly, J.O. *et al.* (2009) Multicenter analysis of glucocerebrosidase mutations in Parkinson's disease. *N Engl J Med*, **361** (17), 1651–1661.

Sienkiewicz, D., Kułak, W., Okurowska-Zawada, B. and Paszko-Patej, G. (2012) Neurologic adverse events following vaccination. *Prog Health Sci*, **2** (1).

Simon-Sanchez, J., Schulte, C., Bras, J.M. *et al.* (2009) Genome-wide association study reveals genetic risk underlying Parkinson's disease. *Nat Genet*, **41** (12), 1308–1312.

Simpson, C.L., Lemmens, R., Miskiewicz, K. *et al.* (2009) Variants of the elongator protein 3 (ELP3) gene are associated with motor neuron degeneration. *Hum Mol Genet*, **18** (3), 472–481.

Simpson, S., Blizzard, L., Otahal, P. *et al.* (2011) Latitude is significantly associated with the prevalence of multiple sclerosis: a meta-analysis. *J Neurol Neurosurg Psychiatr*, **82** (10), 1132–1141.

Singer, H.S., Morris, C.M., Williams, P.N. *et al.* (2006) Antibrain antibodies in children with autism and their unaffected siblings. *J Neuroimmunol*, **178** (1–2), 149–155.

Singer, O., Marr, R.A., Rockenstein, E. *et al.* (2005) Targeting BACE1 with siRNAs ameliorates Alzheimer disease neuropathology in a transgenic model. *Nat Neurosci*, **8** (10), 1343–1349.

Siva, K., Covello, G. and Denti, M.A. (2014) Exon-skipping antisense oligonucleotides to correct missplicing in neurogenetic diseases. *Neucleic Acid Ther*, **24** (1), 69–86.

Sleegers, K., Brouwers, N., Maurer-Stroh, S. *et al.* (2008) Progranulin genetic variability contributes to amyotrophic lateral sclerosis. *Neurology*, **71** (4), 253–259.

Smalley, S.L., Asarnow, R.F. and Spence, M. (1988) Autism and genetics: a decade of research. *Arch Gen Psychiatry*, **45** (10), 953–961.

Smith, B.N., Ticozzi, N., Fallini, C. *et al.* (2014) Exome-wide rare variant analysis identifies TUBA4A mutations associated with familial ALS. *Neuron*, **84** (2), 324–331.

Smith, B.N., Vance, C., Scotter, E.L. *et al.* (2015) Novel mutations support a role for Profilin 1 in the pathogenesis of ALS. *Neurobiol Aging*, **36** (3), 1602.e1617–1602.e1627.

Smith, R.G., Siklos, L., Alexianu, M.E. *et al.* (1996) Autoimmunity and ALS. *Neurology*, **47** (4 Suppl. 2), 40S–46S.

Smith, S.E.P., Li, J., Garbett, K. *et al.* (2007) Maternal immune activation alters fetal brain development through interleukin-6. *J Neurosci*, **27** (40), 10695–10702.

Sollid, L.M. (2000) Molecular basis of celiac disease. *Annu Rev Immunol*, **18** (1), 53–81.

Sollid, L.M. and Lie, B.A. (2005) Celiac disease genetics: current concepts and practical applications. *Clin Gastroenterol Hepatol*, **3** (9), 843–851.

Sollid, L.M., Markussen, G., Ek, J. *et al.* (1989) Evidence for a primary association of celiac disease to a particular HLA-DQ alpha/beta heterodimer. *J Exp Med*, **169** (1), 345–350.

Sorenson, E.J., Windbank, A.J., Mandrekar, J.N. *et al.* (2008) Subcutaneous IGF-1 is not beneficial in 2-year ALS trial. *Neurology*, **71** (22), 1770–1775.

Soumiya, H., Fukumitsu, H. and Furukawa, S. (2011) Prenatal immune challenge compromises the normal course of neurogenesis during development of the mouse cerebral cortex. *J Neurosci Res*, **89** (10), 1575–1585.

Spencer, P.S., Nunn, P., Hugon, J. *et al.* (1987) Guam amyotrophic lateral sclerosis-parkinsonism-dementia linked to a plant excitant neurotoxin. *Science*, **237** (4814), 517–522.

Spencer, P.S., Kisby, G., Palmer, V. and Obendorf, P. (2000) Cycasin, methylazoxymethanol and related compounds. *Exp Clin Neurotoxicol*, 436–447.

Spencer, P.S., Palmer, V.S. and Ludolph, A.C. (2005a) On the decline and etiology of high-incidence motor system disease in West Papua (southwest New Guinea). *Mov Disord*, **20** (12)(Suppl, S119–S126).

Spencer, S.J., Heida, J.G. and Pittman, Q.J. (2005b) Early life immune challenge – effects on behavioural indices of adult rat fear and anxiety. *Behav Brain Res*, **164** (2), 231–238.

Spencer, S.J., Hyland, N.P., Sharkey, K.A. and Pittman, Q.J. (2007) Neonatal immune challenge exacerbates experimental colitis in adult rats: potential role for TNF-alpha. *Am J Physiol Regul Integr Comp Physiol*, **292** (1), R308–315.

Spinelli, D. and Jensen, F. (1979) Plasticity: the mirror of experience. *Science*, **203** (4375), 75–78.

Splansky, G.L., Corey, D., Yang, Q. *et al.* (2007) The third generation cohort of the National Heart, Lung, and Blood Institute's Framingham Heart Study: design, recruitment, and initial examination. *Am J Epidemiol*, **165** (11), 1328–1335.

Sreedharan, J., Blair, I.P., Tripathi, V.B. *et al.* (2008) TDP-43 mutations in familial and sporadic amyotrophic lateral sclerosis. *Science*, **319** (5870), 1668–1672.

Staats, K.A., Van Helleputte, L., Jones, A.R. *et al.* (2013) Genetic ablation of phospholipase C delta 1 increases survival in SOD1G93A mice. *Neurobiol Dis*, **60**, 11–17.

Steele, J.C. (2005) Parkinsonism–dementia complex of Guam. *Mov Disord*, **20** (S12), S99–S107.

Steele, J.C. and Williams, D.B. (1995) Calcium and aluminium in the Chamorro diet: unlikely causes of Alzheimer-type neurofibrillary degeneration on Guam, in *Motor Neuron Disease*, (eds P.N. Leigh and M. Swash), Springer, London, pp. 189–200.

Steele, J.C., Richardson, J. and Olszewski, J. (1964) Progressive supranuclear palsy: a heterogeneous degeneration involving the brain stem, basal ganglia and cerebellum with vertical gaze and pseudobulbar palsy, nuchal dystonia and dementia. *Arch Neurol*, **10** (4), 333–359.

Steele, J.C., Richardson, J.C. and Olszewski, J. (2014) Progressive supranuclear palsy: a heterogeneous degeneration involving the brain stem, basal ganglia and cerebellum with vertical gaze and pseudobulbar palsy, nuchal dystonia and dementia. *Semin Neurol*, **34** (2), 129–150.

Steele, J.C., Guella, I., Szu-Tu, C. *et al.* (2015) Defining neurodegeneration on Guam by targeted genomic sequencing. *Ann Neurol*, **77** (3), 458–468.

Steen, E., Terry, B.M., Rivera, E.J. *et al.* (2005) Impaired insulin and insulin-like growth factor expression and signaling mechanisms in Alzheimer's disease – is this type 3 diabetes? *J Alzheimers Dis*, **7**, 63–80.

Stefanis, L. (2012) α-synuclein in Parkinson's disease. *Cold Spring Harb Perspect Med*, **2** (2), a009399.

Steffenburg, S., Gillberg, C., Hellgren, L. *et al.* (1989) A twin study of autism in Denmark, Finland, Iceland, Norway and Sweden. *J Child Psychol Psychiatry*, **30** (3), 405–416.

Steiner, B., Wolf, S.A. and Kempermann, G. (2005) Adult neurogenesis and neurodegenerative disease. *Regen Med*, **1** (1), 15–28.

Stephan, A.H., Barres, B.A. and Stevens, B. (2012) The complement system: an unexpected role in synaptic pruning during development and disease. *Annu Rev Neurosci*, **35**, 369–389.

Stevenson, D.W. (1990) *The biology, structure, and systematics of the cycadales*, Proceedings of the Symposium CYCAD 87, Beaulieu-sur-Mer, France April 17–22, 1987.

Stocchi, F., Rascol, O., Hauser, R. *et al.* (2014) *Phase-3 clinical trial of the adenosine 2a antagonist preladenant, given as monotherapy, in patients with Parkinson's disease Neurology*, **82** (Suppl. 10), S7.004).

Strong, M.J. (2010) The evidence for altered RNA metabolism in amyotrophic lateral sclerosis (ALS). *J Neurol Sci*, **288** (1–2), 1–12.

Strong, M.J. and Garruto, R.M. (1991) Chronic aluminum-induced motor neuron degeneration: clinical, neuropathological and molecular biological aspects. *Can J Neurol Sci*, **18** (Suppl. 3), 428–431.

Strong, M.J. and Rosenfeld, J. (2003) Amyotrophic lateral sclerosis: a review of current concepts. *Amyotroph Lateral Scler*, **4** (3), 136–143.

Strong, M.J., Kesavapany, S. and Pant, H.C. (2005) The pathobiology of amyotrophic lateral sclerosis: a proteinopathy? *J Neuropathol Exp Neurol*, **64** (8), 649–664.

Strunecká, A., Strunecky, O. and Patocka, J. (2002) Fluoride plus aluminum: useful tools in laboratory investigations, but messengers of false information. *Physiol Res*, **51** (6), 557–564.

Sulzer, D. (2007) Multiple hit hypotheses for dopamine neuron loss in Parkinson's disease. *Trends Neurosci*, **30** (5), 244–250.

Sun, J. and Chang, E.B. (2014) Exploring gut microbes in human health and disease: pushing the envelope. *Genes Dis*, **1** (2), 132–139.

Sundström, E. and Samuelsson, E.-B. (1997) Comparison of key steps in 1-methyl-4-phenyl-1,2,3,6-tetrahydropyridine (MPTP) neurotoxicity in rodents. *Pharmacol Toxicol*, **81** (5), 226–231.

Supèr, H., Soriano, E. and Uylings, H.B.M. (1998) The functions of the preplate in development and evolution of the neocortex and hippocampus. *Brain Res Rev*, **27** (1), 40–64.

Swallow, D.M. (2003) Genetics of lactase persistence and lactose intolerance. *Annu Rev Genet*, **37** (1), 197–219.

Swinnen, B. and Robberecht, W. (2014) The phenotypic variability of amyotrophic lateral sclerosis. *Nat Rev Neurol*, **10** (11), 661–670.

Tabakow, P., Jarmundowicz, W., Czapiga, B. *et al.* (2013) Transplantation of autologous olfactory ensheathing cells in complete human spinal cord injury. *Cell Transplant*, **22** (9), 1591–1612.

Tabakow, P., Raisman, G., Fortuna, W. *et al.* (2014) Functional regeneration of supraspinal connections in a patient with transected spinal cord following transplantation of bulbar olfactory ensheathing cells with peripheral nerve bridging. *Cell Transplant*, **23** (12), 1631–1655.

Tabata, R.C. (2008) *Neuropathology induced by sterol glucosides in mice*, University of British Columbia, Vancouver, Canada, MSc thesis.

Tabata, R.C., Wilson, J.M.B., Ly, P. *et al.* (2008) Chronic exposure to dietary sterol glucosides is neurotoxic to motor neurons and induces an ALS–PDC phenotype. *Neuromolecular Med*, **10** (1), 24–39.

Tam, O.H., Aravin, A.A., Stein, P. *et al.* (2008) Pseudogene-derived small interfering RNAs regulate gene expression in mouse oocytes. *Nature*, **453** (7194), 534–538.

Tanabe, S. (2008) Analysis of food allergen structures and development of foods for allergic patients. *Biosci Biotechnol Biochem*, **72** (3), 649–659.

Tandon, A., Rogaeva, E., Mullan, M. and St George-Hyslop, P.H. (2000) Molecular genetics of Alzheimer's disease: the role of β-amyloid and the presenilins. *Curr Opin Neurol*, **13** (4), 377–384.

Tanner, C.M., Ottman, R., Goldman, S.M. *et al.* (1999) Parkinson disease in twins: an etiologic study. *JAMA*, **281** (4), 341–346.

Tansey, M.G. and Goldberg, M.S. (2010) Neuroinflammation in Parkinson's disease: its role in neuronal death and implications for therapeutic intervention. *Neurobiol Dis*, **37** (3), 510–518.

Tariot, P.N., Schneider, L.S., Cummings, J. *et al.* (2011) Chronic divalproex sodium to attenuate agitation and clinical progression of Alzheimer disease. *Arch Gen Psychiatry*, **68** (8), 853–861.

Theise, N.D. (2005) Now you see it, now you don't. *Nature*, **435** (7046), 1165–1165.

Theise, N.D. and d'Inverno, M. (2004) Understanding cell lineages as complex adaptive systems. *Blood Cells Mol Dis*, **32** (1), 17–20.

Theise, N.D. and Krause, D.S. (2002) Toward a new paradigm of cell plasticity. *Leukemia*, **16** (4), 542–548.

Theoharides, T.C. and Zhang, B. (2011) Neuro-inflammation, blood-brain barrier, seizures and autism. *J Neuroinflammation*, **8** (1), 168.

Theoharides, T.C., Kempuraj, D. and Redwood, L. (2009) Autism: an emerging "neuroimmune disorder" in search of therapy. *Expert Opin Pharmacother*, **10** (13), 2127–2143.

Therrien, M., Rouleau, G.A., Dion, P.A. and Parker, J.A. (2013) *Deletion of C9ORF72 results in motor neuron degeneration and stress sensitivity in C. elegans. PLoS ONE*, **8** (12), e83450.

Thesleff, S. and Sellin, L.C. (1980) Denervation supersensitivity. *Trends Neurosci*, **3** (5), 122–126.

Thiruchelvam, M., Brockel, B.J., Richfield, E.K. *et al.* (2000) Potentiated and preferential effects of combined paraquat and maneb on nigrostriatal dopamine systems: environmental risk factors for Parkinson's disease? *Brain Res*, **873** (2), 225–234.

Thomasson, H.R., Edenberg, H.J., Crabb, D.W. *et al.* (1991) Alcohol and aldehyde dehydrogenase genotypes and alcoholism in Chinese men. *Am J Hum Genet*, **48** (4), 677–681.

Ticozzi, N., Vance, C., LeClerc, A.L. *et al.* (2011) Mutational analysis reveals the FUS homolog TAF15 as a candidate gene for familial amyotrophic lateral sclerosis. *Am J Med Genet B Neuropsychiatr Genet*, **156** (3), 285–290.

Tishkoff, S.A., Reed, F.A., Ranciaro, A. *et al.* (2007) Convergent adaptation of human lactase persistence in Africa and Europe. *Nat Genet*, **39** (1), 31–40.

Toma, J.S., Shettar, B.C., Chipman, P.H. *et al.* (2015) Motoneurons derived from induced pluripotent stem cells develop mature phenotypes typical of endogenous spinal motoneurons. *J Neurosci*, **35** (3), 1291–1306.

Tomasetti, C. and Vogelstein, B. (2015) Variation in cancer risk among tissues can be explained by the number of stem cell divisions. *Science*, **347** (6217), 78–81.

Tomljenovic, L. (2011) Aluminum and Alzheimer's disease: after a century of controversy, is there a plausible link? *J Alzheimers Dis*, **23** (4), 567–598.

Tomljenovic, L. and Shaw, C.A. (2011a) Aluminum vaccine adjuvants: are they safe? *Curr Med Chem*, **18** (17), 2630–2637.

Tomljenovic, L. and Shaw, C.A. (2011b) Do aluminum vaccine adjuvants contribute to the rising prevalence of autism? *J Inorg Biochem*, **105** (11), 1489–1499.

Tomljenovic, L. and Shaw, C.A. (2012) Mechanisms of aluminum adjuvant toxicity and autoimmunity in pediatric populations. *Lupus*, **21** (2), 223–230.

Tomljenovic, L., Blaylock, R.L. and Shaw, C.A. (2014) Autism spectrum disorders and aluminum vaccine adjuvants, in *Comprehensive Guide to Autism*, (eds V.B. Patel, V.R. Preedy and C.R. Martin), Springer, New York, pp. 1585–1609.

Torrente, F., Ashwood, P., Day, R. *et al.* (2002) Small intestinal enteropathy with epithelial IgG and complement deposition in children with regressive autism. *Mol Psychiatry*, **7** (4), 375–382, 334.

Tosto, G. and Reitz, C. (2013) Genome-wide association studies in Alzheimer's disease: a review. *Curr Neurol Neurosci Rep*, **13** (10), 1–7.

Traynor, B.J., Codd, M.B., Corr, B. *et al.* (2000) Clinical features of amyotrophic lateral sclerosis according to the El Escorial and Airlie House diagnostic criteria: a population-based study. *Arch Neurol*, **57** (8), 1171–1176.

Tsao, W., Jeong, Y.H., Lin, S. *et al.* (2012) Rodent models of TDP-43: recent advances. *Brain Res*, **1462**, 26–39.

Tschopp, J., Martinon, F. and Burns, K. (2002) The inflammasome: a molecular platform triggering activation of inflammatory caspases and processing of proIL-beta. *Mol Cell*, **10**, 417–426.

Tsumiyama, K., Miyazaki, Y. and Shiozawa, S. (2009) Self-organized criticality theory of autoimmunity. *PLoS ONE*, **4** (12), e8382.

Tu, P.H., Gurney, M.E., Julien, J.P. *et al.* (1997) Oxidative stress, mutant SOD1, and neurofilament pathology in transgenic mouse models of human motor neuron disease. *Lab Invest*, **76** (4), 441–456.

Tuchman, R. and Rapin, I. (2002) Epilepsy in autism. *Lancet Neurol*, **1** (6), 352–358.

Uhl, G.R., Hedreen, J.C. and Price, D.L. (1985) Parkinson's disease: loss of ineurons from the ventral tegmental area contralateral to therapeutic surgical lesions. *Neurology*, **35** (8), 1215.

UKMND-LiCALS Study Group (2013) Lithium in patients with amyotrophic lateral sclerosis (LiCALS): a phase 3 multicentre, randomised, double-blind, placebo-controlled trial. *Lancet Neurol*, **12** (4), 339–345.

Valente, E.M., Abou-Sleiman, P.M., Caputo, V. *et al.* (2004) Hereditary early-onset Parkinson's disease caused by mutations in PINK1. *Science*, **304** (5674), 1158–1160.

van Blitterswijk, M., DeJesus-Hernandez, M. and Rademakers, R. (2012) How do C9ORF72 repeat expansions cause amyotrophic lateral sclerosis and frontotemporal dementia: can we learn from other noncoding repeat expansion disorders? *Curr Opin Neurol*, **25** (6), 689–700.

van Dellen, A., Blakemore, C., Deacon, R. *et al.* (2000) Delaying the onset of Huntington's in mice. *Nature*, **404** (6779), 721–722.

van der Walt, J.M., Noureddine, M.A., Kittappa, R. *et al.* (2004) Fibroblast growth factor 20 polymorphisms and haplotypes strongly influence risk of Parkinson disease. *Am J Hum Genet*, **74** (6), 1121–1127.

van der Worp, H.B., Howells, D.W., Sena, E.S. *et al.* (2010) Can animal models of disease reliably inform human studies? *PLoS Med*, **7** (3) e1000245.

van Es, M.A., Van Vught, P.W., Blauw, H.M. *et al.* (2007) ITPR2 as a susceptibility gene in sporadic amyotrophic lateral sclerosis: a genome-wide association study. *Lancet Neurol*, **6** (10), 869–877.

van Es, M.A., van Vught, P.W.J., Blauw, H.M. *et al.* (2008) Genetic variation in DPP6 is associated with susceptibility to amyotrophic lateral sclerosis. *Nat Genet*, **40** (1), 29–31.

van Es, M.A., Veldink, J.H., Saris, C.G.J. *et al.* (2009) Genome-wide association study identifies 19p13.3 (UNC13A) and 9p21.2 as susceptibility loci for sporadic amyotrophic lateral sclerosis. *Nat Genet*, **41** (10), 1083–1087.

van Es, M.A., Schelhaas, H.J., van Vught, P.W.J. *et al.* (2011) Angiogenin variants in Parkinson disease and amyotrophic lateral sclerosis. *Ann Neurol*, **70** (6), 964–973.

van Heel, D.A., Franke, L., Hunt, K.A. *et al.* (2007) A genome-wide association study for celiac disease identifies risk variants in the region harboring IL2 and IL21. *Nat Genet*, **39** (7), 827–829.

Van Horn, J.D., Irimia, A., Torgerson, C.M. *et al.* (2012) Mapping connectivity damage in the case of Phineas Gage. *PLoS ONE*, **7** (5), e37454.

Van Kampen, J.M., Baranowski, D. and Kay, D.G. (2014a) Progranulin gene delivery protects dopaminergic neurons in a mouse model of Parkinson's disease. *PLoS ONE*, **9** (5), e97032.

Van Kampen, J.M., Baranowski, D.B., Shaw, C.A. and Kay, D.G. (2014b) Panax ginseng is neuroprotective in a novel progressive model of Parkinson's disease. *Exp Gerontol*, **50**, 95–105.

Van Kampen, J.M., Baranowski, D.C., Robertson, H.A. *et al.* (2015) The progressive BSSG rat model of Parkinson's: recapitulating multiple key features of the human disease. *PLoS ONE*, **10** (10), e0139694.

Vance, C., Rogelj, B., Hortobágyi, T. *et al.* (2009) Mutations in FUS, an RNA processing protein, cause familial amyotrophic lateral sclerosis type 6. *Science*, **323** (5918), 1208–1211.

Vanmierlo, T., Bogie, J.F.J., Mailleux, J. *et al.* (2015) Plant sterols: friend or foe in CNS disorders? *Prog Lipid Res*, **58**, 26–39.

Vargas, D.L., Nascimbene, C., Krishnan, C. *et al.* (2005) Neuroglial activation and neuroinflammation in the brain of patients with autism. *Ann Neurol*, **57** (1), 67–81.

Vargas, M.R. and Johnson, J.A. (2010) Astrogliosis in amyotrophic lateral sclerosis: role and therapeutic potential of astrocytes. *Neurotherapeutics*, **7** (4), 471–481.

Varner, J.A., Jensen, K.F., Horvath, W. and Isaacson, R.L. (1998) Chronic administration of aluminum–fluoride or sodium–fluoride to rats in drinking water: alterations in neuronal and cerebrovascular integrity. *Brain Res*, **784** (1–2), 284–298.

Veen, N.D., Selten, J.-P., Tweel, I.v.d. *et al.* (2004) Cannabis use and age at onset of schizophrenia. *Am J Psychiatry*, **161** (3), 501–506.

Vega, A. and Bell, E.A. (1967) α-amino-β-methylaminopropionic acid, a new amino acid from seeds of Cycas circinalis. *Phytochemistry*, **6** (5), 759–762.

Vehviläinen, P., Koistinaho, J. and Gundars, G. (2014) Mechanisms of mutant SOD1 induced mitochondrial toxicity in amyotrophic lateral sclerosis. *Front Cell Neurosci*, **8**, 126.

Velayudhan, L. (2015) Smell identification function and Alzheimer's disease: a selective review. *Curr Opin Psychiatry*, **28** (2), 173–179.

Vellozzi, C., Iqbal, S. and Broder, K. (2014) Guillain-Barré syndrome, influenza, and influenza vaccination: the epidemiologic evidence. *Clin Infect Dis*, **58** (8), 1149–1155.

Viezeliene, D., Beekhof, P., Gremmer, E. *et al.* (2013) Selective induction of IL-6 by aluminum-induced oxidative stress can be prevented by selenium. *J Trace Elem Med Biol*, **27** (3), 226–229.

Vilariño-Güell, C., Wider, C., Ross, O.A. *et al.* (2011) VPS35 mutations in Parkinson disease. *Am J Hum Genet*, **89** (1), 162–167.

Viola, M.V., Frazier, M., White, L. *et al.* (1975) RNA-instructed DNA polymerase activity in a cytoplasmic particulate fraction in brains from Guamanian patients. *J Exp Med*, **142** (2), 483–494.

Vojdani, A., Campbell, A.W., Anyanwu, E. *et al.* (2002) Antibodies to neuron-specific antigens in children with autism: possible cross-reaction with encephalitogenic proteins from milk, Chlamydia pneumoniae and Streptococcus group A. *J Neuroimmunol*, **129** (1–2), 168–177.

Volta, U. and De Giorgio, R. (2012) New understanding of gluten sensitivity. *Nat Rev Gastroenterol Hepatol*, **9** (5), 295–299.

Von Frisch, K. (1950) *Bees: Their Vision, Chemical Senses, and Language*, Cornell University Press, Ithaca, NY.

Wærhaug, O. and Lømo, T. (1994) Factors causing different properties at neuromuscular junctions in fast and slow rat skeletal muscles. *Anat Embryol*, **190** (2), 113–125.

Wagey, R., Pelech, S.L., Duronio, V. and Krieger, C. (1998) Phosphatidylinositol 3-kinase: increased activity and protein level in amyotrophic lateral sclerosis. *J Neurochem*, **71** (2), 716–722.

Wakayama, I., Nerurkar, V.R., Strong, M.J. and Garruto, R.M. (1996) Comparative study of chronic aluminum-induced neurofilamentous aggregates with intracytoplasmic inclusions of amyotrophic lateral sclerosis. *Acta Neuropathol*, **92** (6), 545–554.

Wall, T.L., Carr, L.G. and Ehlers, C.L. (2003) Protective association of genetic variation in alcohol dehydrogenase with alcohol dependence in Native American Mission Indians. *Am J Psychiatry*, **160** (1), 41–46.

Walloe, S., Pakkenberg, B. and Fabricius, K. (2014) Stereological estimation of total brain numbers in humans. *Front Hum Neurosci*, **8**, 508.

Walsh, J.G., Muruve, D.A. and Power, C. (2014) Inflammasomes in the CNS. *Nat Rev Neurosci*, **15** (2), 84–97.

Walton, J.R. (2006) Aluminum in hippocampal neurons from humans with Alzheimer's disease. *NeuroToxicology*, **27** (3), 385–394.

Walton, J.R. (2007) A longitudinal study of rats chronically exposed to aluminum at human dietary levels. *Neurosci Lett*, **412** (1), 29–33.

Walton, J.R. (2009a) Brain lesions comprised of aluminum-rich cells that lack microtubules may be associated with the cognitive deficit of Alzheimer's disease. *NeuroToxicology*, **30** (6), 1059–1069.

Walton, J.R. (2009b) Functional impairment in aged rats chronically exposed to human range dietary aluminum equivalents. *NeuroToxicology*, **30** (2), 182–193.

Walton, J.R. and Wang, M.X. (2009) APP expression, distribution and accumulation are altered by aluminum in a rodent model for Alzheimer's disease. *J Inorg Biochem*, **103** (11), 1548–1554.

Wang, G., Zhang, J., Hu, X. *et al.* (2013) Microglia/macrophage polarization dynamics in white matter after traumatic brain injury. *J Cereb Blood Flow Metab*, **33** (12), 1864–1874.

Wang, L., Popko, B., Tixier, E. and Roos, R.P. (2014) Guanabenz, which enhances the unfolded protein response, ameliorates mutant SOD1-induced amyotrophic lateral sclerosis. *Neurobiol Dis*, **71**, 317–324.

Wang, Q.L., Wang, S.R., Ding, Y. *et al.* (2005) Age-related changes of the redox state of glutathione in plasma. *Chin Med J*, **118**, 1560–1563.

Wang, X., Su, B., Zheng, L. *et al.* (2009) The role of abnormal mitochondrial dynamics in the pathogenesis of Alzheimer's disease. *J Neurochem*, **109**, 153–159.

Ward, A.C. (2009) The role of causal criteria in causal inferences: Bradford Hill's. *Epidemiol Perspect Innov*, **6** (1), 2.

Warnefors, M., Pereira, V. and Eyre-Walker, A. (2010) Transposable elements: insertion pattern and impact on gene expression evolution in hominids. *Mol Biol Evol*, **27** (8), 1955–1962.

Watanabe, T., Totoki, Y., Toyoda, A. *et al.* (2008) Endogenous siRNAs from naturally formed dsRNAs regulate transcripts in mouse oocytes. *Nature*, **453** (7194), 539–543.

Weaver, F.M., Follett, K., Stern, M. *et al.* (2009) Bilateral deep brain stimulation vs best medical therapy for patients with advanced Parkinson disease: a randomized controlled trial. *JAMA*, **301** (1), 63–73.

Webb, S.J., Monk, C.S. and Nelson, C.A. (2001) Mechanisms of postnatal neurobiological development: implications for human development. *Dev Neuropsychol*, **19** (2), 147–171.

Wei, H., Zou, H., Sheikh, A.M. *et al.* (2011) IL-6 is increased in the cerebellum of autistic brain and alters neural cell adhesion, migration and synaptic formation. *J Neuroinflammation*, **8** (52.10), 1186.

Wei, H., Chadman, K.K., McCloskey, D.P. *et al.* (2012a) Brain IL-6 elevation causes neuronal circuitry imbalances and mediates autism-like behaviors. *Biochim Biophys Acta*, **1822** (6), 831–842.

Wei, H., Mori, S., Hua, K. and Li, X. (2012b) Alteration of brain volume in IL-6 overexpressing mice related to autism. *Int J Dev Neurosci*, **30** (7), 554–559.

Weiss, J.H., Koh, J.-Y. and Choi, D.W. (1989) Neurotoxicity of β-N-methylamino-l-alanine (BMAA) and β-N-oxalylamino-l-alamine (BOAA) on cultured cortical neurons. *Brain Res*, **497** (1), 64–71.

Weisskopf, M.G., McCullough, M.L., Calle, E.E. *et al.* (2004) Prospective study of cigarette smoking and amyotrophic lateral sclerosis. *Am J Epidemiol*, **160** (1), 26–33.

Weisskopf, M.G., O'Reilly, E.J., McCullough, M.L. *et al.* (2005) Prospective study of military service and mortality from ALS. *Neurology*, **64** (1), 32–37.

Werry, J. (1992) Child and adolescent (early onset) schizophrenia: a review in light of DSM-III-R. *J Autism Dev Disord*, **22** (4), 601–624.

White, J.F. (2003) Intestinal pathophysiology in autism. *Exp Biol Med*, **228** (6), 639–649.

White, S.W., Bray, B.C. and Ollendick, T.H. (2012) Examining Shared and Unique Aspects of Social Anxiety Disorder and Autism Spectrum Disorder Using Factor Analysis. *J Autism Dev Disord*, **42** (5), 874–884.

Whiting, M.G. (1963) Toxicity of cycads. *Econ Bot*, **17** (4), 270–302.

Whitney, K.D. and McNamara, J.O. (1999) Autoimmunity and neurological disease: antibody modulation of synaptic transmission. *Annu Rev Neurosci*, **22** (1), 175–195.

Wiesel, T.N. and Hubel, D.H. (1963) Single-cell responses in striate cortex of kittens deprived of vision in one eye. *J Neurophysiol*, **26** (6), 1003–1017.

Wilder, R.L. (1995) Neuroendocrine-immune system interactions and autoimmunity. *Annu Rev Immunol*, **13** (1), 307–338.

Wilkins, H., Bouchard, R., Lorenzon, N. and Linseman, D. (2011) Poor correlation netween drug efficacies in the mutant SOD1 mouse model versus clinical trials of ALS necessitates the development of novel animal models for sporadic motor neuron disease, in *Horizons in Neuroscience Research*, vol. **5**, (eds A. Costa and E. Villalba), Nova Science, Hauppauge, NY.

Williams, A.H., Valdez, G., Moresi, V. *et al.* (2009) MicroRNA-206 delays ALS progression and promotes regeneration of neuromuscular synapses in mice. *Science*, **326** (5959), 1549–1554.

Williams, A., Gill, S., Varma, T. *et al.* (2010) Deep brain stimulation plus best medical therapy versus best medical therapy alone for advanced Parkinson's disease (PD SURG trial): a randomised, open-label trial. *Lancet Neurol*, **9** (6), 581–591.

Williams, J.R., Trias, E., Beilby, P.R. *et al.* (2016) Copper delivery to the CNS by CuATSM effectively treats motor neuron disease in SOD G93A mice co-expressing the Copper-Chaperone-for-SOD. *Neurobiol Dis*, **89**, 1–9.

Wilson, J.M.B., Khabazian, I., Wong, M. *et al.* (2002) Behavioral and neurological correlates of ALS-parkinsonism dementia complex in adult mice fed washed cycad flour. *Neuromolecular Med*, **1** (3), 207–221.

Wilson, J.M.B., Petrik, M.S., Moghadasian, M. and Shaw, C.A. (2005) Examining the role of apoE in neurodegenerative disorders using an environmentally-induced murine model of ALS-PDC. *Can J Physiol Pharmacol*, **83**, 131–141.

Winblad, B., Giacobini, E., Frölich, L. *et al.* (2010) Phenserine efficacy in Alzheimer's disease. *J Alzheimers Dis*, **22** (4), 1201–1208.

Winner, B. and Winkler, J. (2015) Adult neurogenesis in neurodegenerative diseases. *Cold Spring Harb Perspect Biol*, **7** (4), a021287.

Winner, B., Kohl, Z. and Gage, F.H. (2011) Neurodegenerative disease and adult neurogenesis. *Eur J Neurosci*, **33**, 1139–1151.

Wirdefeldt, K., Gatz, M., Reynolds, C.A. *et al.* (2011) Heritability of Parkinson disease in Swedish twins: a longitudinal study. *Neurobiol Aging*, **32** (10), 1923.e1921–1923.e1928.

Wolf, P.A. (2012) Contributions of the Framingham Heart Study to stroke and dementia epidemiologic research at 60 years. *Arch Neurol*, **59** (5), 567–571.

Wolters, V.M. and Wijmenga, C. (2008) Genetic background of celiac disease and its clinical implications. *Am J Gastroenterol*, **103** (1), 190–195.

Wong, P.C., Pardo, C.A., Borchelt, D.R. *et al.* (1995) An adverse property of a familial ALS-linked SOD1 mutation causes motor neuron disease characterized by vacuolar degeneration of mitochondria. *Neuron*, **14** (6), 1105–1116.

Woodhouse, A., Shepherd, C., Sokolova, A. *et al.* (2009) Cytoskeletal alterations differentiate presenilin-1 and sporadic Alzheimer's disease. *Acta Neuropathol*, **117** (1), 19–29.

World Health Organization. (2014). Global Status Report on Alcohol and Health 2014. Available from: http://www.who.int/substance_abuse/publications/global_alcohol_ report/en/ (last accessed September 23, 2016).

World Health Organization and Alzheimer's Disease International. (2012). Dementia: A Public Health Priority. Available from: http://apps.who.int/iris/bitstream/10665/75263/ 1/9789241564458_eng.pdf?ua=1 (last accessed September 23, 2016).

Worrall, B.B., Rowland, L.P., Chin, S.S.-M. and Mastrianni, J.A. (2000) Amyotrophy in prion diseases. *Arch Neurol*, **57** (1), 33–38.

Wu, C.-H., Fallini, C., Ticozzi, N. *et al.* (2012) Mutations in the profilin 1 gene cause familial amyotrophic lateral sclerosis. *Nature*, **488** (7412), 499–503.

Wu, S., Yi, J., Zhang, Y.G. *et al.* (2015) Leaky intestine and impaired microbiome in an amyotrophic lateral sclerosis mouse model. *Physiol Rep*, **3** (4) pii: e12356.

Xu, J., Xilouri, M., Bruban, J. *et al.* (2011) Extracellular progranulin protects cortical neurons from toxic insults by activating survival signaling. *Neurobiol Aging*, **32** (12), 2326.e5–e16.

Xu, Y., Day, T.A. and Buller, K.M. (1999) The central amygdala modulates hypothalamic–pituitary–adrenal axis responses to systemic interleukin-1β administration. *Neuroscience*, **94** (1), 175–183.

Xuan, I.C.Y. and Hampson, D.R. (2014) Gender-dependent effects of maternal immune activation on the behavior of mouse offspring. *PLoS ONE*, **9** (8) e104433.

Yachnis, A.T. and Rivera-Zengotita, M.L. (2014) *Neuropathology: A Volume in the High Yield Pathology Series*, Saunders, Philadelphia, PA.

Yanagihara, R., Garruto, R.M., Gajdusek, D.C. *et al.* (1984) Calcium and vitamin D metabolism in guamanian chamorros with amyotrophic lateral sclerosis and parkinsonism–dementia. *Ann Neurol*, **15** (1), 42–48.

Yen, A.A., Simpson, E.P., Henkel, J.S. *et al.* (2004) HFE mutations are not strongly associated with sporadic ALS. *Neurology*, **62** (9), 1611–1612.

Yokel, R.A. (2002) Brain uptake, retention, and efflux of aluminum and manganese. *Environ Health Perspect*, **110** (5)(Suppl, 699–704.

Yokel, R.A. (2006) Blood-brain barrier flux of aluminum, manganese, iron and other metals suspected to contribute to metal-induced neurodegeneration. *J Alzheimers Dis*, **10** (2–3), 223–253.

Yokel, R.A. and McNamara, P.J. (2001) Aluminium toxicokinetics: an updated mini review. *Pharmacol Toxicol*, **88** (4), 159–167.

Young, N.S., Ioannidis, J.P.A. and Al-Ubaydli, O. (2008) Why current publication practices may distort science. *PLoS Med*, **5** (10), e201.

Young-Wolff, K.C., Enoch, M.-A. and Prescott, C.A. (2011) The influence of gene–environment interactions on alcohol consumption and alcohol use disorders: a comprehensive review. *Clin Psychol Rev*, **31** (5), 800–816.

Yuen, R.K.C., Thiruvahindrapuram, B., Merico, D. *et al.* (2015) Whole-genome sequencing of quartet families with autism spectrum disorder. *Nat Med*, **21** (2), 185–191.

Zafrir, Y., Agmon-Levin, N., Paz, Z. *et al.* (2012) Autoimmunity following hepatitis B vaccine as part of the spectrum of "autoimmune (auto-inflammatory) syndrome induced by adjuvants" (ASIA): analysis of 93 cases. *Lupus*, **21** (2), 146–152.

Zhang, Q., Mao, C., Jin, J. *et al.* (2014) Side of limb-onset predicts laterality of gray matter loss in amyotrophic lateral sclerosis. *Biomed Res Int*, **2014**, 11.

Zhou, R., Yazdi, A.S., Menu, P. and Tschopp, J. (2011) A role for mitochondria in NLRP3 inflammasome activation. *Nature*, **469** (7329), 221–225.

Zhu, X., Raina, A.K., Perry, G. and Smith, M.A. (2004) Alzheimer's disease: the two-hit hypothesis. *Lancet Neurol*, **3** (4), 219–226.

Zhu, X., Lee, H.-g., Perry, G. and Smith, M.A. (2007) Alzheimer disease, the two-hit hypothesis: an update. *Biochim Biophys Acta*, **1772** (4), 494–502.

Zigman, W.B. and Lott, I.T. (2007) Alzheimer's disease in Down syndrome: neurobiology and risk. *Ment Retard Dev Disabil Res Rev*, **13** (3), 237–246.

Zimmerman, H. (1945) *Progress report of work in the laboratory of pathology during May, 1945, Guam*, US Naval Medical Research Unit, Washington, DC.

Zimprich, A., Biskup, S., Leitner, P. *et al.* (2004) Mutations in LRRK2 cause autosomal-dominant parkinsonism with pleomorphic pathology. *Neuron*, **44** (4), 601–607.

Zimprich, A., Benet-Pagès, A., Struhal, W. *et al.* (2011) A mutation in VPS35, encoding a subunit of the retromer complex, causes late-onset Parkinson disease. *Am J Hum Genet*, **89** (1), 168–175.

Zwiegers, P. and Shaw, C.A. (2015) Disparity of outcomes: the limits of modeling amyotrophic lateral sclerosis in murine models and translating results clinically. *J Controv Biomed Res*, **1** (1), 4–22.

Zwiegers, P., Lee, G. and Shaw, C.A. (2014) Reduction in hSOD1 copy number significantly impacts ALS phenotype presentation in G37R (line 29) mice: implications for the assessment of putative therapeutic agents. *J Neg Results Biomed*, **13** (1), 14.

Index

Page numbers in *italics* refer to illustrations; those in **bold** refer to tables

Neural Dynamics of Neurological Disease, First Edition. Christopher A. Shaw.
© 2017 John Wiley & Sons, Inc. Published 2017 by John Wiley & Sons, Inc.